# Dynamical Systems in Neuroscience

# Computational Neuroscience
Terrence J. Sejnowski and Tomaso A. Poggio, editors

*Neural Nets in Electric Fish*, Walter Heiligenberg, 1991

*The Computational Brain*, Patricia S. Churchland and Terrence J. Sejnowski, 1992

*Dynamic Biological Networks: The Stomatogastric Nervous System*, edited by Ronald M. Harris-Warrick, Eve Marder, Allen I. Selverston, and Maurice Maulins, 1992

*The Neurobiology of Neural Networks*, edited by Daniel Gardner, 1993

*Large-Scale Neuronal Theories of the Brain*, edited by Christof Koch and Joel L. Davis, 1994

*The Theoretical Foundations of Dendritic Function: Selected Papers of Wilfrid Rall with Commentaries*, edited by Idan Segev, John Rinzel, and Gordon M. Shepherd, 1995

*Models of Information Processing in the Basal Ganglia*, edited by James C. Houk, Joel L. Davis, and David G. Beiser, 1995

*Spikes: Exploring the Neural Code*, Fred Rieke, David Warland, Rob de Ruyter van Stevenick, and William Bialek, 1997

*Neurons, Networks, and Motor Behavior*, edited by Paul S. Stein, Sten Grillner, Allen I. Selverston, and Douglas G. Stuart, 1997

*Methods in Neuronal Modeling: From Ions to Networks*, second edition, edited by Christof Koch and Idan Segev, 1998

*Fundamentals of Neural Network Modeling: Neuropsychology and Cognitive Neuroscience*, edited by Randolph W. Parks, Daniel S. Levin, and Debra L. Long, 1998

*Neural Codes and Distributed Representations: Foundations of Neural Computation*, edited by Laurence Abbott and Terrence J. Sejnowski, 1999

*Unsupervised Learning: Foundations of Neural Computation*, edited by Geoffrey Hinton and Terrence J. Sejnowski, 1999

*Fast Oscillations in Cortical Circuits*, Roger D. Traub, John G.R. Jefferys, and Miles Al Whittington, 1999

*Computational Vision: Information Processing in Perception and Visual Behavior*, Hanspeter A. Mallot, 2000

*Graphical Models: Foundations of Neural Computation*, edited by Michael I. Jordan and Terrence J. Sejnowski, 2001

*Self-Organizing Map Formation: Foundation of Neural Computation*, edited by Klaus Obermayer and Terrence J. Sejnowski, 2001

*Theoretical Neuroscience: Computational and Mathematical Modeling of Neural Systems*, Peter Dayan and L. F. Abbott, 2001

*Neural Engineering: Computation, Representation, and Dynamics in Neurobiological Systems*, Chris Eliasmith and Charles H. Anderson, 2003

*The Computational Neurobiology of Reaching and Pointing*, edited by Reza Shadmehr and Steven P. Wise, 2005

*Dynamical Systems in Neuroscience: The Geometry of Excitability and Bursting*, Eugene M. Izhikevich, 2007

# Dynamical Systems in Neuroscience:
## The Geometry of Excitability and Bursting

Eugene M. Izhikevich

The MIT Press
Cambridge, Massachusetts
London, England

First MIT Press paperback edition, 2010

© 2007 Massachusetts Institute of Technology

This book was set in LaTeX by the author.

Library of Congress Cataloging-in-Publication Data

Izhikevich, Eugene M., 1967–

    Dynamical systems in neuroscience: the geometry of excitability and bursting / Eugene M. Izhikevich.
       p. cm. — (Computational neuroscience)
    Includes bibliographical references and index.
    ISBN 978-0-262-09043-8 (hc. : alk. paper), 978-0-262-51420-0, (pb. : alk. paper)
    1. Neural networks (Neurobiology) 2. Neurons - computer simulation. 3. Dynamical systems. 4. Computational neuroscience. I. Izhikevich, E. M. II Title. III. Series.

QP363.3.I94    2007
573.8'01'13—DC21                                 2006040349

To my beautiful daughters, Liz and Kate.

# Contents

Preface                                                                          xv

1  Introduction                                                                    1
   1.1  Neurons  . . . . . . . . . . . . . . . . . . . . . . . . . . . . . . . . .   1
        1.1.1  What Is a Spike?  . . . . . . . . . . . . . . . . . . . . . . . .     2
        1.1.2  Where Is the Threshold?  . . . . . . . . . . . . . . . . . . . . .    3
        1.1.3  Why Are Neurons Different, and Why Do We Care?  . . . . . . .         6
        1.1.4  Building Models . . . . . . . . . . . . . . . . . . . . . . . . .     6
   1.2  Dynamical Systems . . . . . . . . . . . . . . . . . . . . . . . . . . .      8
        1.2.1  Phase Portraits  . . . . . . . . . . . . . . . . . . . . . . . . .    8
        1.2.2  Bifurcations  . . . . . . . . . . . . . . . . . . . . . . . . . . .  11
        1.2.3  Hodgkin Classification  . . . . . . . . . . . . . . . . . . . . .    14
        1.2.4  Neurocomputational properties  . . . . . . . . . . . . . . . . .     16
        1.2.5  Building Models (Revisited)  . . . . . . . . . . . . . . . . . .     20
   Review of Important Concepts . . . . . . . . . . . . . . . . . . . . . . . .     21
   Bibliographical Notes . . . . . . . . . . . . . . . . . . . . . . . . . . . .    21

2  Electrophysiology of Neurons                                                    25
   2.1  Ions  . . . . . . . . . . . . . . . . . . . . . . . . . . . . . . . . . .   25
        2.1.1  Nernst Potential  . . . . . . . . . . . . . . . . . . . . . . . .    26
        2.1.2  Ionic Currents and Conductances . . . . . . . . . . . . . . . .      27
        2.1.3  Equivalent Circuit  . . . . . . . . . . . . . . . . . . . . . . .    28
        2.1.4  Resting Potential and Input Resistance . . . . . . . . . . . . .     29
        2.1.5  Voltage-Clamp and I-V Relation . . . . . . . . . . . . . . . . .     30
   2.2  Conductances . . . . . . . . . . . . . . . . . . . . . . . . . . . . . .    32
        2.2.1  Voltage-Gated Channels  . . . . . . . . . . . . . . . . . . . . .    33
        2.2.2  Activation of Persistent Currents . . . . . . . . . . . . . . . .    34
        2.2.3  Inactivation of Transient Currents . . . . . . . . . . . . . . . .   35
        2.2.4  Hyperpolarization-Activated Channels  . . . . . . . . . . . . .      36
   2.3  The Hodgkin-Huxley Model . . . . . . . . . . . . . . . . . . . . . . .      37
        2.3.1  Hodgkin-Huxley Equations . . . . . . . . . . . . . . . . . . . .     37
        2.3.2  Action Potential  . . . . . . . . . . . . . . . . . . . . . . . .    41
        2.3.3  Propagation of the Action Potentials . . . . . . . . . . . . . .     42

|  | 2.3.4 | Dendritic Compartments | 43 |
|  | 2.3.5 | Summary of Voltage-Gated Currents | 44 |
|  | Review of Important Concepts | | 49 |
|  | Bibliographical Notes | | 50 |
|  | Exercises | | 50 |

**3 One-Dimensional Systems** — **53**

| 3.1 | Electrophysiological Examples | 53 |
|  | 3.1.1 I-V Relations and Dynamics | 54 |
|  | 3.1.2 Leak + Instantaneous $I_{Na,p}$ | 55 |
| 3.2 | Dynamical Systems | 57 |
|  | 3.2.1 Geometrical Analysis | 59 |
|  | 3.2.2 Equilibria | 60 |
|  | 3.2.3 Stability | 60 |
|  | 3.2.4 Eigenvalues | 61 |
|  | 3.2.5 Unstable Equilibria | 61 |
|  | 3.2.6 Attraction Domain | 62 |
|  | 3.2.7 Threshold and Action Potential | 63 |
|  | 3.2.8 Bistability and Hysteresis | 66 |
| 3.3 | Phase Portraits | 67 |
|  | 3.3.1 Topological Equivalence | 68 |
|  | 3.3.2 Local Equivalence and the Hartman-Grobman Theorem | 69 |
|  | 3.3.3 Bifurcations | 70 |
|  | 3.3.4 Saddle-Node (Fold) Bifurcation | 74 |
|  | 3.3.5 Slow Transition | 75 |
|  | 3.3.6 Bifurcation Diagram | 77 |
|  | 3.3.7 Bifurcations and I-V Relations | 77 |
|  | 3.3.8 Quadratic Integrate-and-Fire Neuron | 80 |
|  | Review of Important Concepts | 82 |
|  | Bibliographical Notes | 83 |
|  | Exercises | 83 |

**4 Two-Dimensional Systems** — **89**

| 4.1 | Planar Vector Fields | 89 |
|  | 4.1.1 Nullclines | 92 |
|  | 4.1.2 Trajectories | 94 |
|  | 4.1.3 Limit Cycles | 96 |
|  | 4.1.4 Relaxation Oscillators | 98 |
| 4.2 | Equilibria | 99 |
|  | 4.2.1 Stability | 100 |
|  | 4.2.2 Local Linear Analysis | 101 |
|  | 4.2.3 Eigenvalues and Eigenvectors | 102 |
|  | 4.2.4 Local Equivalence | 103 |

        4.2.5   Classification of Equilibria . . . . . . . . . . . . . . . . . . 103
        4.2.6   Example: FitzHugh-Nagumo Model . . . . . . . . . . . . . 106
    4.3   Phase Portraits . . . . . . . . . . . . . . . . . . . . . . . . . . . 108
        4.3.1   Bistability and Attraction Domains . . . . . . . . . . . . . 108
        4.3.2   Stable/Unstable Manifolds . . . . . . . . . . . . . . . . . . 109
        4.3.3   Homoclinic/Heteroclinic Trajectories . . . . . . . . . . . . 111
        4.3.4   Saddle-Node Bifurcation . . . . . . . . . . . . . . . . . . . 113
        4.3.5   Andronov-Hopf Bifurcation . . . . . . . . . . . . . . . . . 116
    Review of Important Concepts . . . . . . . . . . . . . . . . . . . . . 121
    Bibliographical Notes . . . . . . . . . . . . . . . . . . . . . . . . . . 122
    Exercises . . . . . . . . . . . . . . . . . . . . . . . . . . . . . . . . . 122

5   **Conductance-Based Models and Their Reductions**                           **127**
    5.1   Minimal Models . . . . . . . . . . . . . . . . . . . . . . . . . . . 127
        5.1.1   Amplifying and Resonant Gating Variables . . . . . . . . . 129
        5.1.2   $I_{Na,p}+I_K$-Model . . . . . . . . . . . . . . . . . . . . . . 132
        5.1.3   $I_{Na,t}$-model . . . . . . . . . . . . . . . . . . . . . . . . . 133
        5.1.4   $I_{Na,p}+I_h$-Model . . . . . . . . . . . . . . . . . . . . . . 136
        5.1.5   $I_h+I_{Kir}$-Model . . . . . . . . . . . . . . . . . . . . . . . 138
        5.1.6   $I_K+I_{Kir}$-Model . . . . . . . . . . . . . . . . . . . . . . . 140
        5.1.7   $I_A$-Model . . . . . . . . . . . . . . . . . . . . . . . . . . 142
        5.1.8   $Ca^{2+}$-Gated Minimal Models . . . . . . . . . . . . . . . . 147
    5.2   Reduction of Multidimensional Models . . . . . . . . . . . . . . 147
        5.2.1   Hodgkin-Huxley model . . . . . . . . . . . . . . . . . . . . 147
        5.2.2   Equivalent Potentials . . . . . . . . . . . . . . . . . . . . . 151
        5.2.3   Nullclines and I-V Relations . . . . . . . . . . . . . . . . . 151
        5.2.4   Reduction to Simple Model . . . . . . . . . . . . . . . . . 153
    Review of Important Concepts . . . . . . . . . . . . . . . . . . . . . 156
    Bibliographical Notes . . . . . . . . . . . . . . . . . . . . . . . . . . 156
    Exercises . . . . . . . . . . . . . . . . . . . . . . . . . . . . . . . . . 157

6   **Bifurcations**                                                             **159**
    6.1   Equilibrium (Rest State) . . . . . . . . . . . . . . . . . . . . . . 159
        6.1.1   Saddle-Node (Fold) . . . . . . . . . . . . . . . . . . . . . . 162
        6.1.2   Saddle-Node on Invariant Circle . . . . . . . . . . . . . . . 164
        6.1.3   Supercritical Andronov-Hopf . . . . . . . . . . . . . . . . . 168
        6.1.4   Subcritical Andronov-Hopf . . . . . . . . . . . . . . . . . . 174
    6.2   Limit Cycle (Spiking State) . . . . . . . . . . . . . . . . . . . . . 178
        6.2.1   Saddle-Node on Invariant Circle . . . . . . . . . . . . . . . 180
        6.2.2   Supercritical Andronov-Hopf . . . . . . . . . . . . . . . . . 181
        6.2.3   Fold Limit Cycle . . . . . . . . . . . . . . . . . . . . . . . 181
        6.2.4   Homoclinic . . . . . . . . . . . . . . . . . . . . . . . . . . 185
    6.3   Other Interesting Cases . . . . . . . . . . . . . . . . . . . . . . . 190

      6.3.1   Three-Dimensional Phase Space . . . . . . . . . . . . . . . 190

      6.3.2   Cusp and Pitchfork . . . . . . . . . . . . . . . . . . . . . 192

      6.3.3   Bogdanov-Takens . . . . . . . . . . . . . . . . . . . . . . 194

      6.3.4   Relaxation Oscillators and Canards . . . . . . . . . . . . 198

      6.3.5   Bautin . . . . . . . . . . . . . . . . . . . . . . . . . . . . 200

      6.3.6   Saddle-Node Homoclinic Orbit . . . . . . . . . . . . . . . 201

      6.3.7   Hard and Soft Loss of Stability . . . . . . . . . . . . . . 204

  Bibliographical Notes . . . . . . . . . . . . . . . . . . . . . . . . . . 205

  Exercises . . . . . . . . . . . . . . . . . . . . . . . . . . . . . . . . . 210

**7  Neuronal Excitability**                                                **215**

  7.1  Excitability . . . . . . . . . . . . . . . . . . . . . . . . . . . . . 215

      7.1.1   Bifurcations . . . . . . . . . . . . . . . . . . . . . . . . . 216

      7.1.2   Hodgkin's Classification . . . . . . . . . . . . . . . . . . 218

      7.1.3   Classes 1 and 2 . . . . . . . . . . . . . . . . . . . . . . . 221

      7.1.4   Class 3 . . . . . . . . . . . . . . . . . . . . . . . . . . . . 222

      7.1.5   Ramps, Steps, and Shocks . . . . . . . . . . . . . . . . . 224

      7.1.6   Bistability . . . . . . . . . . . . . . . . . . . . . . . . . . 226

      7.1.7   Class 1 and 2 Spiking . . . . . . . . . . . . . . . . . . . . 228

  7.2  Integrators vs. Resonators . . . . . . . . . . . . . . . . . . . . 229

      7.2.1   Fast Subthreshold Oscillations . . . . . . . . . . . . . . 230

      7.2.2   Frequency Preference and Resonance . . . . . . . . . . . 232

      7.2.3   Frequency Preference in Vivo . . . . . . . . . . . . . . . 237

      7.2.4   Thresholds and Action Potentials . . . . . . . . . . . . . 238

      7.2.5   Threshold manifolds . . . . . . . . . . . . . . . . . . . . 240

      7.2.6   Rheobase . . . . . . . . . . . . . . . . . . . . . . . . . . . 242

      7.2.7   Postinhibitory Spike . . . . . . . . . . . . . . . . . . . . 242

      7.2.8   Inhibition-Induced Spiking . . . . . . . . . . . . . . . . . 244

      7.2.9   Spike Latency . . . . . . . . . . . . . . . . . . . . . . . . 246

      7.2.10  Flipping from an Integrator to a Resonator . . . . . . . . . 248

      7.2.11  Transition Between Integrators and Resonators . . . . . . 251

  7.3  Slow Modulation . . . . . . . . . . . . . . . . . . . . . . . . . 252

      7.3.1   Spike Frequency Modulation . . . . . . . . . . . . . . . . 255

      7.3.2   I-V Relation . . . . . . . . . . . . . . . . . . . . . . . . . 256

      7.3.3   Slow Subthreshold Oscillation . . . . . . . . . . . . . . . 258

      7.3.4   Rebound Response and Voltage Sag . . . . . . . . . . . . 259

      7.3.5   AHP and ADP . . . . . . . . . . . . . . . . . . . . . . . 260

  Review of Important Concepts . . . . . . . . . . . . . . . . . . . . 264

  Bibliographical Notes . . . . . . . . . . . . . . . . . . . . . . . . . . 264

  Exercises . . . . . . . . . . . . . . . . . . . . . . . . . . . . . . . . . 265

**8  Simple Models**                                                         **267**
  8.1  Simplest Models . . . . . . . . . . . . . . . . . . . . . . . 267
      8.1.1  Integrate-and-Fire . . . . . . . . . . . . . . . . 268
      8.1.2  Resonate-and-Fire . . . . . . . . . . . . . . . . 269
      8.1.3  Quadratic Integrate-and-Fire . . . . . . . . . . . 270
      8.1.4  Simple Model of Choice . . . . . . . . . . . . . 272
      8.1.5  Canonical Models . . . . . . . . . . . . . . . . 278
  8.2  Cortex . . . . . . . . . . . . . . . . . . . . . . . . . . . 281
      8.2.1  Regular Spiking (RS) Neurons . . . . . . . . . . 282
      8.2.2  Intrinsically Bursting (IB) Neurons . . . . . . . . 288
      8.2.3  Multi-Compartment Dendritic Tree . . . . . . . . 292
      8.2.4  Chattering (CH) Neurons . . . . . . . . . . . . 294
      8.2.5  Low-Threshold Spiking (LTS) Interneurons . . . . . . 296
      8.2.6  Fast Spiking (FS) Interneurons . . . . . . . . . 298
      8.2.7  Late Spiking (LS) Interneurons . . . . . . . . . 300
      8.2.8  Diversity of Inhibitory Interneurons . . . . . . . 301
  8.3  Thalamus . . . . . . . . . . . . . . . . . . . . . . . . . 304
      8.3.1  Thalamocortical (TC) Relay Neurons . . . . . . . 305
      8.3.2  Reticular Thalamic Nucleus (RTN) Neurons . . . . . . 306
      8.3.3  Thalamic Interneurons . . . . . . . . . . . . . 308
  8.4  Other Interesting Cases . . . . . . . . . . . . . . . . . . 308
      8.4.1  Hippocampal CA1 Pyramidal Neurons . . . . . . . 308
      8.4.2  Spiny Projection Neurons of Neostriatum and Basal Ganglia . . 311
      8.4.3  Mesencephalic V Neurons of Brainstem . . . . . . . 313
      8.4.4  Stellate Cells of Entorhinal Cortex . . . . . . . 314
      8.4.5  Mitral Neurons of the Olfactory Bulb . . . . . . . 316
  Review of Important Concepts . . . . . . . . . . . . . . . . 319
  Bibliographical Notes . . . . . . . . . . . . . . . . . . . . 319
  Exercises . . . . . . . . . . . . . . . . . . . . . . . . . . 321

**9  Bursting**                                                              **325**
  9.1  Electrophysiology . . . . . . . . . . . . . . . . . . . . . 325
      9.1.1  Example: The $I_{\mathrm{Na,p}}+I_{\mathrm{K}}+I_{\mathrm{K(M)}}$-Model . . . . . . . . . . . . . 327
      9.1.2  Fast-Slow Dynamics . . . . . . . . . . . . . . . 329
      9.1.3  Minimal Models . . . . . . . . . . . . . . . . . 332
      9.1.4  Central Pattern Generators and Half-Center Oscillators . . . . 334
  9.2  Geometry . . . . . . . . . . . . . . . . . . . . . . . . . 335
      9.2.1  Fast-Slow Bursters . . . . . . . . . . . . . . . 336
      9.2.2  Phase Portraits . . . . . . . . . . . . . . . . . 336
      9.2.3  Averaging . . . . . . . . . . . . . . . . . . . . 339
      9.2.4  Equivalent Voltage . . . . . . . . . . . . . . . 341
      9.2.5  Hysteresis Loops and Slow Waves . . . . . . . . . 342
      9.2.6  Bifurcations "Resting $\leftrightarrow$ Bursting $\leftrightarrow$ Tonic Spiking" . . . . . . 344

9.3    Classification . . . . . . . . . . . . . . . . . . . . . . . . 347
       9.3.1   Fold/Homoclinic . . . . . . . . . . . . . . . . . . . 350
       9.3.2   Circle/Circle . . . . . . . . . . . . . . . . . . . . . 354
       9.3.3   SubHopf/Fold Cycle . . . . . . . . . . . . . . . . . 359
       9.3.4   Fold/Fold Cycle . . . . . . . . . . . . . . . . . . . . 364
       9.3.5   Fold/Hopf . . . . . . . . . . . . . . . . . . . . . . . 365
       9.3.6   Fold/Circle . . . . . . . . . . . . . . . . . . . . . . 366
9.4    Neurocomputational Properties . . . . . . . . . . . . . . . 367
       9.4.1   How to Distinguish? . . . . . . . . . . . . . . . . . 367
       9.4.2   Integrators vs. Resonators . . . . . . . . . . . . . . 368
       9.4.3   Bistability . . . . . . . . . . . . . . . . . . . . . . . 368
       9.4.4   Bursts as a Unit of Neuronal Information . . . . . . . 371
       9.4.5   Chirps . . . . . . . . . . . . . . . . . . . . . . . . . 372
       9.4.6   Synchronization . . . . . . . . . . . . . . . . . . . . 373
Review of Important Concepts . . . . . . . . . . . . . . . . . . . . 375
Bibliographical Notes . . . . . . . . . . . . . . . . . . . . . . . . . 376
Exercises . . . . . . . . . . . . . . . . . . . . . . . . . . . . . . . . 378

**10 Synchronization                                                   385**

**Solutions to Exercises                                               387**

**References                                                           419**

**Index                                                                435**

**10 Synchronization (www.izhikevich.com)                              443**
10.1   Pulsed Coupling . . . . . . . . . . . . . . . . . . . . . . . . 444
       10.1.1  Phase of Oscillation . . . . . . . . . . . . . . . . . 444
       10.1.2  Isochrons . . . . . . . . . . . . . . . . . . . . . . . 445
       10.1.3  PRC . . . . . . . . . . . . . . . . . . . . . . . . . . 446
       10.1.4  Type 0 and Type 1 Phase Response . . . . . . . . . . 450
       10.1.5  Poincare Phase Map . . . . . . . . . . . . . . . . . 452
       10.1.6  Fixed points . . . . . . . . . . . . . . . . . . . . . . 453
       10.1.7  Synchronization . . . . . . . . . . . . . . . . . . . . 454
       10.1.8  Phase-Locking . . . . . . . . . . . . . . . . . . . . . 456
       10.1.9  Arnold Tongues . . . . . . . . . . . . . . . . . . . . 456
10.2   Weak Coupling . . . . . . . . . . . . . . . . . . . . . . . . . 458
       10.2.1  Winfree's Approach . . . . . . . . . . . . . . . . . . 459
       10.2.2  Kuramoto's Approach . . . . . . . . . . . . . . . . . 460
       10.2.3  Malkin's Approach . . . . . . . . . . . . . . . . . . 461
       10.2.4  Measuring PRCs Experimentally . . . . . . . . . . . 462
       10.2.5  Phase Model for Coupled Oscillators . . . . . . . . . 465
10.3   Synchronization . . . . . . . . . . . . . . . . . . . . . . . . 467

     10.3.1  Two Oscillators . . . . . . . . . . . . . . . . . . . . . . . 469
     10.3.2  Chains . . . . . . . . . . . . . . . . . . . . . . . . . . . 471
     10.3.3  Networks  . . . . . . . . . . . . . . . . . . . . . . . . . 473
     10.3.4  Mean-Field Approximations . . . . . . . . . . . . . . . . 474
 10.4  Examples  . . . . . . . . . . . . . . . . . . . . . . . . . . . . . 475
     10.4.1  Phase Oscillators . . . . . . . . . . . . . . . . . . . . . 475
     10.4.2  SNIC Oscillators  . . . . . . . . . . . . . . . . . . . . . 477
     10.4.3  Homoclinic Oscillators . . . . . . . . . . . . . . . . . . 482
     10.4.4  Relaxation Oscillators and FTM . . . . . . . . . . . . . 484
     10.4.5  Bursting Oscillators . . . . . . . . . . . . . . . . . . . . 486
Review of Important Concepts . . . . . . . . . . . . . . . . . . . . . 488
Bibliographical Notes . . . . . . . . . . . . . . . . . . . . . . . . . 489
Solutions . . . . . . . . . . . . . . . . . . . . . . . . . . . . . . . . 497

# Preface

Historically, much of theoretical neuroscience research concerned neuronal circuits and synaptic organization. The neurons were divided into excitatory and inhibitory types, but their electrophysiological properties were largely neglected or taken to be identical to those of Hodgkin-Huxley's squid axon. The present awareness of the importance of the electrophysiology of individual neurons is best summarized by David McCormick in the fifth edition of Gordon Shepherd's book *The Synaptic Organization of the Brain*:

> Information-processing depends not only on the *anatomical* substrates of synaptic circuits but also on the *electrophysiological* properties of neurons... Even if two neurons in different regions of the nervous system possess identical morphological features, they may respond to the same synaptic input in very different manners because of each cell's intrinsic properties.
> McCormick (2004)

Much of present neuroscience research concerns voltage- and second-messenger-gated currents in individual cells, with the goal of understanding the cell's intrinsic neurocomputational properties. It is widely accepted that knowing the currents suffices to determine what the cell is doing and why it is doing it. This, however, contradicts a half-century-old observation that cells having similar currents can nevertheless exhibit quite different dynamics. Indeed, studying isolated axons having presumably similar electrophysiology (all are from the crustacean *Carcinus maenas*), Hodgkin (1948) injected a DC-current of varying amplitude, and discovered that some preparations could exhibit repetitive spiking with arbitrarily low frequencies, while the others discharged in a narrow frequency band. This observation was largely ignored by the neuroscience community until the seminal paper by Rinzel and Ermentrout (1989), who showed that the difference in behavior is due to different *bifurcation* mechanisms of excitability.

Let us treat the amplitude of the injected current in Hodgkin's experiments as a bifurcation parameter: When the amplitude is small, the cell is quiescent; when the amplitude is large, the cell fires repetitive spikes. When we change the amplitude of the injected current, the cell undergoes a transition from quiescence to repetitive spiking. From the dynamical systems point of view, the transition corresponds to a bifurcation from equilibrium to a limit cycle attractor. The type of bifurcation determines the most fundamental computational properties of neurons, such as the class of excitability, the existence or nonexistence of threshold, all-or-none spikes, subthreshold oscillations, the ability to generate postinhibitory rebound spikes, bistability of resting and spiking states, whether the neuron is an integrator or a resonator, and so on.

This book is devoted to a systematic study of the relationship between electrophysiology, bifurcations, and computational properties of neurons. The reader will learn why cells having nearly identical currents may undergo distinct bifurcations, and hence they will have fundamentally different neurocomputational properties. (Conversely, cells having quite different currents may undergo identical bifurcations, and hence they will have similar neurocomputational properties.) The major message of the book can be summarized as follows (compare with the McCormick statement above):

> Information-processing depends not only on the electrophysiological properties of neurons but also on their *dynamical properties*. Even if two neurons in the same region of the nervous system possess similar electrophysiological features, they may respond to the same synaptic input in very different manners because of each cell's bifurcation dynamics.

Nonlinear dynamical system theory is a core of computational neuroscience research, but it is not a standard part of the graduate neuroscience curriculum. Neither is it taught in most math/physics departments in a form suitable for a general biological audience. As a result, many neuroscientists fail to grasp such fundamental concepts as equilibrium, stability, limit cycle attractor, and bifurcations, even though neuroscientists constantly encounter these nonlinear phenomena.

This book introduces dynamical systems starting with simple one- and two-dimensional spiking models and continuing all the way to bursting systems. Each chapter is organized from simple to complex, so everybody can start reading the book; only the reader's background will determine where he or she stops. The book emphasizes the geometrical approach, so there are few equations but a lot of figures. Half of them are simulations of various neural models, so there are hundreds of possible exercises such as "Use MATLAB (GENESIS, NEURON, XPPAUT, etc.) and parameters in the caption of figure $X$ to simulate the figure." Additional problems are provided at the end of each chapter; the reader is encouraged to solve at least some of them and to look at the solutions of the others at the end of the book. Problems marked [**M.S.**] or [**Ph.D.**] are suggested thesis topics.

**Acknowledgments.** I thank the scientists who reviewed the first draft of the book: Pablo Achard, Jose M. Amigo, Vlatko Becanovic, Brent Doiron, George Bard Ermentrout, Richard FitzHugh, David Golomb, Andrei Iacob, Paul Kulchenko, Maciej Lazarewicz, Georgi Medvedev, John Rinzel, Anil K. Seth, Gautam C Sethia, Arthur Sherman, Klaus M. Stiefel, and Takashi Tateno. I also thank the anonymous referees who peer-reviewed the book and made quite a few valuable suggestions instead of just rejecting it. Special thanks go to Niraj S. Desai, who made most of the in vitro recordings used in the book (the data are available on the author's Web page www.izhikevich.com), and to Bruno van Swinderen, who drew the cartoons. I enjoyed the hospitality of The Neurosciences Institute – a monastery of interdisciplinary science – and I benefited greatly from the expertise and support of its fellows.

Finally, I thank my wife, Tatyana, and my wonderful daughters, Elizabeth and Kate, for their support and patience during the five-year gestation of this book.

Eugene M. Izhikevich                                              www.izhikevich.com
San Diego, California                                              December 19, 2005

# Chapter 1

# Introduction

This chapter highlights some of the most important concepts developed in the book. First, we discuss several common misconceptions regarding the spike generation mechanism of neurons. Our goal is to motivate the reader to think of a neuron not only in terms of ions and channels, as many biologists do, and not only in terms of an input/output relationship, as many theoreticians do, but also as a nonlinear dynamical system that looks at the input through the prism of its own intrinsic dynamics. We ask such questions as "What makes a neuron fire?" or "Where is the threshold?", and then outline the answers, using the geometrical theory of dynamical systems.

From a dynamical systems point of view, neurons are excitable because they are near a transition, called bifurcation, from resting to sustained spiking activity. While there is a huge number of possible ionic mechanisms of excitability and spike generation, there are only four bifurcation mechanisms that can result in such a transition. Considering the geometry of phase portraits at these bifurcations, we can understand many computational properties of neurons, such as the nature of threshold and all-or-none spiking, the coexistence of resting and spiking states, the origin of spike latencies, postinhibitory spikes, and the mechanism of integration and resonance. Moreover, we can understand how these properties are interrelated, why some are equivalent, and why some are mutually exclusive.

## 1.1  Neurons

If somebody were to put a gun to the head of the author of this book and ask him to name the single most important concept in brain science, he would say it is the concept of a *neuron*. There are only $10^{11}$ or so neurons in the human brain, much fewer than the number of non-neural cells such as glia. Yet neurons are unique in the sense that only they can transmit electrical signals over long distances. From the neuronal level we can go down to cell biophysics and to the molecular biology of gene regulation. From the neuronal level we can go up to neuronal circuits, to cortical structures, to the whole brain, and finally to the behavior of the organism. So let us see how much we understand of what is going on at the level of individual neurons.

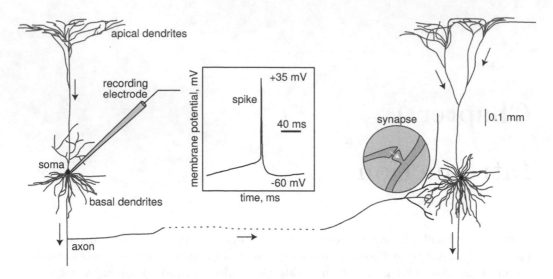

Figure 1.1: Two interconnected cortical pyramidal neurons (hand drawing) and in vitro recorded spike.

### 1.1.1   What Is a Spike?

A typical neuron receives inputs from more than $10,000$ other neurons through the contacts on its dendritic tree called synapses; see Fig.1.1. The inputs produce electrical transmembrane currents that change the membrane potential of the neuron. Synaptic currents produce changes, called postsynaptic potentials (PSPs). Small currents produce small PSPs; larger currents produce significant PSPs that can be amplified by the voltage-sensitive channels embedded in the neuronal membrane and lead to the generation of an *action potential* or *spike* – an abrupt and transient change of membrane voltage that propagates to other neurons via a long protrusion called an axon.

Such spikes are the main means of communication between neurons. In general, neurons do not fire on their own; they fire as a result of incoming spikes from other neurons. One of the most fundamental questions of neuroscience is *What, exactly, makes neurons fire?* What is it in the incoming pulses that elicits a response in one neuron but not in another? Why can two neurons have different responses to exactly the same input and identical responses to completely different inputs? To answer these questions, we need to understand the dynamics of spike generation mechanisms of neurons.

Most introductory neuroscience books describe neurons as integrators with a threshold: neurons sum incoming PSPs and "compare" the integrated PSP with a certain voltage value, called the firing threshold. If it is below the threshold, the neuron remains quiescent; when it is above the threshold, the neuron fires an all-or-none spike, as in Fig.1.3, and resets its membrane potential. To add theoretical plausibility to this argument, the books refer to the Hodgkin-Huxley model of spike generation in squid

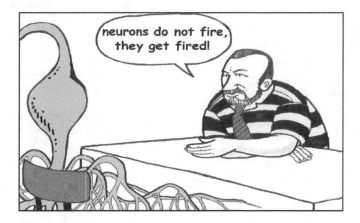

Figure 1.2: What makes a neuron fire?

giant axons, which we study in chapter 2. The irony is that the Hodgkin-Huxley model does not have a well-defined threshold; it does not fire all-or-none spikes; and it is not an integrator, but a resonator (i.e., it prefers inputs having certain frequencies that resonate with the frequency of subthreshold oscillations of the neuron). We consider these and other properties in detail in this book.

## 1.1.2   Where Is the Threshold?

Much effort has been spent trying to experimentally determine the firing thresholds of neurons. Here, we challenge the classical view of a threshold. Let us consider two typical experiments, depicted in Fig.1.4, that are designed to measure the threshold. in Fig.1.4a, we shock a cortical neuron (i.e., we inject brief but strong pulses of current of various amplitudes to depolarize the membrane potential to various values). Is there a clear-cut voltage value, as in Fig.1.3, above which the neuron fires but below which no spikes occur? If you find one, let the author know! In Fig.1.4b we inject long but weak pulses of current of various amplitudes, which results in slow depolarization and a spike. The firing threshold, if it exists, must be somewhere in the shaded region, but where? Where does the slow depolarization end and the spike start? Is it meaningful to talk about firing thresholds at all?

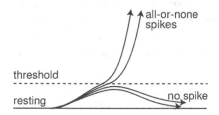

Figure 1.3: The concept of a firing threshold.

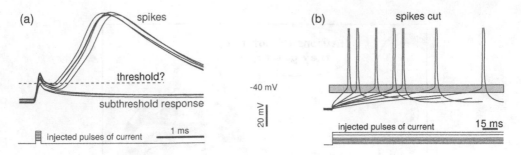

Figure 1.4: Where is the firing threshold? Shown are in vitro recordings of two layer 5 rat pyramidal neurons. Notice the differences of voltage and time scales.

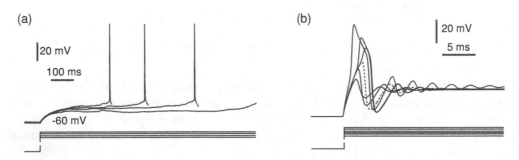

Figure 1.5: Where is the rheobase (i.e., the minimal current that fires the cell)? (a) in vitro recordings of the pyramidal neuron of layer 2/3 of a rat's visual cortex show increasing latencies as the amplitude of the injected current decreases. (b) Simulation of the $I_{\text{Na,p}}+I_{\text{K}}$ – model (pronounced: *persistent sodium plus potassium model*) shows spikes of graded amplitude.

Perhaps, we should measure current thresholds instead of voltage thresholds. The current threshold (i.e., the minimal amplitude of injected current of infinite duration needed to fire a neuron) is called the *rheobase*. In Fig.1.5 we decrease the amplitudes of injected pulses of current to find the minimal one that still elicits a spike or the maximal one that does not. In Fig.1.5a, progressively weaker pulses result in longer latencies to the first spike. Eventually the neuron does not fire because the latency is longer than the duration of the pulse, which is 1 second in the figure. Did we really measure the neuronal rheobase? What if we waited a bit longer? How long is long enough? In Fig.1.5b the latencies do not grow, but the spike amplitudes decrease until the spikes do not look like spikes at all. To determine the current threshold, we need to draw the line and separate spike responses from "subthreshold" ones. How can we do that if the spikes are not all-or-none? Is the response denoted by the dashed line a spike?

Risking adding more confusion to the notion of a threshold, consider the following. If excitatory inputs depolarize the membrane potential (i.e., bring it closer to

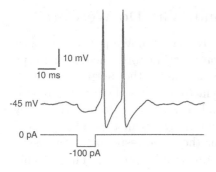

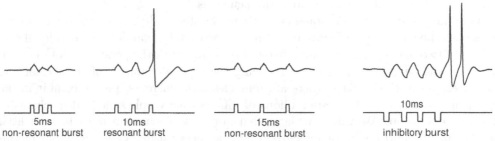

Figure 1.6: In vitro recording of rebound spikes of a rat's brainstem mesV neuron in response to a brief hyperpolarizing pulse of current.

Figure 1.7: Resonant response of the mesencephalic V neuron of a rat's brainstem to pulses of injected current having a 10 ms period (in vitro).

the "firing threshold"), and inhibitory inputs hyperpolarize the potential and move it away from the threshold, then *how can the neuron in Fig.1.6 fire in response to the inhibitory input?* This phenomenon, also observed in the Hodgkin-Huxley model, is called anodal break excitation, rebound spike, or postinhibitory spike. Many biologists say that rebound responses are due to the activation and inactivation of certain slow currents, which bring the membrane potential over the threshold or, equivalently, lower the threshold upon release from the hyperpolarization – a phenomenon called a low-threshold spike in thalamocortical neurons. The problem with this explanation is that neither the Hodgkin-Huxley model nor the neuron in Fig.1.6 has these currents, and even if they did, the hyperpolarization is too short and too weak to affect the currents.

Another interesting phenomenon is depicted in Fig.1.7. The neuron is stimulated with brief pulses of current mimicking an incoming burst of three spikes. When the stimulation frequency is high (5 ms period), presumably reflecting a strong input, the neuron does not fire at all. However, stimulation with a lower frequency (10 ms period) that resonates with the frequency of subthreshold oscillation of the neuron evokes a spike response, regardless of whether the stimulation is excitatory or inhibitory. Stimulation with even lower frequency (15 ms period) cannot elicit spike response again. Thus, the neuron is sensitive only to the inputs having resonant frequency. The same pulses applied to a cortical pyramidal neuron evoke a response only in the first case (small period), but not in the other cases.

### 1.1.3   Why Are Neurons Different, and Why Do We Care?

Why would two neurons respond completely differently to the same input? A biologist would say that the response of a neuron depends on many factors, such as the type of voltage- and $Ca^{2+}$-gated channels expressed by the neuron, the morphology of its dendritic tree, the location of the input, and other factors. These factors are indeed important, but they do not determine the neuronal response per se. Rather they determine the rules that govern dynamics of the neuron. Different conductances and currents can result in the same rules, and hence in the same responses; conversely, similar currents can result in different rules and in different responses. The currents define what kind of dynamical system the neuron is.

We study ionic transmembrane currents in chapter 2. In subsequent chapters we investigate how the types of currents determine neuronal dynamics. We divide all currents into two major classes: amplifying and resonant, with the persistent $Na^+$ current $I_{Na,p}$ and the persistent $K^+$ current $I_K$ being the typical examples of the former and the latter, respectively. Since there are tens of known currents, purely combinatorial argument implies that there are millions of different electrophysiological mechanisms of spike generation. We will show later that any such mechanism must have at least one amplifying and one resonant current. Some mechanisms, called minimal in this book, have one resonant and one amplifying current. They provide an invaluable tool in classifying and understanding the electrophysiology of spike generation.

Many illustrations in this book are based on simulations of the reduced $I_{Na,p} + I_K$-model (pronounced *persistent sodium plus potassium model*), which consists of a fast persistent $Na^+$ (amplifying) current and a slower persistent $K^+$ (resonant) current. It is equivalent to the famous and widely used Morris-Lecar $I_{Ca} + I_K$-model (Morris and Lecar 1981). We show that the model exhibits quite different dynamics, depending on the values of the parameters, e.g., the half-activation voltage of the $K^+$ current: in one case, it can fire in a narrow frequency range, it can exhibit coexistence of resting and spiking states, and it has damped subthreshold oscillations of membrane potential. In another case, it can fire in a wide frequency range and show no coexistence of resting and spiking and no subthreshold oscillations. Thus, seemingly inessential differences in parameter values could result in drastically distinct behaviors.

### 1.1.4   Building Models

To build a good model of a neuron, electrophysiologists apply different pharmacological blockers to tease out the currents that the neuron has. Then they apply different stimulation protocols to measure the kinetic parameters of the currents, such as the Boltzmann activation function, time constants, and maximal conductances. We consider all these functions in chapter 2. Next, they create a Hodgkin-Huxley-type model and simulate it using the NEURON, GENESIS, or XPP environment or MATLAB (the first two are invaluable tools for simulating realistic dendritic structures).

The problem is that the parameters are measured in different neurons and then put together into a single model. As an illustration, consider two neurons having the same

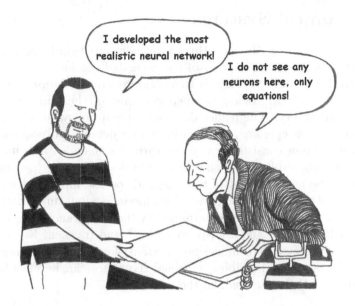

Figure 1.8: Neurons are dynamical systems.

currents, say $I_{\text{Na,p}}$ and $I_{\text{K}}$, and exhibiting excitable behavior; that is, both neurons are quiescent but can fire a spike in response to a stimulation. Suppose the second neuron has stronger $I_{\text{Na,p}}$, which is balanced by stronger $I_{\text{K}}$. If we measure $\text{Na}^+$ conductance using the first neuron and $\text{K}^+$ conductance using the second neuron, the resulting $I_{\text{Na,p}} + I_{\text{K}}$-model will have an excess of $\text{K}^+$ current and probably will not be able to fire spikes at all. Conversely, if we measure $\text{Na}^+$ and $\text{K}^+$ conductances using the second neuron and then the first neuron, respectively, the model would have too much $\text{Na}^+$ current and probably would exhibit sustained pacemaking activity. In any case, the model fails to reproduce the excitable behavior of the neurons whose parameters we measured.

Some of the parameters cannot be measured at all, so many arbitrary choices are made via a process called "fine-tuning". Navigating in the dark, possibly with the help of some biological intuition, the researcher modifies parameters, compares simulations with experiment, and repeats this trial-and-error procedure until he or she is satisfied with the results. Since seemingly similar values of parameters can result in drastically different behaviors, and quite different parameters can result in seemingly similar behaviors, how do we know that the resulting model is correct? How do we know that its behavior is equivalent to that of the neuron we want to study? And what is *equivalent* in this case? Now, you are primed to consider dynamical systems. If not, see Fig.1.8.

## 1.2 Dynamical Systems

In chapter 2 we introduce the Hodgkin-Huxley formalism to describe neuronal dynamics in terms of activation and inactivation of voltage-gated conductances. An important result of the Hodgkin-Huxley studies is that *neurons are dynamical systems*, so they should be studied as such. Below we mention some of the important concepts of dynamical systems theory. The reader does not have to follow all the details of this section because the concepts are explained in greater detail in subsequent chapters.

A dynamical system consists of a set of variables that describe its state and a law that describes the evolution of the state variables with time (i.e., how the state of the system in the next moment of time depends on the input and its state in the previous moment of time). The Hodgkin-Huxley model is a four-dimensional dynamical system because its state is uniquely determined by the membrane potential, $V$, and so-called gating variables $n, m$, and $h$ for persistent $K^+$ and transient $Na^+$ currents. The evolution law is given by a four-dimensional system of ordinary differential equations.

Typically, all variables describing neuronal dynamics can be classified into four classes, according to their function and the time scale.

1. *Membrane potential.*

2. *Excitation variables*, such as activation of a $Na^+$ current. These variables are responsible for the upstroke of the spike.

3. *Recovery variables*, such as inactivation of a $Na^+$ current and activation of a fast $K^+$ current. These variables are responsible for the repolarization (downstroke) of the spike.

4. *Adaptation variables*, such as activation of slow voltage- or $Ca^{2+}$-dependent currents. These variables build up during prolonged spiking and can affect excitability in the long run.

The Hodgkin-Huxley model does not have variables of the fourth type, but many neuronal models do, especially those exhibiting bursting dynamics.

### 1.2.1 Phase Portraits

The power of the dynamical systems approach to neuroscience, as well as to many other sciences, is that we can tell something, or many things, about a system without knowing all the details that govern the system evolution. We do not even use equations to do that! Some may even wonder why we call it a mathematical theory.

As a start, let us consider a quiescent neuron whose membrane potential is resting. From the dynamical systems point of view, there are no changes of the state variables of such a neuron; hence it is at an equilibrium point. All the inward currents that depolarize the neuron are balanced, or equilibrated, by the outward currents that hyperpolarize it. If the neuron remains quiescent despite small disturbances and membrane noise, as in Fig.1.9a (top), then we conclude that the equilibrium is stable. Isn't

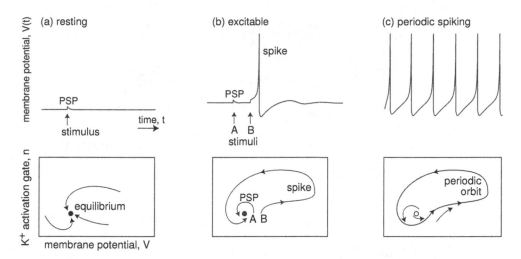

Figure 1.9: Resting, excitable, and periodic spiking activity correspond to a stable equilibrium (a and b) or limit cycle (c), respectively.

it amazing that we can reach such a conclusion without knowing the equations that describe the neuron's dynamics? We do not even know the number of variables needed to describe the neuron; it could be infinite, for all we care.

In this book we introduce the notions of equilibria, stability, threshold, and attraction domains using one- and two-dimensional dynamical systems, e.g., the $I_{\mathrm{Na,p}}+I_{\mathrm{K}}$-model with instantaneous Na$^+$ kinetics. The state of this model is described by the membrane potential, $V$, and the activation variable, $n$, of the persistent K$^+$ current, so it is a two-dimensional vector $(V, n)$. Instantaneous activation of the Na$^+$ current is a function of $V$, so it does not result in a separate variable of the model. The evolution of the model is a trajectory $(V(t), n(t))$ on the $V \times n$–plane. Depending on the initial point, the system can have many trajectories, such as those depicted in Fig.1.9a (bottom). Time is not explicitly present in the figure, but units of time may be thought of as plotted along each trajectory. All of the trajectories in the figure are attracted to the stable equilibrium denoted by the black dot, called an *attractor*. The overall qualitative description of dynamics can be obtained through the study of the *phase portrait* of the system, which depicts certain special trajectories (equilibria, separatrices, limit cycles) that determine the topological behavior of all the other trajectories in the phase space. Probably 50 percent of illustrations in this book are phase portraits.

A fundamental property of neurons is *excitability*, illustrated in Fig.1.9b. The neuron is resting, i.e., its phase portrait has a stable equilibrium. Small perturbations, such as A, result in small excursions from the equilibrium, denoted as PSP (postsynaptic potential). Larger perturbations, such as B, are amplified by the neuron's intrinsic dynamics and result in the spike response. To understand the dynamic mechanism of such amplification, we need to consider the geometry of the phase portrait near the resting equilibrium, i.e., in the region where the decision to fire or not to fire is made.

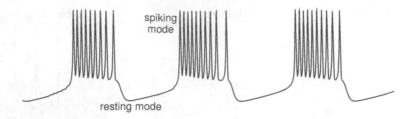

Figure 1.10: Rhythmic transitions between resting and spiking modes result in bursting behavior.

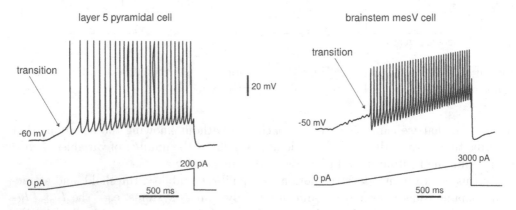

Figure 1.11: As the magnitude of the injected current slowly increases, the neurons bifurcate from resting (equilibrium) mode to tonic spiking (limit cycle) mode.

If we inject a sufficiently strong current into the neuron, we bring it to a pacemaking mode, so that it exhibits periodic spiking activity, as in Fig.1.9c. From the dynamical systems point of view, the state of such a neuron has a stable limit cycle, also known as a stable periodic orbit. The electrophysiological details of the neuron (i.e., the number and the type of currents it has, their kinetics, etc.) determine only the location, the shape, and the period of the limit cycle. As long as the limit cycle exists, the neuron can have periodic spiking activity. Of course, equilibria and limit cycles can coexist, so a neuron can be switched from one mode to another by a transient input. The famous example is the permanent extinguishing of ongoing spiking activity in the squid giant axon by a brief transient depolarizing pulse of current applied at a proper phase (Guttman et al. 1980) – a phenomenon predicted by John Rinzel (1978) purely on the basis of theoretical analysis of the Hodgkin-Huxley model. The transition between resting and spiking modes could be triggered by intrinsic slow conductances, resulting in the bursting behavior in Fig.1.10.

## 1.2.2    Bifurcations

Now suppose that the magnitude of the injected current is a parameter that we can control, e.g., we can ramp it up, as in Fig.1.11. Each cell in the figure is quiescent at the beginning of the ramps, so its phase portrait has a stable equilibrium and it may look like the one in Fig.1.9a or Fig.1.9b. Then it starts to fire tonic spikes, so its phase portrait has a limit cycle attractor and it may look like the one in Fig.1.9c, with a white circle denoting an unstable resting equilibrium. Apparently there is some intermediate level of injected current that corresponds to the transition from resting to sustained spiking, i.e., from the phase portrait in Fig.1.9b to Fig.1.9c. What does the transition look like?

From the dynamical systems point of view, the transition corresponds to a *bifurcation* of neuron dynamics, i.e., a qualitative change of phase portrait of the system. For example, there is no bifurcation going from the phase portrait in Fig.1.9a to that in Fig.1.9b, since both have one globally stable equilibrium; the difference in behavior is quantitative but not qualitative. In contrast, there is a bifurcation going from Fig.1.9b to Fig.1.9c, since the equilibrium is no longer stable and another attractor, limit cycle, has appeared. The neuron is not excitable in Fig.1.9a but it is in Fig.1.9b, simply because the former phase portrait is far from the bifurcation and the latter is near.

In general, neurons are excitable *because* they are near bifurcations from resting to spiking activity, so the type of the bifurcation determines the excitable properties of the neuron. Of course, the type depends on the neuron's electrophysiology. An amazing observation is that there could be millions of different electrophysiological mechanisms of excitability and spiking, but there are only four – yes, *four* – different types of bifurcations of equilibrium that a system can undergo without any additional constraints, such as symmetry. Thus, considering these four bifurcations in a general setup, we can understand excitable properties of many models, even those that have not been invented yet. What is even more amazing, we can understand excitable properties of neurons whose currents are not measured and whose models are not known, provided we can experimentally identify which of the four bifurcations the resting state of the neuron undergoes.

The four bifurcations are summarized in Fig.1.12, which plots the phase portrait before (left), at (center), and after (right) a particular bifurcation occurs. Mathematicians refer to these bifurcations as being of codimension-1 because we need to vary only one parameter, e.g., the magnitude of the injected DC current $I$, to observe the bifurcations reliably in simulations or experiments. There are many more codimension-2, 3, (etc.), bifurcations, but they need special conditions to be observed. We discuss these in chapter 6.

Let us consider the four bifurcations and their phase portraits in Fig.1.12. The horizontal and vertical axes are the membrane potential with instantaneous activation variable and a recovery variable, respectively. At this stage, the reader is not required to fully understand the intricacies of the phase portraits in the figure, since they will be explained systematically in later chapters.

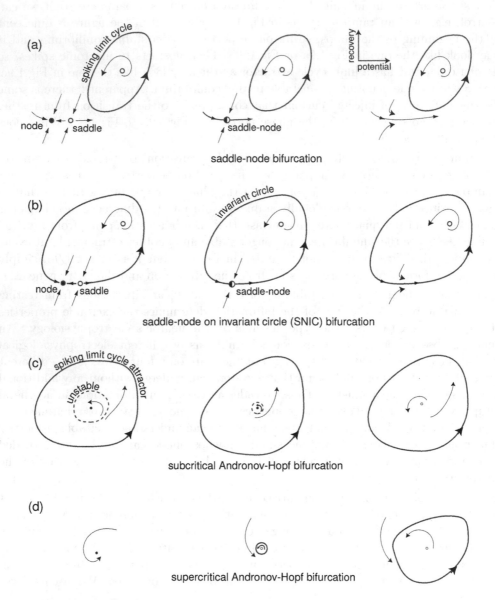

Figure 1.12: Four generic (codimension-1) bifurcations of an equilibrium state leading to the transition from resting to periodic spiking behavior in neurons.

- *Saddle-node bifurcation.* As the magnitude of the injected current or any other bifurcation parameter changes, a stable equilibrium corresponding to the resting state (black circle marked "node" in Fig.1.12a) is approached by an unstable equilibrium (white circle marked "saddle"); they coalesce and annihilate each other, as in Fig.1.12a (middle). Since the resting state no longer exists, the trajectory describing the evolution of the system jumps to the limit cycle attractor, indicating that the neuron starts to fire tonic spikes. Notice that the limit cycle, or some other attractor, must coexist with the resting state in order for the transition resting → spiking to occur.

- *Saddle-node on invariant circle bifurcation* is similar to the saddle-node bifurcation except that there is an invariant circle at the moment of bifurcation, which then becomes a limit cycle attractor, as in Fig.1.12b.

- *Subcritical Andronov-Hopf bifurcation.* A small unstable limit cycle shrinks to a stable equilibrium and makes it lose stability, as in Fig.1.12c. Because of instabilities, the trajectory diverges from the equilibrium and approaches a large-amplitude spiking limit cycle or some other attractor.

- *Supercritical Andronov-Hopf bifurcation.* The stable equilibrium loses stability and gives birth to a small-amplitude limit cycle attractor, as in Fig.1.12d. As the magnitude of the injected current increases, the amplitude of the limit cycle increases and it becomes a full-size spiking limit cycle.

Notice that there is a coexistence of resting and spiking states in the case of saddle-node and subcritical Andronov-Hopf bifurcations, but not in the other two cases. Such a coexistence reveals itself via a hysteresis behavior when the injected current slowly increases and then decreases past the bifurcation value, because the transitions "resting → spiking" and "spiking → resting" occur at different values of the current. In addition, brief stimuli applied at the appropriate times can switch the activity from spiking to resting and back. There are also spontaneous noise-induced transitions between the two modes that result in the stuttering spiking that, for instance, is exhibited by the so-called fast spiking (FS) cortical interneurons when they are kept close to the bifurcation (Tateno et al. 2004). Some bistable neurons have a slow adaptation current that activates during the spiking mode and impedes spiking, often resulting in bursting activity.

Systems undergoing Andronov-Hopf bifurcations, whether subcritical or supercritical, exhibit damped oscillations of membrane potential, whereas systems near saddle-node bifurcations, whether on or off an invariant circle, do not. The existence of small amplitude oscillations creates the possibility of resonance to the frequency of the incoming pulses, as in Fig.1.7, and other interesting features.

We refer to neurons with damped subthreshold oscillations as *resonators* and to those that do not have this property as *integrators*. We refer to the neurons that exhibit the coexistence of resting and spiking states, at least near the transition from

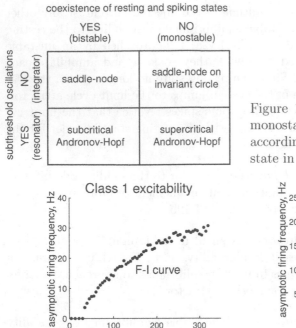

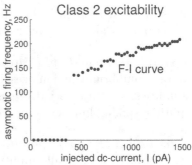

Figure 1.13: Classification of neurons into monostable/bistable integrators/resonators according to the bifurcation of the resting state in Fig.1.12.

Figure 1.14: Frequency-current (F-I) curves of cortical pyramidal neuron and brainstem mesV neuron from Fig.7.3. These are the same neurons used in the ramp experiment in Fig.1.11.

resting to spiking, as *bistable*, and to those that do not, *monostable*. The four bifurcations in Fig.1.12 are uniquely defined by these two features. For example, a bistable resonator is a neuron undergoing subcritical Andronov-Hopf bifurcation, and a monostable integrator is a neuron undergoing saddle-node on invariant circle bifurcation (see Fig.1.13). Cortical fast spiking (FS) and regular spiking (RS) neurons, studied in chapter 8, are typical examples of the former and the latter, respectively.

### 1.2.3  Hodgkin Classification

Hodgkin (1948) was the first to study bifurcations in neuronal dynamics, years before the mathematical theory of bifurcations was developed. He stimulated squid axons with pulses of various amplitudes and identified three classes of responses:

- *Class 1 neural excitability.* Action potentials can be generated with arbitrarily low frequency, depending on the strength of the applied current.

- *Class 2 neural excitability.* Action potentials are generated in a certain frequency band that is relatively insensitive to changes in the strength of the applied current.

- *Class 3 neural excitability.* A single action potential is generated in response to a pulse of current. Repetitive (tonic) spiking can be generated only for extremely strong injected currents or not at all.

The qualitative distinction between the classes is that the frequency-current relation (the F-I curve in Fig.1.14) starts from zero and continuously increases for Class 1 neurons, is discontinuous for Class 2 neurons, and is not defined at all for Class 3 neurons.

Obviously, neurons belonging to different classes have different neurocomputational properties. Class 1 neurons, which include cortical excitatory pyramidal neurons, can smoothly encode the strength of the input into the output firing frequency, as in Fig.1.11 (left). In contrast, Class 2 neurons, such as fast-spiking (FS) cortical inhibitory interneurons, cannot do that; instead, they fire in a relatively narrow frequency band, as in Fig.1.11 (right). Class 3 neurons cannot exhibit sustained spiking activity, so Hodgkin regarded them as "sick" or "unhealthy". There are other distinctions between the classes, which we discuss later.

Different classes of excitability occur because neurons have different bifurcations of resting and spiking states – a phenomenon first explained by Rinzel and Ermentrout (1989). If ramps of current are injected to measure the F-I curves, then Class 1 excitability occurs when the neuron undergoes the saddle-node bifurcation on an invariant circle depicted in Fig.1.12b. Indeed, the period of the limit cycle attractor is infinite at the bifurcation point, and then it decreases as the bifurcation parameter – say, the magnitude of the injected current – increases. The other three bifurcations result in Class 2 excitability. Indeed, the limit cycle attractor exists and has a finite period when the resting state in Fig.1.12 undergoes a subcritical Andronov-Hopf bifurcation, so emerging spiking has a nonzero frequency. The period of the small limit cycle attractor appearing via supercritical Andronov-Hopf bifurcation is also finite, so the frequency of oscillations is nonzero, but their amplitudes are small. In contrast to the common and erroneous folklore, the saddle-node bifurcation (off-limit cycle) also results in Class 2 excitability because the limit cycle has a finite period at the bifurcation. There is a considerable latency (delay) to the first spike in this case, but the subsequent spiking has nonzero frequency. Thus, the simple scheme "Class 1 = saddle-node, Class 2 = Hopf" that permeates many publications is unfortunately incorrect.

When pulses of current are used to measure the F-I curve, as in Hodgkin's experiments, the firing frequency depends on factors besides the type of the bifurcation of the resting state. In particular, low-frequency firing can be observed in systems near Andronov-Hopf bifurcations, as we show in chapter 7. To avoid possible confusion, we define the class of excitability only on the basis of slow ramp experiments.

Hodgkin's classification has an important historical value, but it is of little use for the dynamic description of a neuron, since naming a class of excitability of a neuron does not tell much about the bifurcations of the resting state. Indeed, it says only that saddle-node on invariant circle bifurcation (Class 1) is different from the other three bifurcations (Class 2), and only when ramps are injected. Dividing neurons into integrators and resonators with bistable or monostable activity is more informative, so we adopt the classification in Fig.1.13 in this book. In this classification, a Class 1 neuron is a monostable integrator, whereas a Class 2 neuron can be a bistable integrator or a resonator.

## 1.2.4   Neurocomputational properties

Using the same arrangement as in Fig.1.13, we depict typical geometry of phase portraits near the four bifurcations in Fig.1.15. Let us use the portraits to explain what happens "near the threshold", i.e., near the place where the decision to fire or not to fire is made. To simplify our geometrical analysis, we assume here that neurons receive shock inputs, i.e., brief but strong pulses of current that do not change the phase portraits, but only push or reset the state of the neuron into various regions of the phase space. We consider these and other cases in detail in chapter 7.

The horizontal axis in each plot in Fig.1.15 corresponds to the membrane potential $V$ with instantaneous $Na^+$ current, and the vertical axis corresponds to a recovery variable, say activation of $K^+$ current. Black circles denote stable equilibria corresponding to the neuronal resting state. Spiking limit cycle attractors correspond to sustained spiking states, which exist in the two cases depicted in the left half of the figure corresponding to the bistable dynamics. The limit cycles are surrounded by shaded regions – their attraction domains. The white region is the attraction domain of the equilibrium. To initiate spiking, the external input should push the state of the system into the shaded region, and to extinguish spiking, the input should push the state back into the white region.

There are no limit cycles in the two cases depicted in the right half of the figure, so the entire phase space is the attraction domain of the stable equilibrium, and the dynamics are monostable. However, if the trajectory starts in the shaded region, it makes a large-amplitude rotation before returning to the equilibrium – a transient spike. Apparently, to elicit such a spike, the input should push the state of the system into the shaded region.

Now let us contrast the upper and lower halves of the figure, corresponding to integrators and resonators, respectively. We distinguish these two modes of operation on the basis of the existence of subthreshold oscillations near the equilibrium.

First, let us show that *inhibition impedes spiking in integrators, but can promote it in resonators*. In the integrator, the shaded region is in the depolarized voltage range, i.e., to the right of the equilibrium. Excitatory inputs push the state of the system toward the shaded region, while inhibitory inputs push it away. In resonators, both excitation and inhibition push the state toward the shaded region, because the region wraps around the equilibrium and can be reached along any direction. This explains the rebound spiking phenomenon depicted in Fig.1.6.

*Integrators have all-or-none spikes; resonators may not.* Indeed, any trajectory starting in the shaded region in the upper half of Fig.1.15 has to rotate around the

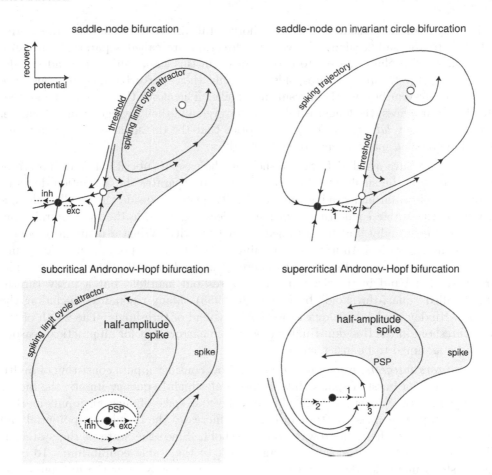

Figure 1.15: The geometry of phase portraits of excitable systems near four bifurcations can explain many neurocomputational properties (see section 1.2.4 for details).

white circle at the top that corresponds to an unstable equilibrium. Moreover, the state of the system is quickly attracted to the spiking trajectory and moves along that trajectory, thereby generating a stereotypical spike. A resonator neuron also can fire large amplitude spikes when its state is pushed to or beyond the trajectory denoted "spike". Such neurons generate subthreshold responses when the state slides along the smaller trajectory denoted PSP; they also can generate spikes of an intermediate amplitude when the state is pushed between the PSP and "spike" trajectories, which explains the partial-amplitude spiking in Fig.1.5b or in the squid axon in Fig.7.26. The set of initial conditions corresponding to such spiking is quite small, so typical spikes have large amplitudes and partial spikes are rare.

*Integrators have well-defined thresholds; resonators may not.* The white circles near the resting states of integrators in Fig.1.15 are called saddles. They are stable along the vertical direction and unstable along the horizontal direction. The two trajectories that lead to the saddle along the vertical direction are called separatrices because they separate the phase space into two regions – in this case, white and shaded. The separatrices play the role of thresholds since only those perturbations that push the state of the system beyond them result in a spike. The closer the state of the system is to the separatrices, the longer it takes to converge and then diverge from the saddle, resulting in a long *latency to the spike*. Notice that the threshold is not a point, but a tilted curve that spans a range of voltage values.

Resonators have a well-defined threshold in the case of subcritical Andronov-Hopf bifurcation: it is the small unstable limit cycle that separates the attraction domains of stable equilibrium and spiking limit cycle. Trajectories inside the small cycle spiral toward the stable equilibrium, whereas trajectories outside the cycle spiral away from it and eventually lead to sustained spiking activity. When a neuronal model is far from the subcritical Andronov-Hopf bifurcation, its phase portrait may look similar to the one corresponding to the supercritical Andronov-Hopf bifurcation. The narrow shaded band in the figure is not a threshold manifold but a fuzzy threshold set called "quasi-threshold" by FitzHugh (1955). Many resonators, including the Hodgkin-Huxley model, have quasi-thresholds instead of thresholds. The width of the quasi-threshold in the Hodgkin-Huxley model is so narrow that for all practical reasons it may be assumed to be just a curve.

*Integrators integrate, resonators resonate.* Now consider inputs consisting of multiple pulses, e.g., a burst of spikes. Integrators prefer high-frequency inputs; the higher the frequency, the sooner they fire. Indeed, the first spike of such an input, marked "1" in the top-right phase portrait in Fig.1.15, increases the membrane potential and shifts the state to the right, toward the threshold. Since the state of the system is still in the white area, it slowly converges back to the stable equilibrium. To cross the threshold manifold, the second pulse must arrive shortly after the first one. The reaction of a resonator to a pair of pulses is quite different. The first pulse initiates a damped subthreshold oscillation of the membrane potential, which looks like a spiral in the bottom-right phase portrait in Fig.1.15. The effect of the second pulse depends on its timing. If it arrives after the trajectory makes half a rotation, marked "2" in the figure, it cancels the effect of the first pulse. If it arrives after the trajectory makes a full rotation, marked "3" in the figure, it adds to the first pulse and either increases the amplitude of subthreshold oscillation or evokes a spike response. Thus, the response of the resonator neuron depends on the frequency content of the input, as in Fig.1.7.

Integrators and resonators constitute two major modes of activity of neurons. Most cortical pyramidal neurons, including the regular spiking (RS), intrinsically bursting (IB), and chattering (CH) types considered in Chap. 8, are integrators. So are thalamocortical neurons in the relay mode of firing, and neostriatal spiny projection neurons. Most cortical inhibitory interneurons, including the FS type, are resonators. So are brainstem mesencephalic V neurons and stellate neurons of the entorhinal cortex. Some cortical pyramidal neurons and low-threshold spiking (LTS) interneurons can be at the border of transition between integrator and resonator modes. Such a transition corre-

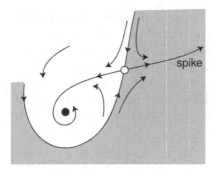

Figure 1.16: Phase portrait of a system near a Bogdanov-Takens bifurcation that corresponds to the transition from integrator to resonator mode.

sponds to another bifurcation, which has codimension-2, and hence it is less likely to be encountered experimentally. We consider this and other uncommon bifurcations in detail later. The phase portrait near the bifurcation is depicted in Fig.1.16, and it is a good exercise for the reader to explain why such a system has damped oscillations and postinhibitory responses, yet a well-defined threshold, all-or-none spikes, and possibly long latencies.

Of course, figures 1.15 and 1.16 cannot encompass all the richness of neuronal behavior, otherwise this book would be only 19pages long (this book is actually quite short; most of the space is taken by figures, exercises, and solutions). Many aspects of neuronal dynamics depend on other bifurcations, e.g., those corresponding to appearance and disappearance of spiking limit cycles. These bifurcations describe the transitions from spiking to resting, and they are especially important when we consider bursting activity. In addition, we need to take into account the relative geometry of equilibria, limit cycles, and other relevant trajectories, and how they depend on the parameters of the system, such as maximal conductances, and activation time constants. We explore all these issues systematically in subsequent chapters.

In chapter 2 we review some of the most fundamental concepts of neuron electrophysiology, culminating with the Hodgkin-Huxley model. This chapter is aimed at mathematicians learning neuroscience. In chapters 3 and 4 we use one- and two-dimensional neuronal models, respectively, to review some of the most fundamental concepts of dynamical systems, such as equilibria, limit cycles, stability, attraction domain, nullclines, phase portrait, and bifurcation. The material in these chapters, aimed at biologists learning the language of dynamical systems, is presented with the emphasis on geometrical rather than mathematical intuition. In fact, the spirit of the entire book is to explain concepts by using pictures, not equations. Chapter 5 explores phase portraits of various conductance-based models and the relations between ionic currents and dynamic behavior. In Chapter 6 we use the $I_{\text{Na,p}}+I_{\text{K}}$-model to systematically introduce the geometric bifurcation theory. Chapter 7, probably the most important chapter of the book, applies the theory to explain many computational properties of neurons. In fact, all the material in the previous chapters is given so that the reader can understand this chapter. In chapter 8 we use a simple phenomenological model to simulate many cortical, hippocampal, and thalamic neurons. This chapter contains probably the most comprehensive up-to-date review of various firing patterns exhibited by mammalian neurons. In chapter 9 we introduce the electrophysiological and topological classification of bursting dynamics, as well as some useful methods to study the bursters. Finally, the last and the most mathematically advanced chapter of the book, Chap. 10, deals with coupled neurons. There we show how the details of the spike generation mechanism of neurons affect neurons' collective properties, such as synchronization.

## 1.2.5   Building Models (Revisited)

To have a good model of a neuron, it is not enough to put the right kind of currents together and tune the parameters so that the model can fire spikes. It is not even enough to reproduce the right input resistance, rheobase, and firing frequencies. The model has to reproduce all the neurocomputational features of the neuron, starting with the coexistence of resting and spiking states, spike latencies, subthreshold oscillations, and rebound spikes, among others.

A good way to start is to determine what kind of bifurcations the neuron under consideration undergoes and how the bifurcations depend on neuromodulators and pharmacological blockers. Instead of or in addition to measuring neuronal responses to get the kinetic parameters, we need to measure them to get the right bifurcation behavior. Only in this case we can be sure that the behavior of the model is *equivalent* to that of the neuron, even if we omitted a current or guessed some of the parameters incorrectly.

Implementation of this research program is still a pipe dream. The people who understand the mathematical aspects of neuron dynamics – those who see beyond conductances and currents – usually do not have the opportunity to do experiments. Conversely, those who study neurons in vitro or in vivo on a daily basis – those who see spiking, bursting, and oscillations; those who can manipulate the experimental setup to test practically any aspect of neuronal activity – do not usually see the value of studying phase portraits, bifurcations, and nonlinear dynamics in general. One of the goals of this book is to change this state and bring these two groups of people closer together.

# Review of Important Concepts

- Neurons are dynamical systems.

- The resting state of neurons corresponds to a stable equilibrium; the tonic spiking state corresponds to a limit cycle attractor.

- Neurons are excitable because the equilibrium is near a bifurcation.

- There are many ionic mechanisms of spike generation, but only four generic bifurcations of equilibria.

- These bifurcations divide neurons into four categories: integrators or resonators, monostable or bistable.

- Analyses of phase portraits at bifurcations explain why some neurons have well-defined thresholds, all-or-none spikes, postinhibitory spikes, frequency preference, hysteresis, and so on, while others do not.

- These features, and not ionic currents per se, determine the neuronal responses, i.e., the kind of computations neurons do.

- A good neuronal model must reproduce not only electrophysiology but also the bifurcation dynamics of neurons.

# Bibliographical Notes

Richard FitzHugh at the National Institutes of Health (NIH) pioneered the phase plane analysis of neuronal models with the view to understanding their neurocomputational properties. He was the first to analyze the Hodgkin-Huxley model (FitzHugh 1955; years before they received the Nobel Prize) and to prove that it has neither threshold nor all-or-none spikes. FitzHugh (1961) introduced the simplified model of excitability (see Fig.1.18) and showed that one can get the right kind of neuronal dynamics in models lacking conductances and currents. Nagumo et al. (1962) designed a corresponding tunnel diode circuit, so the model is called the FitzHugh-Nagumo oscillator. Chapter 8 deals with such simplified models. The history of the development of FitzHugh-Nagumo model is reviewed by Izhikevich and FitzHugh (2006).

FitzHugh's research program was further developed by John Rinzel and G. Bard Ermentrout (see Fig.1.19 and Fig.1.20). In their 1989 seminal paper, Rinzel and Ermentrout revived Hodgkin's classification of excitability and pointed out the connection between the behavior of neuronal models and the bifurcations they exhibit. (They also referred to the excitability as "type I" or "type II"). Unfortunately, many people treat

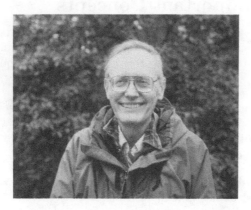

Figure 1.17: Richard FitzHugh in 1984.

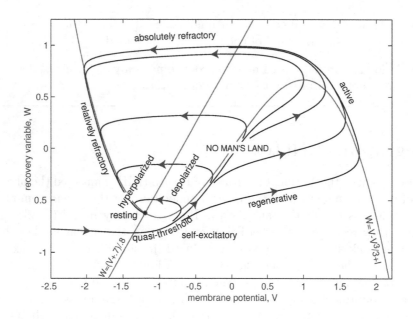

Figure 1.18: Phase portrait and physiological state diagram of FitzHugh-Nagumo model $\dot{V} = V - V^3/3 - W + I$, $\dot{W} = 0.08(V + 0.7 - 0.8W)$. The meaning of curves and trajectories is explained in chapter 4. (Reproduced from Izhikevich and FitzHugh (2006) with permission.)

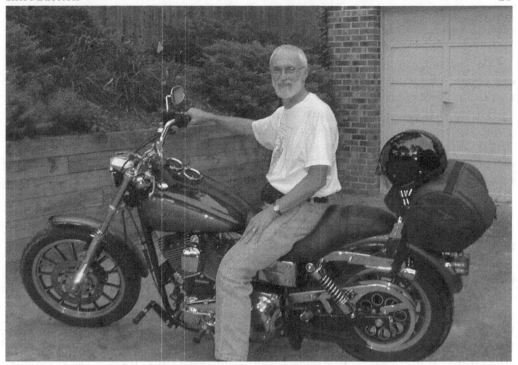

Figure 1.19: John Rinzel in 2004. Depicted on his T-shirt is the cover of the first issue of *Journal of Computational Neuroscience*, in which the Pinsky-Rinzel (1994) model appeared.

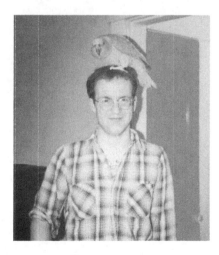

Figure 1.20: G. Bard Ermentrout (G. stands for George) with his parrot, Junior, in 1983.

the connection in a simpleminded fashion and incorrectly identify "type I = saddle-node, type II = Hopf". If only life were so simple!

The geometrical analysis of neuronal models was further developed by, among others, Izhikevich (2000a), who stressed the integrator and resonator modes of operation and made connections to other neurocomputational properties.

The neuroscience and mathematics parts of this book are standard, though many connections are new. The literature sources are listed at the end of each chapter. Among many outstanding books on computational neuroscience, the author especially recommends *Spikes, Decisions, and Actions* by Wilson (1999), *Biophysics of Computation* by Koch (1999), *Theoretical Neuroscience* by Dayan and Abbott (2001), and *Foundations of Cellular Neurophysiology* by Johnston and Wu (1995). The present volume complements these excellent books in the sense that it is more ambitious, focused, and thorough in dealing with neurons as dynamical systems. Though its views may be biased by the author's philosophy and taste, the payoffs in understanding neuronal dynamics are immense, provided the reader has enough patience and perseverance to follow the author's line of thought.

The NEURON simulation environment is described by Hines (1989) and Carnevale and Hines (2006) (http://www.neuron.yale.edu); the GENESIS environment, by Bower and Beeman (1995) (http://www.genesis-sim.org); the XPP environment, by Ermentrout (2002). The author of this book uses MATLAB, which has become a standard computational tool in science and engineering. MATLAB is the registered trademark of The MathWorks, Inc. (http://www.mathworks.com).

# Chapter 2

# Electrophysiology of Neurons

In this chapter we remind the reader of some fundamental concepts of neuronal electrophysiology that are necessary to understand the rest of the book. We start with ions and currents, and move quickly toward the dynamics of the Hodgkin-Huxley model. If the reader is already familiar with the Hodgkin-Huxley formalism, this chapter can be skipped. Our exposition is brief, and it cannot substitute for a good introductory neuroscience course or the reading of such excellent textbooks as *Theoretical Neuroscience* by Dayan and Abbott (2001), *Foundations of Cellular Neurophysiology* by Johnston and Wu (1995), *Biophysics of Computation* by Koch (1999), or *Ion Channels of Excitable Membranes* by Hille (2001).

## 2.1 Ions

Electrical activity in neurons is sustained and propagated via ionic currents through neuron membranes. Most of these transmembrane currents involve one of four ionic species: sodium ($Na^+$), potassium ($K^+$), calcium ($Ca^{2+}$), or chloride ($Cl^-$). The first three have a positive charge (cations) and the fourth has a negative charge (anion). The concentrations of these ions are different on the inside and the outside of a cell, which creates electrochemical gradients – the major driving forces of neural activity. The extracellular medium has a high concentration of $Na^+$ and $Cl^-$ (salty, like seawater) and a relatively high concentration of $Ca^{2+}$. The intracellular medium has high concentrations of $K^+$ and negatively charged molecules (denoted by $A^-$), as we illustrate in Fig.2.1.

The cell membrane has large protein molecules forming channels through which ions (but not $A^-$) can flow according to their electrochemical gradients. The flow of $Na^+$ and $Ca^{2+}$ ions is not significant, at least at rest, but the flow of $K^+$ and $Cl^-$ ions is. This, however, does not eliminate the concentration asymmetry for two reasons.

- *Passive redistribution.* The impermeable anions $A^-$ attract more $K^+$ into the cell (opposites attract) and repel more $Cl^-$ out of the cell, thereby creating concentration gradients.

- *Active transport.* Ions are pumped in and out of the cell via ionic pumps. For example, the $Na^+$-$K^+$ pump depicted in Fig.2.1 pumps out three $Na^+$ ions for every two $K^+$ ions pumped in, thereby maintaining concentration gradients.

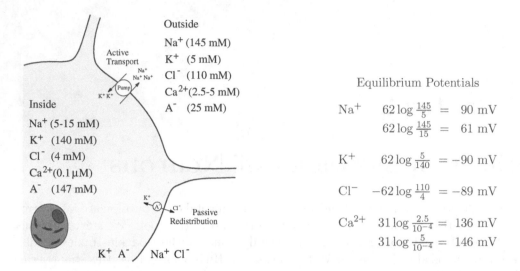

Figure 2.1: Ion concentrations and Nernst equilibrium potentials (2.1) in a typical mammalian neuron (modified from Johnston and Wu 1995). $A^-$ are membrane-impermeant anions. Temperature $T = 37°C$ (310°K).

## 2.1.1  Nernst Potential

There are two forces that drive each ion species through the membrane channel: concentration and electric potential gradients. First, the ions diffuse down the concentration gradient. For example, the $K^+$ ions depicted in Fig.2.2a diffuse out of the cell because $K^+$ concentration inside is higher than that outside. While exiting the cell, $K^+$ ions carry a positive charge and leave a net negative charge inside the cell (consisting mostly of impermeable anions $A^-$), thereby producing the outward current. The positive and negative charges accumulate on the opposite sides of the membrane surface, creating an electric potential gradient across the membrane – *transmembrane potential* or *membrane voltage.*  This potential slows the diffusion of $K^+$, since $K^+$ ions are attracted to the negatively charged interior and repelled from the positively charged exterior of the membrane, as we illustrate in Fig.2.2b. At some point an equilibrium is achieved: the concentration gradient and the electric potential gradient exert equal and opposite forces that counterbalance each other, and the net cross-membrane current is zero, as in Fig.2.2c. The value of such an *equilibrium potential* depends on the ionic species, and it is given by the Nernst equation (Hille 2001):

$$E_{\text{ion}} = \frac{RT}{zF} \ln \frac{[\text{Ion}]_{\text{out}}}{[\text{Ion}]_{\text{in}}} , \qquad (2.1)$$

where $[\text{Ion}]_{\text{in}}$ and $[\text{Ion}]_{\text{out}}$ are concentrations of the ions inside and outside the cell, respectively; $R$ is the universal gas constant ($8,315$ mJ/(K°·Mol)); $T$ is temperature in degrees Kelvin (K° = $273.16 + $C°); $F$ is Faraday's constant ($96,480$ coulombs/Mol),

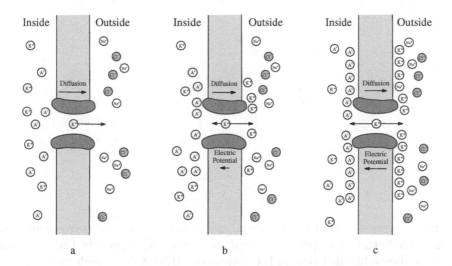

Figure 2.2: Diffusion of $K^+$ ions down the concentration gradient though the membrane (a) creates an electric potential force pointing in the opposite direction (b) until the diffusion and electrical forces counter each other (c). The resulting transmembrane potential (2.1) is referred to as the Nernst equilibrium potential for $K^+$.

$z$ is the valence of the ion ($z = 1$ for $Na^+$ and $K^+$; $z = -1$ for $Cl^-$; and $z = 2$ for $Ca^{2+}$). Substituting the numbers, taking $\log_{10}$ instead of natural $\ln$ and using body temperature $T = 310°K$ (37°C) results in

$$E_{ion} \approx 62 \log \frac{[\text{Ion}]_{out}}{[\text{Ion}]_{in}} \quad (\text{mV})$$

for monovalent ($z = 1$) ions. Nernst equilibrium potentials in a typical mammalian neuron are summarized in Fig.2.1.

## 2.1.2   Ionic Currents and Conductances

In the rest of the book $V$ denotes the membrane potential and $E_{Na}$, $E_{Ca}$, $E_K$, and $E_{Cl}$ denote the Nernst equilibrium potentials. When the membrane potential equals the equilibrium potential, say $E_K$, the net $K^+$ current, denoted as $I_K$ ($\mu A/cm^2$), is zero (this is the definition of the Nernst equilibrium potential for $K^+$). Otherwise, the net $K^+$ current is proportional to the difference of potentials; that is,

$$I_K = g_K (V - E_K),$$

where the positive parameter $g_K$ ($mS/cm^2$) is the $K^+$ conductance and $(V - E_K)$ is the $K^+$ *driving force*. The other major ionic currents,

$$I_{Na} = g_{Na} (V - E_{Na}), \qquad I_{Ca} = g_{Ca} (V - E_{Ca}), \qquad I_{Cl} = g_{Cl} (V - E_{Cl}),$$

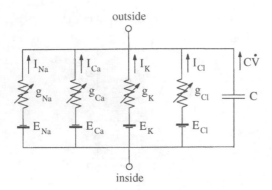

Figure 2.3: Equivalent circuit representation of a patch of cell membrane.

could also be expressed as products of nonlinear conductances and corresponding driving forces. A better description of membrane currents, especially $Ca^{2+}$ current, is provided by the Goldman-Hodgkin-Katz equation (Hille 2001), which we do not use in this book.

When the conductance is constant, the current is said to be *Ohmic*. In general, ionic currents in neurons are not Ohmic, since the conductances may depend on time, membrane potential, and pharmacological agents, e.g., neurotransmitters, neuromodulators, second-messengers, etc. It is the time-dependent variation in conductances that allows a neuron to generate an action potential, or spike.

### 2.1.3  Equivalent Circuit

It is traditional to represent electrical properties of membranes in terms of equivalent circuits similar to the one depicted in Fig.2.3. According to Kirchhoff's law, the total current, $I$, flowing across a patch of a cell membrane is the sum of the membrane capacitive current $C\dot{V}$ (the capacitance $C \approx 1.0\,\mu\mathrm{F/cm^2}$ in the squid axon) and all the ionic currents

$$I = C\dot{V} + I_{\mathrm{Na}} + I_{\mathrm{Ca}} + I_{\mathrm{K}} + I_{\mathrm{Cl}} \,,$$

where $\dot{V} = dV/dt$ is the derivative of the voltage variable $V$ with respect to time $t$. The derivative arises because it takes time to charge the membrane. This is the first *dynamic* term in the book! We write this equation in the standard "dynamical system" form

$$C\dot{V} = I - I_{\mathrm{Na}} - I_{\mathrm{Ca}} - I_{\mathrm{K}} - I_{\mathrm{Cl}} \tag{2.2}$$

or

$$C\dot{V} = I - g_{\mathrm{Na}}\left(V - E_{\mathrm{Na}}\right) - g_{\mathrm{Ca}}\left(V - E_{\mathrm{Ca}}\right) - g_{\mathrm{K}}\left(V - E_{\mathrm{K}}\right) - g_{\mathrm{Cl}}\left(V - E_{\mathrm{Cl}}\right) . \tag{2.3}$$

If there are no additional current sources or sinks, such as synaptic current, axial current, or tangential current along the membrane surface, or current injected via an electrode, then $I = 0$. In this case, the membrane potential is typically bounded by the equilibrium potentials in the order (see Fig.2.4)

$$E_{\mathrm{K}} < E_{\mathrm{Cl}} < V_{(\text{at rest})} < E_{\mathrm{Na}} < E_{\mathrm{Ca}} ,$$

so that $I_{\mathrm{Na}}, I_{\mathrm{Ca}} < 0$ (inward currents) and $I_{\mathrm{K}}, I_{\mathrm{Cl}} > 0$ (outward currents). From (2.2) it follows that inward currents increase the membrane potential, that is, make it more positive (depolarization), whereas outward currents decrease it, that is, make it more negative (hyperpolarization). Note that $I_{\mathrm{Cl}}$ is called an outward current even though the flow of $\mathrm{Cl}^-$ ions is inward; the ions bring negative charge inside the membrane, which is equivalent to positively charged ions leaving the cell, as in $I_{\mathrm{K}}$.

## 2.1.4 Resting Potential and Input Resistance

If there were only $\mathrm{K}^+$ channels, as in Fig.2.2, the membrane potential would quickly approach the $\mathrm{K}^+$ equilibrium potential, $E_{\mathrm{K}}$, which is around $-90$ mV. Indeed,

$$C\dot{V} = -I_{\mathrm{K}} = -g_{\mathrm{K}}(V - E_{\mathrm{K}})$$

in this case. However, most membranes contain a diversity of channels. For example, $\mathrm{Na}^+$ channels would produce an inward current and pull the membrane potential toward the $\mathrm{Na}^+$ equilibrium potential, $E_{\mathrm{Na}}$, which could be as large as $+90$ mV. The value of the membrane potential at which all inward and outward currents balance each other so that the net membrane current is zero corresponds to the *resting membrane potential*. It can be found from (2.3) with $I = 0$, by setting $\dot{V} = 0$. The resulting expression,

$$V_{\mathrm{rest}} = \frac{g_{\mathrm{Na}}E_{\mathrm{Na}} + g_{\mathrm{Ca}}E_{\mathrm{Ca}} + g_{\mathrm{K}}E_{\mathrm{K}} + g_{\mathrm{Cl}}E_{\mathrm{Cl}}}{g_{\mathrm{Na}} + g_{\mathrm{Ca}} + g_{\mathrm{K}} + g_{\mathrm{Cl}}} \tag{2.4}$$

has a nice mechanistic interpretation: $V_{\mathrm{rest}}$ is the center of mass of the balance depicted in Fig.2.4. Incidentally, the entire equation (2.3) can be written in the form

$$C\dot{V} = I - g_{\mathrm{inp}}(V - V_{\mathrm{rest}}) , \tag{2.5}$$

where

$$g_{\mathrm{inp}} = g_{\mathrm{Na}} + g_{\mathrm{Ca}} + g_{\mathrm{K}} + g_{\mathrm{Cl}}$$

is the total membrane conductance, called *input conductance*. The quantity $R_{\mathrm{inp}} = 1/g_{\mathrm{inp}}$ is the *input resistance* of the membrane, and it measures the asymptotic sensitivity of the membrane potential to injected or intrinsic currents. Indeed, from (2.5) it follows that

$$V \to V_{\mathrm{rest}} + IR_{\mathrm{inp}} , \tag{2.6}$$

so greater values of $R_{\mathrm{inp}}$ imply greater steady-state displacement of $V$ due to the injection of DC current $I$.

A remarkable property of neuronal membranes is that ionic conductances, and hence the input resistance, are functions of $V$ and time. We can use (2.6) to trace an action

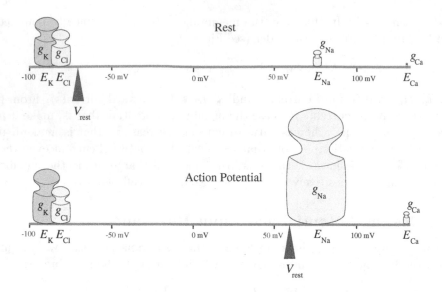

Figure 2.4: Mechanistic interpretation of the resting membrane potential (2.4) as the center of mass. Na$^+$ conductance increases during the action potential.

potential in a quasi-static fashion, i.e., assuming that time is frozen. When a neuron is quiescent, Na$^+$ and Ca$^{2+}$ conductances are relatively small, $V_{\text{rest}}$ is near $E_K$ and $E_{Cl}$, as in Fig.2.4 (top), and so is $V$. During the upstroke of an action potential, the Na$^+$ or Ca$^{2+}$ conductance becomes very large; $V_{\text{rest}}$ is near $E_{Na}$, as in Fig.2.4 (bottom), and $V$ increases, trying to catch $V_{\text{rest}}$. This event is, however, quite brief, for the reasons explained in subsequent sections.

## 2.1.5   Voltage-Clamp and I-V Relation

In section 2.2 we will study how the membrane potential affects ionic conductances and currents, assuming that the potential is fixed at certain value $V_c$ controlled by an experimenter. To maintain the membrane potential constant (clamped), one inserts a metallic conductor to short-circuit currents along the membrane (space-clamp), and then injects a current proportional to the difference $V_c - V$ (voltage-clamp), as in Fig.2.5. From (2.2) and the clamp condition $\dot{V} = 0$, it follows that the injected current $I$ equals the net current generated by the membrane conductances.

In a typical voltage-clamp experiment the membrane potential is held at a certain resting value $V_c$ and then reset to a new value $V_s$, as in Fig.2.6a. The injected membrane current needed to stabilize the potential at the new value is a function of time, the pre-step holding potential $V_c$, and the step potential $V_s$. First, the current jumps to a new value to accommodate the instantaneous voltage change from $V_c$ to $V_s$. From (2.5) we find that the amplitude of the jump is $g_{\text{inp}}(V_s - V_c)$. Then, time- and voltage-

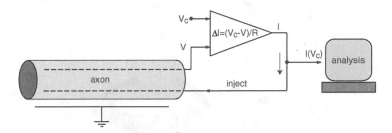

Figure 2.5: Two-wire voltage-clamp experiment on the axon. The top wire is used to monitor the membrane potential $V$. The bottom wire is used to inject the current $I$, proportional to the difference $V_c - V$, to keep the membrane potential at $V_c$.

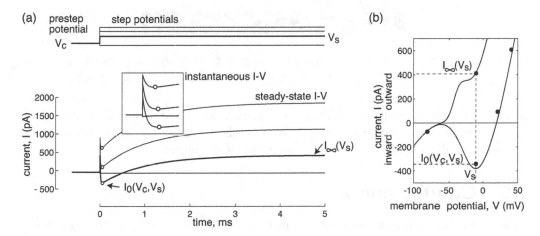

Figure 2.6: Voltage-clamp experiment to measure instantaneous and steady-state I-V relation. Shown are simulations of the $I_{Na}+I_K$-model (see Fig.4.1b); the continuous curves are theoretically found I-V relations.

dependent processes start to occur and the current decreases and then increases. The value at the negative peak, marked by the open circle "o" in Fig.2.6, depends only on $V_c$ and $V_s$, and it is called *the instantaneous current-voltage (I-V) relation*, or $I_0(V_c, V_s)$. The asymptotic $(t \to \infty)$ value depends only on $V_s$ and it is called the *steady-state current-voltage (I-V) relation*, or $I_\infty(V_s)$.

Both relations, depicted in Fig.2.6b, can be found experimentally (black circles) or theoretically (curves). The instantaneous I-V relation usually has a non-monotone N-shape reflecting nonlinear autocatalytic (positive feedback) transmembrane processes, which are fast enough on the time scale of the action potential that they can be assumed to have instantaneous kinetics. The steady-state I-V relation measures the asymptotic values of all transmembrane processes, and it may be monotone (as in the figure) or not, depending on the properties of the membrane currents. Both I-V relations provide invaluable quantitative information about the currents operating on fast and slow time

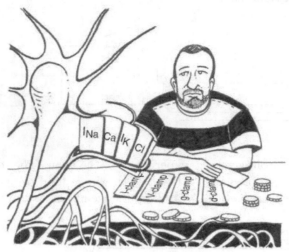

Figure 2.7: To tease out neuronal currents, biologists employ an arsenal of sophisticated "clamp" methods, such as current-, voltage-, conductance-, and dynamic-clamp.

scales, and both are useful in building mathematical models of neurons. Finally, when $I_\infty(V) = 0$, the net membrane current is zero, and the potential is at rest or equilibrium, which may still be unstable, as we discuss in the next chapter.

## 2.2   Conductances

Ionic channels are large transmembrane proteins having aqueous pores through which ions can flow down their electrochemical gradients. The electrical conductance of individual channels may be controlled by gating particles (gates), which switch the channels between open and closed states. The gates may be sensitive to the following factors:

- *Membrane potential.* Example: voltage-gated $Na^+$ or $K^+$ channels

- *Intracellular agents* (second-messengers). Example: $Ca^{2+}$-gated $K^+$ channels

- *Extracellular agents* (neurotransmitters and neuromodulators). Examples: AMPA, NMDA, or GABA receptors.

Despite the stochastic nature of transitions between open and closed states in individual channels, the net current generated by a large population or ensemble of identical channels can reasonably be described by the equation

$$I = \bar{g}\, p\,(V - E)\,, \tag{2.7}$$

where $p$ is the average proportion of channels in the open state, $\bar{g}$ is the *maximal conductance* of the population, and $E$ is the *reverse potential* of the current, i.e., the potential at which the current reverses its direction.   If the channels are selective

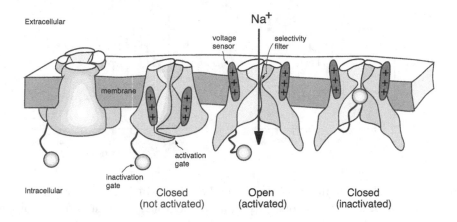

Figure 2.8: Structure of voltage-gated ion channels. Voltage sensors open an activation gate and allow selected ions to flow through the channel according to their electrochemical gradients. The inactivation gate blocks the channel. (Modified from Armstrong and Hille 1998.)

for a single ionic species, then the reverse potential $E$ equals the Nernst equilibrium potential (2.1) for that ionic species (see exercise 2).

## 2.2.1  Voltage-Gated Channels

When the gating particles are sensitive to the membrane potential, the channels are said to be *voltage-gated*. The gates are divided into two types: those that *activate* or open the channels, and those that *inactivate* or close them (see Fig.2.8). According to the tradition initiated in the middle of the twentieth century by Hodgkin and Huxley, the probability of an activation gate being in the open state is denoted by the variable $m$ (sometimes the variable $n$ is used for $K^+$ and $Cl^-$ channels). The probability of an inactivation gate being in the open state is denoted by the variable $h$. The proportion of open channels in a large population is

$$p = m^a \, h^b \, , \tag{2.8}$$

where $a$ is the number of activation gates and $b$ is the number of inactivation gates per channel.      The channels can be partially ($0 < m < 1$) or completely *activated* ($m = 1$); not activated or *deactivated* ($m = 0$); *inactivated* ($h = 0$); released from inactivation or *deinactivated* ($h = 1$). Some channels do not have inactivation gates ($b = 0$), hence $p = m^a$. Such channels do not inactivate, and they result in *persistent* currents. In contrast, channels that do inactivate result in *transient* currents.

Below we describe voltage- and time-dependent kinetics of gates. This description is often referred to as the *Hodgkin-Huxley gate model* of membrane channels.

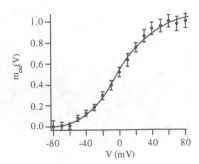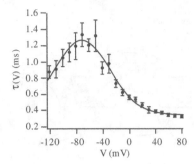

Figure 2.9: The activation function $m_\infty(V)$ and the time constant $\tau(V)$ of the fast transient $K^+$ current in layer 5 neocortical pyramidal neurons. (Modified from Korngreen and Sakmann 2000.)

## 2.2.2 Activation of Persistent Currents

The dynamics of the activation variable $m$ is described by the first-order differential equation

$$\dot{m} = (m_\infty(V) - m)/\tau(V) \,, \tag{2.9}$$

where the voltage-sensitive steady-state *activation function* $m_\infty(V)$ and the *time constant* $\tau(V)$ can be measured experimentally. They have sigmoid and unimodal shapes, respectively, as in Fig.2.9 (see also Fig.2.20). The steady-state activation function $m_\infty(V)$ gives the asymptotic value of $m$ when the potential is fixed (voltage-clamp). Smaller values of $\tau(V)$ result in faster dynamics of $m$.

In Fig.2.10 we depict a typical experiment to determine $m_\infty(V)$ of a persistent current, i.e., a current having no inactivation variable. Initially we hold the membrane potential at a hyperpolarized value $V_0$ so that all activation gates are closed and $I \approx 0$. Then we step-increase $V$ to a greater value $V_s$ ($s = 1, \ldots, 7$; see Fig.2.10a) and hold it there until the current is essentially equal to its asymptotic value, which is denoted here as $I_s$ ($s$ stands for "step"; see Fig.2.10b). Repeating the experiment for various stepping potentials $V_s$, one can easily determine the corresponding $I_s$, and hence the entire steady-state I-V relation, which we depict in Fig.2.10c. According to (2.7), $I(V) = \bar{g}m_\infty(V)(V - E)$, and the steady-state activation curve $m_\infty(V)$ depicted in Fig.2.10d is $I(V)$ divided by the driving force $(V - E)$ and normalized so that max $m_\infty(V) = 1$. To determine the time constant $\tau(V)$, one needs to analyze the convergence rates. In exercise 6 we describe an efficient method to determine $m_\infty(V)$ and $\tau(V)$.

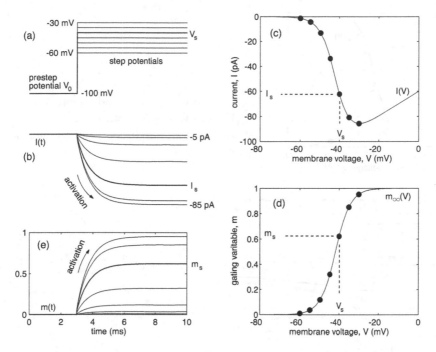

Figure 2.10: An experiment to determine $m_\infty(V)$. Shown are simulations of the persistent $Na^+$ current in Purkinje cells (see section 2.3.5).

### 2.2.3 Inactivation of Transient Currents

The dynamics of the inactivation variable $h$ can be described by the first-order differential equation

$$\dot{h} = (h_\infty(V) - h)/\tau(V) , \qquad (2.10)$$

where $h_\infty(V)$ is the voltage-sensitive steady-state *inactivation function* depicted in Fig.2.11. In Fig.2.12 we present a typical voltage-clamp experiment to determine $h_\infty(V)$ in the presence of activation $m_\infty(V)$. It relies on the observation that inactivation kinetics is usually slower than activation kinetics. First, we hold the membrane potential at a certain pre-step potential $V_s$ for a long enough time that the activation and inactivation variables are essentially equal to their steady-state values $m_\infty(V_s)$ and $h_\infty(V_s)$, respectively, which have yet to be determined. Then we step-increase $V$ to a sufficiently high value $V_0$, chosen so that $m_\infty(V_0) \approx 1$. If activation is much faster than inactivation, $m$ approaches 1 after the first few milliseconds, while $h$ continues to be near its asymptotic value $h_s = h_\infty(V_s)$, which can be found from the peak value of the current $I_s \approx \bar{g} \cdot 1 \cdot h_s(V_0 - E)$. Repeating this experiment for various pre-step potentials, one can determine the steady-state inactivation curve $h_\infty(V)$ in Fig.2.11. In exercise 6 we describe a better method to determine $h_\infty(V)$ that does not rely on the difference between the activation and inactivation time scales.

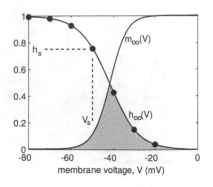

Figure 2.11: Steady-state activation function $m_\infty(V)$ from Fig.2.10, and inactivation function $h_\infty(V)$ and values $h_s$ from Fig.2.12. Their overlap (shaded region) produces a noticeable, persistent "window" current.

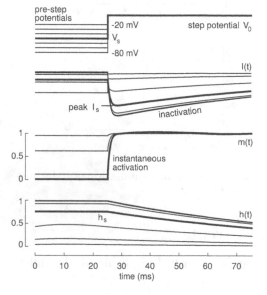

Figure 2.12: Dynamics of the current ($I$), activation ($m$), and inactivation ($h$) variables in the voltage-clamp experiment aimed at measuring $h_\infty(V)$ in Fig.2.11.

The voltage-sensitive steady-state activation and inactivation functions overlap in a shaded window depicted in Fig.2.11. Depending on the size of the shaded area in the figure, the overlap may result in a noticeable "window" current.

## 2.2.4  Hyperpolarization-Activated Channels

Many neurons in various parts of the brain have channels that are opened by hyperpolarization. These channels produce currents that are turned on by hyperpolarization and turned off by depolarization. Biologists refer to such currents as "exceptional" or "weird", and denote them as $I_Q$ (queer), $I_f$ (funny), $I_h$ (hyperpolarization-activated), or $I_{Kir}$ (K$^+$ inward rectifier). (We will consider the last two currents in detail in the next chapter). Most neuroscience textbooks classify these currents in a special category – *hyperpolarization-activated currents*. However, from the theoretical point of view, it is inconvenient to create special categories. In this book we treat these currents as "normal" transient currents with the understanding that they are always activated (either $a = 0$ or variable $m = 1$ in (2.8)), but can be inactivated by depolarization (variable $h \to 0$) or deinactivated by hyperpolarization (variable $h \to 1$). Moreover, there is biophysical evidence suggesting that closing/opening of $I_{\text{Kir}}$ is indeed related to the inactivation/deinactivation process (Lopatin et al. 1994).

## 2.3   The Hodgkin-Huxley Model

In section 2.1 we studied how the membrane potential depends on the membrane currents, assuming that ionic conductances are fixed. In section 2.2 we used the Hodgkin-Huxley gate model to study how the conductances and currents depend on the membrane potential, assuming that the potential is clamped at different values. In this section we put it all together and study how the potential $\leftrightarrow$ current nonlinear interactions lead to many interesting phenomena, such as generation of action potentials.

### 2.3.1   Hodgkin-Huxley Equations

One of the most important models in computational neuroscience is the Hodgkin-Huxley model of the squid giant axon. Using pioneering experimental techniques of that time, Hodgkin and Huxley (1952) determined that the squid axon carries three major currents: voltage-gated persistent K$^+$ current with four activation gates (resulting in the term $n^4$ in the equation below, where $n$ is the activation variable for K$^+$); voltage-gated transient Na$^+$ current with three activation gates and one inactivation gate (the term $m^3 h$ below), and Ohmic leak current, $I_{\text{L}}$, which is carried mostly by Cl$^-$ ions. The complete set of space-clamped Hodgkin-Huxley equations is

$$
C\dot{V} = I - \overbrace{\bar{g}_{\text{K}} n^4 (V - E_{\text{K}})}^{I_{\text{K}}} - \overbrace{\bar{g}_{\text{Na}} m^3 h (V - E_{\text{Na}})}^{I_{\text{Na}}} - \overbrace{g_{\text{L}}(V - E_{\text{L}})}^{I_{\text{L}}}
$$
$$
\dot{n} = \alpha_n(V)(1 - n) - \beta_n(V) n
$$
$$
\dot{m} = \alpha_m(V)(1 - m) - \beta_m(V) m
$$
$$
\dot{h} = \alpha_h(V)(1 - h) - \beta_h(V) h \, ,
$$

where

$$
\alpha_n(V) = 0.01 \frac{10 - V}{\exp(\frac{10-V}{10}) - 1} \, ,
$$
$$
\beta_n(V) = 0.125 \exp\left(\frac{-V}{80}\right) \, ,
$$
$$
\alpha_m(V) = 0.1 \frac{25 - V}{\exp(\frac{25-V}{10}) - 1} \, ,
$$
$$
\beta_m(V) = 4 \exp\left(\frac{-V}{18}\right) \, ,
$$

$$\alpha_h(V) = 0.07 \exp\left(\frac{-V}{20}\right) ,$$

$$\beta_h(V) = \frac{1}{\exp(\frac{30-V}{10}) + 1} .$$

These parameters, provided in the original Hodgkin and Huxley paper, correspond to the membrane potential shifted by approximately 65 mV, so that the resting potential is at $V \approx 0$. Hodgkin and Huxley did that for the sake of convenience, but the shift has led to a lot of confusion over the years. The shifted Nernst equilibrium potentials are

$$E_K = -12 \text{ mV} , \qquad E_{Na} = 120 \text{ mV} , \qquad E_L = 10.6 \text{ mV};$$

(see also exercise 1). Typical values of maximal conductances are

$$\bar{g}_K = 36 \text{ mS/cm}^2 , \qquad \bar{g}_{Na} = 120 \text{ mS/cm}^2 , \qquad g_L = 0.3 \text{ mS/cm}^2.$$

$C = 1\,\mu\text{F/cm}^2$ is the membrane capacitance and $I = 0\,\mu\text{A/cm}^2$ is the applied current. The functions $\alpha(V)$ and $\beta(V)$ describe the transition rates between open and closed states of the channels. We present this notation only for historical reasons. In the rest of the book, we use the standard form

$$\dot{n} = (n_\infty(V) - n)/\tau_n(V) ,$$
$$\dot{m} = (m_\infty(V) - m)/\tau_m(V) ,$$
$$\dot{h} = (h_\infty(V) - h)/\tau_h(V) ,$$

where

$$n_\infty = \alpha_n/(\alpha_n + \beta_n) , \qquad \tau_n = 1/(\alpha_n + \beta_n) ,$$
$$m_\infty = \alpha_m/(\alpha_m + \beta_m) , \qquad \tau_m = 1/(\alpha_m + \beta_m) ,$$
$$h_\infty = \alpha_h/(\alpha_h + \beta_h) , \qquad \tau_h = 1/(\alpha_h + \beta_h)$$

as depicted in Fig.2.13. These functions can be approximated by the Boltzmann and Gaussian functions; see Ex. 4. We also shift the membrane potential back to its true value, so that the resting state is near -65 mV.

The membrane of the squid giant axon carries only two major currents: transient $Na^+$ and persistent $K^+$. Most neurons in the central nervous system have additional currents with diverse activation and inactivation dynamics, which we summarize in section 2.3.5. The Hodgkin-Huxley formalism is the most accepted model to describe their kinetics.

Since we are interested in geometrical and qualitative methods of analysis of neuronal models, we assume that all variables and parameters have appropriate scales and dimensions, but we do not explicitly state them. An exception is the membrane potential $V$, whose mV scale is stated in every figure.

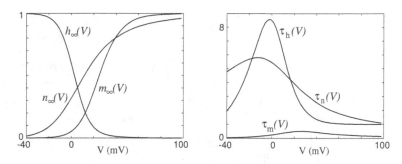

Figure 2.13: Steady-state (in)activation functions (left) and voltage-dependent time constants (right) in the Hodgkin-Huxley model.

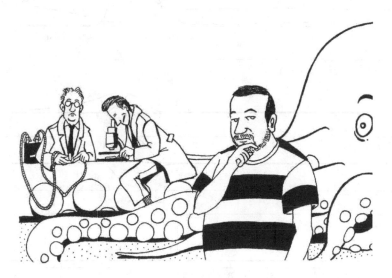

Figure 2.14: Studies of spike-generation mechanism in "giant squid" axons won Alan Hodgkin and Andrew Huxley the 1963 Nobel Prize for physiology or medicine (shared with John Eccles). See also Fig. 4.1 in Keener and Sneyd (1998).

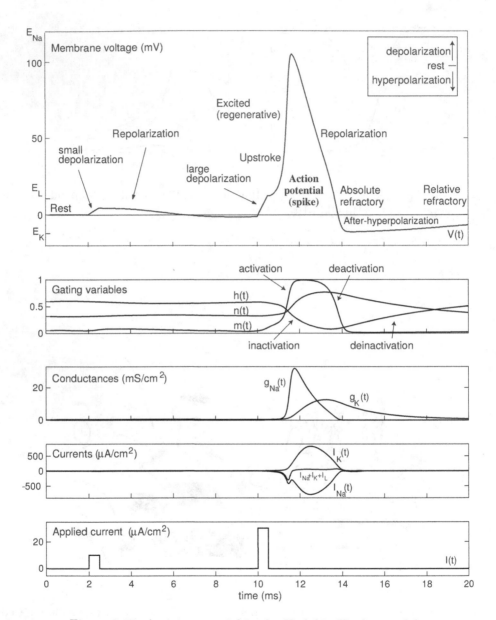

Figure 2.15: Action potential in the Hodgkin-Huxley model.

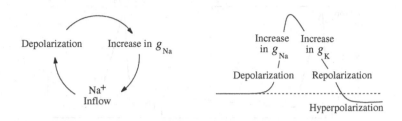

Figure 2.16: Positive and negative feedback loops resulting in excited (regenerative) behavior in neurons.

## 2.3.2 Action Potential

Recall that when $V = V_{\text{rest}}$, which is 0 mV in the Hodgkin-Huxley model, all inward and outward currents balance each other so the net current is zero, as in Fig.2.15. The resting state is stable: a small pulse of current applied via $I(t)$ produces a small positive perturbation of the membrane potential (depolarization), which results in a small net current that drives $V$ back to resting (repolarization). However, an intermediate size pulse of current produces a perturbation that is amplified significantly because membrane conductances depend on $V$. Such a nonlinear amplification causes $V$ to deviate considerably from $V_{\text{rest}}$ – a phenomenon referred to as an *action potential* or *spike*.

In Fig.2.15 we show a typical time course of an action potential in the Hodgkin-Huxley system. Strong depolarization increases activation variables $m$ and $n$ and decreases inactivation variable $h$. Since $\tau_m(V)$ is relatively small, variable $m$ is relatively fast. Fast activation of Na$^+$ conductance drives $V$ toward $E_{\text{Na}}$, resulting in further depolarization and further activation of $g_{\text{Na}}$. This positive feedback loop, depicted in Fig.2.16, results in the *upstroke* of $V$. While $V$ moves toward $E_{\text{Na}}$, the slower gating variables catch up. Variable $h \to 0$, causing inactivation of the Na$^+$ current, and variable $n \to 1$, causing slow activation of the outward K$^+$ current. The latter and the leak current repolarize the membrane potential toward $V_{\text{rest}}$.

When $V$ is near $V_{\text{rest}}$, the voltage-sensitive time constants $\tau_n(V)$ and $\tau_h(V)$ are relatively large, as one can see in Fig.2.13. Therefore, recovery of variables $n$ and $h$ is slow. In particular, the outward K$^+$ current continues to be activated ($n$ is large) even after the action potential downstroke, thereby causing $V$ to go below $V_{\text{rest}}$ toward $E_K$ – a phenomenon known as *afterhyperpolarization*.

In addition, the Na$^+$ current continues to be inactivated ($h$ is small) and not available for any regenerative function. The Hodgkin-Huxley system cannot generate another action potential during this *absolute refractory* period. While the current deinactivates, the system becomes able to generate an action potential, provided the stimulus is relatively strong (*relative refractory* period).

To study the relationship between these refractory periods, we stimulate the Hodgkin-Huxley model with 1-ms pulses of current having various amplitudes and latencies. The

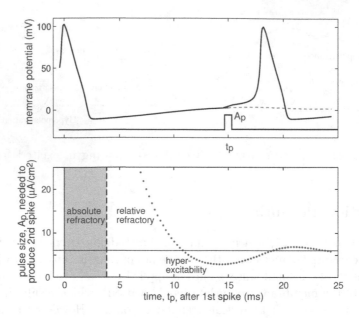

Figure 2.17: Refractory periods in the Hodgkin-Huxley model with $I = 3$.

minimal amplitude of the stimulation needed to evoke a second spike in the model is depicted in Fig.2.17 (bottom). Notice that around 14 ms after the first spike, the model is hyper-excitable, that is, the stimulation amplitude is less than the baseline amplitude $A_p \approx 6$ needed to evoke a spike from the resting state. This occurs because the Hodgkin-Huxley model exhibits damped oscillations of membrane potential (discussed in chapter 7).

### 2.3.3   Propagation of the Action Potentials

The space-clamped Hodgkin-Huxley model of the squid giant axon describes non-propagating action potentials since $V(t)$ does not depend on the location, $x$, along the axon. To describe propagation of action potentials (pulses) along the axon having potential $V(x,t)$, radius $a$ (cm), and intracellular resistivity $R$ ($\Omega \cdot$cm), the partial derivative $V_{xx}$ is added to the voltage equation to account for axial currents along the membrane. The resulting nonlinear parabolic partial differential equation

$$C\,V_t = \frac{a}{2R}\,V_{xx} + I - I_\mathrm{K} - I_\mathrm{Na} - I_\mathrm{L}$$

is often referred to as the Hodgkin-Huxley cable or propagating equation. Its important type of solution, a traveling pulse, is depicted in Fig.2.18. Studying this equation goes beyond the scope of this book; the reader can consult Keener and Sneyd (1998) and references therein.

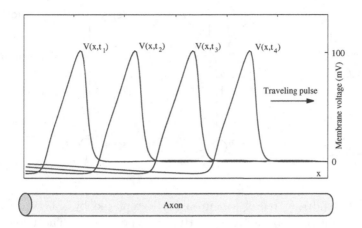

Figure 2.18: Traveling pulse solution of the Hodgkin-Huxley cable equation at four successive moments.

## 2.3.4 Dendritic Compartments

Modifications of the Hodgkin-Huxley model, often called Hodgkin-Huxley-type models or conductance-based models, can describe the dynamics of spike-generation of many, if not all, neurons recorded in nature. However, there is more to the computational property of neurons than just the spike-generation mechanism. Many neurons have an extensive dendritic tree that can sample the synaptic input arriving at different locations and integrate it over space and time.

Many dendrites have voltage-gated currents, so the synaptic integration is non-linear, sometimes resulting in dendritic spikes that can propagate forward to the soma of the neuron or backward to distant dendritic locations. Dendritic spikes are prominent in intrinsically bursting (IB) and chattering (CH) neocortical neurons considered in chapter 8. In that chapter we also model regular spiking (RS) pyramidal neurons, the most numerous class of neurons in mammalian neocortex, and show that their spike-generation mechanism is one of the simplest. The computation complexity of RS neurons must be hidden, then, in the arbors of their dendritic trees.

It is not feasible at present to study the dynamics of membrane potential in dendritic trees either analytically or geometrically (i.e., without resort to computer simulations), unless dendrites are assumed to be passive (linear) and semi-infinite, and to satisfy Rall's branching law (Rall 1959). Much of the insight can be obtained via simulations, which typically replace the continuous dendritic structure in Fig.2.19a with a network of discrete compartments in Fig.2.19b. Dynamics of each compartment is simulated by a Hodgkin-Huxley-type model, and the compartments are coupled via conductances. For example, if $V_s$ and $V_d$ denote the membrane potential at the soma and in the dendritic tree, respectively, as in Fig.2.19c, then

$$C_s \dot{V}_s = -I_s(V_s, t) + g_s(V_d - V_s) , \quad \text{and} \quad C_d \dot{V}_d = -I_d(V_d, t) + g_d(V_s - V_d) ,$$

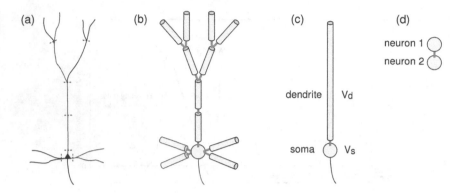

Figure 2.19: A dendritic tree of a neuron (a) is replaced by a network of compartments (b), each modeled by a Hodgkin-Huxley-type model. The two-compartment neuronal model (c) may be equivalent to two neurons coupled via gap junctions (electrical synapse) (d).

where each $I(V,t)$ represents the sum of all voltage-, $Ca^{2+}$-, and time-dependent currents in the compartment, and $g_s$ and $g_d$ are the coupling conductances that depend on the relative sizes of dendritic and somatic compartments. One can obtain many spiking and bursting patterns by changing the conductances and keeping all the other parameters fixed (Pinsky and Rinzel 1994, Mainen and Sejnowski 1996).

Once we understand how to couple two compartments, we can do it for hundreds or thousands of compartments. GENESIS and NEURON simulation environments could be useful here, especially since they contain databases of dendritic trees reconstructed from real neurons.

Interestingly, the somatic-dendritic pair in Fig.2.19c is equivalent to a pair of neurons in Fig.2.19d coupled via *gap-junctions*. These are electrical contacts that allow ions and small molecules to pass freely between the cells. Gap junctions are often called electrical synapses, because they allow potentials to be conducted directly from one neuron to another.

Computational study of multi-compartment dendritic processing is outside of the scope of this book. We consider multi-compartment models of cortical pyramidal neurons in chapter 8 and gap-junction coupled neurons in chapter 10 (which is on the author's webpage).

### 2.3.5 Summary of Voltage-Gated Currents

Throughout this book we model kinetics of various voltage-sensitive currents using the Hodgkin-Huxley gate model

$$I = \bar{g}\, m^a h^b (V - E)$$

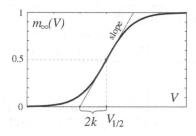 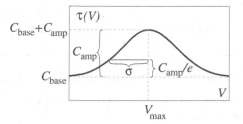

Figure 2.20: Boltzmann (2.11) and Gaussian (2.12) functions and geometrical interpretations of their parameters.

where
$I$ - current , $(\mu A/cm^2)$,
$V$ - membrane voltage, (mV),
$E$ - reverse potential, (mV),
$\bar{g}$ - maximal conductance, $(mS/cm^2)$,
$m$ - probability of activation gate to be open,
$h$ - probability of inactivation gate to be open,
$a$ - the number of activation gates per channel,
$b$ - the number of inactivation gates per channel.

The gating variables $m$ and $n$ satisfy linear first-order differential equations (2.9) and (2.10), respectively. We approximate the steady-state activation curve $m_\infty(V)$ by the Boltzmann function depicted in Fig.2.20,

$$m_\infty(V) = \frac{1}{1 + \exp\left\{(V_{1/2} - V)/k\right\}} \tag{2.11}$$

The parameter $V_{1/2}$ satisfies $m_\infty(V_{1/2}) = 0.5$, and $k$ is the slope factor (negative for the inactivation curve $h_\infty(V)$). Smaller values of $|k|$ result in steeper $m_\infty(V)$.

The voltage-sensitive time constant $\tau(V)$ can be approximated by the Gaussian function

$$\tau(V) = C_{base} + C_{amp} \exp \frac{-(V_{max} - V)^2}{\sigma^2}, \tag{2.12}$$

see Fig.2.20. The graph of the function is above $C_{base}$ with amplitude $C_{amp}$. The maximal value is achieved at $V_{max}$. The parameter $\sigma$ measures the characteristic width of the graph, that is, $\tau(V_{max} \pm \sigma) = C_{base} + C_{amp}/e$. The Gaussian description is often not adequate, so we replace it with other functions whenever appropriate.

Below is the summary of voltage-gated currents whose kinetics were measured experimentally. The division into persistent and transient is somewhat artificial, since most "persistent" currents can still inactivate after seconds of prolonged depolarization. Hyperpolarization-activated currents, such as the h-current or $K^+$ inwardly rectifying current, are mathematically equivalent to currents that are always activated, but can be inactivated by depolarization. To avoid possible confusion, we mark these currents "opened by hyperpolarization".

| $\mathbf{Na^+}$ **currents** | Parameters (Fig.2.20) | | | | | | |
|---|---|---|---|---|---|---|---|
| | Eq. (2.11) | | | Eq. (2.12) | | | |
| | $V_{1/2}$ | $k$ | | $V_{\max}$ | $\sigma$ | $C_{\mathrm{amp}}$ | $C_{\mathrm{base}}$ |
| Fast transient [1] | $I_{\mathrm{Na,t}} = \bar{g}\,m^3 h(V - E_{\mathrm{Na}})$ | | | | | | |
| activation | $-40$ | $15$ | | $-38$ | $30$ | $0.46$ | $0.04$ |
| inactivation | $-62$ | $-7$ | | $-67$ | $20$ | $7.4$ | $1.2$ |
| Fast transient [2] | $I_{\mathrm{Na,t}} = \bar{g}\,m_\infty(V)h(V - E_{\mathrm{Na}})$ | | | | | | |
| activation | $-30$ | $5.5$ | | $-$ | $-$ | $-$ | $-$ |
| inactivation | $-70$ | $-5.8$ | | $\tau_h(V) = 3\exp((-40 - V)/33)$ | | | |
| Fast transient [3] | $I_{\mathrm{Na,t}} = \bar{g}\,m_\infty(V)h(V - E_{\mathrm{Na}})$ | | | | | | |
| activation | $-28$ | $6.7$ | | $-$ | $-$ | $-$ | $-$ |
| inactivation | $-66$ | $-6$ | | $\tau_h(V) = 4\exp((-30 - V)/29)$ | | | |
| Fast persistent [4,a] | $I_{\mathrm{Na,p}} = \bar{g}\,m_\infty(V)h(V - E_{\mathrm{Na}})$ | | | | | | |
| activation | $-50$ | $4$ | | $-$ | $-$ | $-$ | $-$ |
| inactivation | $-49$ | $-10$ | | $-66$ | $35$ | $4.5$ sec | $2$ sec |
| Fast persistent [5,a] | $I_{\mathrm{Na,p}} = \bar{g}\,m_\infty(V)(0.14 + 0.86h)(V - E_{\mathrm{Na}})$ | | | | | | |
| activation | $-50$ | $6$ | | $-$ | $-$ | $-$ | $-$ |
| inactivation | $-56$ | $-7$ | | $\tau_h(V) = 63.2 + 25\exp(-V/25.5)$ | | | |
| Fast persistent [2] | $I_{\mathrm{Na,p}} = \bar{g}\,m(V - E_{\mathrm{Na}})$ | | | | | | |
| activation | $-54$ | $9$ | | $-$ | $-$ | $-$ | $0.8$ |
| Fast persistent [6] | $I_{\mathrm{Na,p}} = \bar{g}\,m(V - E_{\mathrm{Na}})$ | | | | | | |
| activation | $-42$ | $4$ | | $-$ | $-$ | $-$ | $0.8$ |

1. Squid giant axon (Hodgkin and Huxley 1952); see exercise 4.

2. Thalamocortical neurons in rats (Parri and Crunelli 1999).

3. Thalamocortical neurons in cats (Parri and Crunelli 1999).

4. Layer-II principal neurons in entorhinal cortex (Magistretti and Alonso 1999).

5. Large dorsal root ganglion neurons in rats (Baker and Bostock 1997, 1998).

6. Purkinje cells (Kay et al. 1998).

a Very slow inactivation.

| K⁺ currents | Parameters (Fig.2.20) | | | | | |
| | Eq. (2.11) | | Eq. (2.12) | | | |
| | $V_{1/2}$ | $k$ | $V_{max}$ | $\sigma$ | $C_{amp}$ | $C_{base}$ |
| **Delayed rectifier** [1]  $I_K = \bar{g}\,n^4(V - E_K)$ | | | | | | |
| activation | −53 | 15 | −79 | 50 | 4.7 | 1.1 |
| **Delayed rectifier** [2,4]  $I_K = \bar{g}\,mh(V - E_K)$ | | | | | | |
| activation | −3 | 10 | −50 | 30 | 47 | 5 |
| inactivation | −51 | −12 | −50 | 50 | 1000 | 360 |
| **M current** [3]  $I_{K(M)} = \bar{g}\,m(V - E_K)$ | | | | | | |
| activation | −44 | 8 | −50 | 25 | 320 | 20 |
| **Transient** [4]  $I_A = \bar{g}\,mh(V - E_K)$ | | | | | | |
| activation | −3 | 20 | −71 | 60 | 0.92 | 0.34 |
| inactivation | −66 | −10 | −73 | 23 | 50 | 8 |
| **Transient** [5]  $I_A = \bar{g}\,mh(V - E_K)$ | | | | | | |
| activation | −26 | 20 | − | − | − | − |
| inactivation | −72 | −9.6 | − | − | − | 15.5 |
| **Transient** [6]  $I_A = \bar{g}\,m^4h\,(V - E_K)$ | | | | | | |
| Fast component (60% of total conductance) | | | | | | |
| activation | −60 | 8.5 | −58 | 25 | 2 | 0.37 |
| inactivation | −78 | −6 | −78 | 25 | 45 | 19 |
| Slow component (40% of total conductance) | | | | | | |
| activation | −36 | 20 | −58 | 25 | 2 | 0.37 |
| inactivation | −78 | −6 | −78 | 25 | 45 | 19 |
| $\tau_h(V) = 60$ when $V > -73$ | | | | | | |
| **Inward rectifier** [7]  $I_{Kir} = \bar{g}\,h_\infty(V)(V - E_K)$ *(opened by hyperpolarization)* | | | | | | |
| inactivation | −80 | −12 | − | − | − | < 1 |

1. Squid giant axon (Hodgkin and Huxley 1952); see exercise 4.
2. Neocortical pyramidal neurons (Bekkers 2000).
3. Rodent neuroblastoma-glioma hybrid cells (Robbins et al. 1992).
4. Neocortical pyramidal neurons (Korngreen and Sakmann 2000).
5. Hippocampal mossy fiber boutons (Geiger and Jonas 2000).
6. Thalamic relay neurons (Huguenard and McCormick 1992).
7. Horizontal cells in catfish retina (Dong and Werblin 1995); AP cell of leech (Wessel et al. 1999); rat locus coeruleus neurons (Williams et al. 1988, $V_{1/2} = E_K$).

| **Cation currents** | Parameters (Fig.2.20) | | | | | | |
|---|---|---|---|---|---|---|---|
| | Eq. (2.11) | | | Eq. (2.12) | | | |
| | $V_{1/2}$ | $k$ | | $V_{max}$ | $\sigma$ | $C_{amp}$ | $C_{base}$ |
| $I_h$ current [1] | $I_h = \bar{g}\,h\,(V - E_h),$ | | $E_h = -43$ mV | | | | |
| (*opened by hyperpolarization*) | | | | | | | |
| inactivation | $-75$ | $-5.5$ | | $-75$ | 15 | 1000 | 100 |
| $I_h$ current [2] | $I_h = \bar{g}\,h\,(V - E_h),$ | | $E_h = -1$ mV | | | | |
| inact. (soma) | $-82$ | $-9$ | | $-75$ | 20 | 50 | 10 |
| inact. (dendrite) | $-90$ | $-8.5$ | | $-75$ | 20 | 40 | 10 |
| $I_h$ current [3] | $I_h = \bar{g}\,h\,(V - E_h),$ | | $E_h = -21$ mV | | | | |
| fast inact. (65%) | $-67$ | $-12$ | | $-75$ | 30 | 50 | 20 |
| slow inact. (35%) | $-58$ | $-9$ | | $-65$ | 30 | 300 | 100 |

1. Thalamic relay neurons (McCormick and Pape 1990; Huguenard and McCormick 1992).

2. Hippocampal pyramidal neurons in CA1 (Magee 1998).

3. Entorhinal cortex layer II neurons (Dickson et al. 2000).

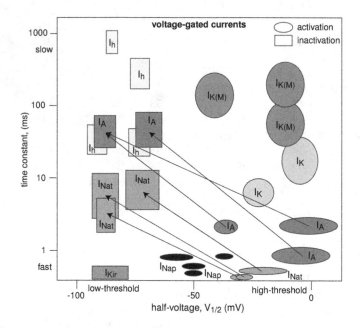

Figure 2.21: Summary of current kinetics. Each oval (rectangle) denotes the voltage and temporal scale of activation (inactivation) of a current. Transient currents are represented by arrows connecting ovals and rectangles.

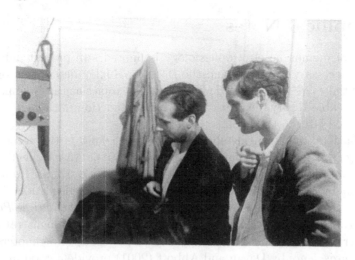

Figure 2.22: Alan Hodgkin (right) and Andrew Huxley (left) in their Plymouth Marine Lab in 1949. (Photo provided by National Marine Biological Library, Plymouth, UK).

## Review of Important Concepts

- Electrical signals in neurons are carried by $Na^+$, $Ca^{2+}$, $K^+$, and $Cl^-$ ions, which move through membrane channels according to their electrochemical gradients.

- The membrane potential $V$ is determined by the membrane conductances $g_i$ and corresponding reversal potentials $E_i$:

$$C\dot{V} = I - \sum_i g_i \cdot (V - E_i).$$

- Neurons are excitable because the conductances depend on the membrane potential and time.

- The most accepted description of kinetics of voltage-sensitive conductances is the Hodgkin-Huxley gate model.

- Voltage-gated activation of inward $Na^+$ or $Ca^{2+}$ current depolarizes (increases) the membrane potential.

- Voltage-gated activation of outward $K^+$ or $Cl^-$ current hyperpolarizes (decreases) the membrane potential.

- An action potential or spike is a brief regenerative depolarization of the membrane potential followed by its repolarization and possibly hyperpolarization, as in Fig.2.16.

## Bibliographical Notes

Our summary of membrane electrophysiology is limited: we present only those concepts that are necessary to understand the Hodgkin-Huxley description of generation of action potentials. We have omitted such important topics as the Goldman-Hodgkin-Katz equation, cable theory, dendritic and synaptic function, although some of those will be introduced later in the book.

The standard textbook on membrane electrophysiology is the second edition of *Ion Channels of Excitable Membranes* by B. Hille (2001). An excellent introductory textbook with an emphasis on the quantitative approach is *Foundations of Cellular Neurophysiology* by D. Johnston and S. Wu (1995). A detailed introduction to mathematical aspects of cellular biophysics can be found in *Mathematical Physiology* by J. Keener and J. Sneyd (1998). The latter two books complement rather than repeat each other. *Biophysics of Computation* by Koch (1999) and chapters 5 and 6 of *Theoretical Neuroscience* by Dayan and Abbott (2001) provide a good introduction to biophysics of excitable membranes.

The first book devoted exclusively to dendrites is *Dendrites* by Stuart et al. (1999). It emphasizes the active nature of dendritic dynamics. Arshavsky et al. (1971; Russian language edition, 1969) make the first, and probably still the best, theoretical attempt to understand the neurocomputational properties of branching dendritic trees endowed with voltage-gated channels and capable of generating action potentials. Had they published their results in the 1990s, they would have been considered classics in the field. Unfortunately, the computational neuroscience community of the 1970s was not ready to accept the "heretic" idea that dendrites can fire spikes, that spikes can propagate backward and forward along the dendritic tree, that EPSPs can be scaled-up with distance, that individual dendritic branches can perform coincidence detection and branching points can perform nonlinear summation, and that different and independent computations can be carried out at different parts of the neuronal dendritic tree. We touch on some of these issues in chapter 8.

## Exercises

1. Determine the Nernst equilibrium potentials for the membrane of the squid giant axon using the following data:

|        | Inside (mM) | Outside (mM) |
|--------|-------------|--------------|
| $K^+$  | 430         | 20           |
| $Na^+$ | 50          | 440          |
| $Cl^-$ | 65          | 560          |

and $T = 20°C$.

2. Show that a nonselective cation current

$$I = \bar{g}_{Na}\, p\,(V - E_{Na}) + \bar{g}_K\, p\,(V - E_K)$$

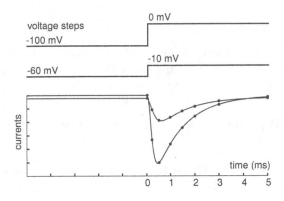

Figure 2.23: Current traces corresponding to voltage steps of various amplitudes; see exercise 6.

can be written in the form (2.7) with

$$\bar{g} = \bar{g}_{Na} + \bar{g}_{K} \qquad \text{and} \qquad E = \frac{\bar{g}_{Na} E_{Na} + \bar{g}_{K} E_{K}}{\bar{g}_{Na} + \bar{g}_{K}} .$$

3. Show that applying a DC current $I$ in the neuronal model

$$C\dot{V} = I - g_{L}(V - E_{L}) - I_{\text{other}}(V)$$

is equivalent to changing the leak reverse potential $E_{L}$.

4. Steady-state (in)activation curves and voltage-sensitive time constants can be approximated by the Boltzmann (2.11) and Gaussian (2.12) functions, respectively, depicted in Fig.2.20. Explain the meaning of the parameters $V_{1/2}, k$, $C_{\text{base}}, C_{\text{amp}}, V_{\text{max}}$, and $\sigma$ and find their values that provide satisfactory fit near the rest state $V = 0$ for the Hodgkin-Huxley functions depicted in Fig.2.13.

5. (Willms et al. 1999) Consider the curve $m_{\infty}^{p}(V)$, where $m_{\infty}(V)$ is the Boltzmann function with parameters $V_{1/2}$ and $k$, and $p > 1$. This curve can be approximated by another Boltzmann function with some parameters $\tilde{V}_{1/2}$ and $\tilde{k}$ (and $p = 1$). Find the formulas that relate $\tilde{V}_{1/2}$ and $\tilde{k}$ to $V_{1/2}$, $k$, and $p$.

6. (Willms et al. 1999) Write a MATLAB program that determines activation and inactivation parameters via a simultaneous fitting of current traces from a voltage-clamp experiment similar to the one in Fig.2.23. Assume that the values of the voltage pairs – e.g., $-60, -10; -100, 0$ (mV) – are in the file v.dat. The values of the current (circles in Fig.2.23) are in the file **current.dat**, and the sampling times – e.g., 0, 0.25, 0.5, 1, 1.5, 2, 3, 5 (ms) – are in the file **times.dat**.

7. Modify the MATLAB program from exercise 6 to handle multi-step (Fig.2.24) and ramp protocols.

8. **[M.S.]** Find the best sequence of step potentials that can determine activation and inactivation parameters (a) in the shortest time, (b) with the highest precision.

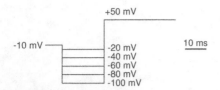

Figure 2.24: Multiple voltage steps are often needed to determine time constants of inactivation; see exercise 7.

9. [**M.S.**]  Modify the MATLAB program from exercise 6 to handle multiple currents.

10. [**M.S.**]  Add a PDE solver to the MATLAB program from exercise 6 to simulate poor space and voltage clamp conditions.

11. [**Ph.D.**]  Introduce numerical optimization into the dynamic clamp protocol to analyze experimentally in real time the (in)activation parameters of membrane currents.

12. [**Ph.D.**]  Use new classification of families of channels (Kv3,1, Na$_v$1.2, etc.; see Hille 2001) to determine the kinetics of each subgroup, and provide a complete table similar to those in section 2.3.5.

# Chapter 3

# One-Dimensional Systems

In this chapter we describe geometrical methods of analysis of one-dimensional dynamical systems, i.e., systems having only one variable. An example of such a system is the space-clamped membrane having Ohmic leak current $I_L$:

$$C\dot{V} = -g_L(V - E_L)\,. \tag{3.1}$$

Here the membrane voltage $V$ is a time-dependent variable, and the capacitance $C$, leak conductance $g_L$, and leak reverse potential $E_L$ are constant parameters described in chapter 2. We use this and other one-dimensional neural models to introduce and illustrate the most important concepts of dynamical system theory: equilibrium, stability, attractor, phase portrait, and bifurcation.

## 3.1 Electrophysiological Examples

The Hodgkin-Huxley description of dynamics of membrane potential and voltage-gated conductances can be reduced to a one-dimensional system when all transmembrane conductances have fast kinetics. For the sake of illustration, let us consider a space-clamped membrane having leak current and a fast voltage-gated current $I_{fast}$ with only one gating variable $p$,

$$
\begin{aligned}
C\dot{V} &= \overbrace{-g_L(V - E_L)}^{\text{Leak } I_L} \overbrace{-g\,p\,(V - E)}^{I_{fast}} \tag{3.2}\\
\dot{p} &= (p_\infty(V) - p)/\tau(V)\,, \tag{3.3}
\end{aligned}
$$

with dimensionless parameters $C = 1$, $g_L = 1$, and $g = 1$. Suppose that the gating kinetics (3.3) is much faster than the voltage kinetics (3.2), which means that the voltage-sensitive time constant $\tau(V)$ is very small, that is, $\tau(V) \ll 1$ in the entire biophysical voltage range. Then the gating process may be treated as being instantaneous, and the asymptotic value $p = p_\infty(V)$ may be used in the voltage equation (3.2)

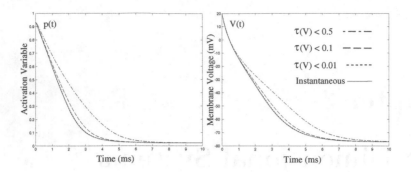

Figure 3.1: Solution of the full system (3.2, 3.3) converges to that of the reduced one-dimensional system (3.4) as $\tau(V) \to 0$.

to reduce the two-dimensional system (3.2, 3.3) to a one-dimensional equation:

$$C\dot{V} = -g_{\mathrm{L}}(V - E_{\mathrm{L}}) - \overbrace{g\,p_{\infty}(V)\,(V - E)}^{\text{instantaneous } I_{\text{fast}}} \; . \tag{3.4}$$

This reduction introduces a small error of the order $\tau(V) \ll 1$, as one can see in Fig.3.1.

Since the hypothetical current $I_{\text{fast}}$ can be either inward $(E > E_{\mathrm{L}})$ or outward $(E < E_{\mathrm{L}})$, and the gating process can be either activation ($p$ is $m$, as in the Hodgkin-Huxley model) or inactivation ($p$ is $h$), there are four fundamentally different choices for $I_{\text{fast}}(V)$, which we summarize in Fig.3.2 and elaborate on below.

|  |  | Current | |
|---|---|---|---|
|  |  | inward | outward |
| Gating | activation | $I_{\mathrm{Na,p}}$ | $I_{\mathrm{K}}$ |
|  | inactivation | $I_{\mathrm{h}}$ | $I_{\mathrm{Kir}}$ |

Figure 3.2: Four fundamental examples of voltage-gated currents with one gating variable. In this book we treat "hyperpolarization-activated" currents $I_{\mathrm{h}}$ and $I_{\mathrm{Kir}}$ as inactivating currents, which are turned off (inactivated via $h$) by depolarization and turned on (deinactivated) by hyperpolarization (see discussion in section 2.2.4).

## 3.1.1   I-V Relations and Dynamics

The four choices in Fig.3.2 result in four simple one-dimensional models of the form (3.4):

$$I_{\mathrm{Na,p}}\text{-model}, \qquad I_{\mathrm{K}}\text{-model}, \qquad I_{\mathrm{h}}\text{-model}, \quad \text{and} \quad I_{\mathrm{Kir}}\text{-model}.$$

These models might seem too simple to biologists, who can easily understand their behavior just by looking at the I-V relations of the currents depicted in Fig.3.3 without

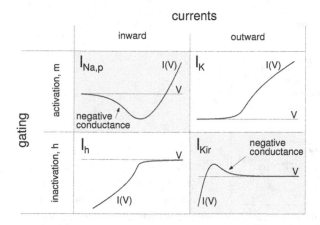

Figure 3.3: Typical current-voltage (I-V) relations of the four currents considered in this chapter. Shaded boxes correspond to nonmonotonic I-V relations having a region of negative conductance ($I'(V) < 0$) in the biophysically relevant voltage range.

using any dynamical systems theory. The models might also appear too simple to mathematicians, who can easily understand their dynamics just by looking at the graphs of the right-hand side of (3.4) without using any electrophysiological intuition. In fact, the models provide an invaluable learning tool, since they establish a bridge between electrophysiology and dynamical systems.

In Fig.3.3 we plot typical steady-state current-voltage (I-V) relations of the four currents considered above. Note that the I-V curve is nonmonotonic for $I_{\text{Na,p}}$ and $I_{\text{Kir}}$ but monotonic for $I_{\text{K}}$ and $I_{\text{h}}$, at least in the biophysically relevant voltage range. This subtle difference is an indication of the fundamentally different roles these currents play in neuron dynamics. The I-V relation in the first group has a region of "negative conductance" (i.e., $I'(V) < 0$), which creates positive feedback between the voltage and the gating variable (Fig.3.4), and plays an amplifying role in neuron dynamics. We refer to such currents as *amplifying currents*. In contrast, the currents in the second group have negative feedback between voltage and gating variable, and they often result in damped oscillation of the membrane potential, as we show in chapter 4. We refer to such currents as *resonant currents*. Most neural models involve a combination of at least one amplifying and one resonant current, as we discuss in chapter 5. The way these currents are combined determines whether the neuron is an *integrator* or a *resonator*.

## 3.1.2   Leak + Instantaneous $I_{\text{Na,p}}$

To ease our introduction into dynamical systems, we will use the $I_{\text{Na,p}}$-model

$$C\,\dot{V} = I - g_{\text{L}}(V - E_{\text{L}}) - \overbrace{g_{\text{Na}}\,m_\infty(V)\,(V - E_{\text{Na}})}^{\text{instantaneous } I_{\text{Na,p}}}, \tag{3.5}$$

called *persistent sodium model*, with

$$m_\infty(V) = 1/(1 + \exp\{(V_{1/2} - V)/k\})$$

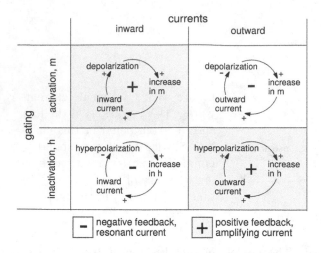

Figure 3.4: Feedback loops between voltage and gating variables in the four models presented above (see also Fig.5.2).

throughout the rest of this chapter. (Some biologists refer to transient Na$^+$ currents with very slow inactivation as being persistent, since the current does not change much on the time scale of 1 sec.) We obtain the experimental parameter values

$$C = 10 \ \mu\text{F}, \qquad I = 0 \ \text{pA}, \qquad g_\text{L} = 19 \ \text{mS}, \qquad E_\text{L} = -67 \ \text{mV},$$
$$g_\text{Na} = 74 \ \text{mS}, \qquad V_{1/2} = 1.5 \ \text{mV}, \qquad k = 16 \ \text{mV}, \qquad E_\text{Na} = 60 \ \text{mV}$$

using whole-cell patch-clamp recordings of a layer 5 pyramidal neuron in the visual cortex of a rat at room temperature. We prove in exercise 3.3.8 and illustrate in Fig.3.15 that the model approximates the action potential upstroke dynamics of this neuron.

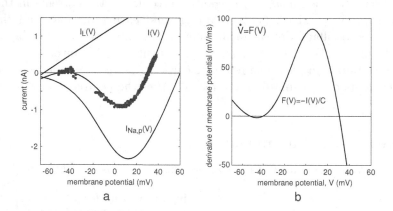

Figure 3.5: (a) I-V relations of the leak current $I_\text{L}$, fast Na$^+$ current $I_\text{Na}$, and combined current $I(V) = I_\text{L}(V) + I_\text{Na}(V)$ in the $I_\text{Na,p}$-model (3.5). Dots denote $I_0(V)$ data from layer 5 pyramidal cell in rat visual cortex. (b) The right-hand side of the $I_\text{Na,p}$-model (3.5).

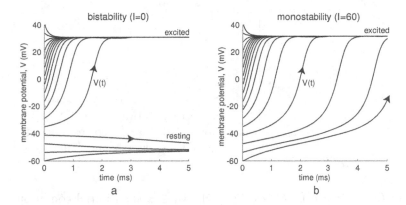

Figure 3.6: Typical voltage trajectories of the $I_{Na,p}$-model (3.5) having different values of $I$.

The model's I-V relation, $I(V)$, is depicted in Fig.3.5a. Due to the negative conductance region in the I-V curve, this one-dimensional model can exhibit a number of interesting nonlinear phenomena, such as bistability, i.e. coexistence of resting and excited states. From a mathematical point of view, bistability occurs because the right-hand-side function in the differential equation (3.5), depicted in Fig.3.5b, is not monotonic. In Fig.3.6 we depict typical voltage time courses of the model (3.5) with two values of injected DC current $I$ and 16 different initial conditions. The qualitative behavior in Fig.3.6a is clearly bistable: depending on the initial condition, the trajectory of the membrane potential goes either up to the excited state or down to the resting state. In contrast, the behavior in Fig.3.6b is monostable, since the resting state does not exist. The goal of the dynamical system theory reviewed in this chapter is to understand why and how the behavior depends on the initial conditions and the parameters of the system.

## 3.2 Dynamical Systems

In general, dynamical systems can be continuous or discrete, depending on whether they are described by differential or difference equations. Continuous one-dimensional dynamical systems are usually written in the form

$$\dot{V} = F(V) , \qquad V(0) = V_0 \in \mathbb{R} . \tag{3.6}$$

For example,

$$\dot{V} = -80 - V , \qquad V(0) = -20 ,$$

where $V$ is a scalar time-dependent variable denoting the current state of the system, $\dot{V} = V_t = dV/dt$ is its derivative with respect to time $t$, $F$ is a scalar function (its output is one-dimensional) that determines the evolution of the system, e.g., the right-

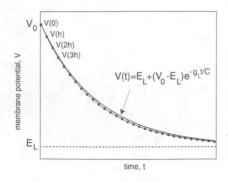

Figure 3.7: Explicit analytical solution ($V(t) = E_L + (V_0 - E_L)e^{-g_L t/C}$) of the linear equation (3.1) and corresponding numerical approximation (dots) using Euler's method (3.7).

hand side of (3.5) divided by $C$; see Fig.3.5b. $V_0 \in \mathbb{R}$ is an initial condition, and $\mathbb{R}$ is the real line, that is, a line of real numbers ($\mathbb{R}^n$ would be the $n$-dimensional real space).

In the context of dynamical systems, the real line $\mathbb{R}$ is called the *phase line* or *state line* (phase space or state space for $\mathbb{R}^n$) to stress the fact that each point in $\mathbb{R}$ corresponds to a certain, possibly inadmissible state of the system, and each state of the system corresponds to a certain point in $\mathbb{R}$. For example, the state of the Ohmic membrane (3.1) is its membrane potential $V \in \mathbb{R}$. The state of the Hodgkin-Huxley model (see section 2.3) is the four-dimensional vector $(V, m, n, h) \in \mathbb{R}^4$. The state of the $I_{Na,p}$-model (3.5) is its membrane potential $V \in \mathbb{R}$, because the value $m = m_\infty(V)$ is unequivocally defined by $V$.

When all parameters are constant, the dynamical system is called *autonomous*. When at least one of the parameters is time-dependent, the system is nonautonomous, denoted as $\dot{V} = F(V, t)$.

"To solve equation (3.6)" means to find a function $V(t)$ whose initial value is $V(0) = V_0$ and whose derivative is $F(V(t))$ at each moment $t \geq 0$. For example, the function $V(t) = V_0 + at$ is an explicit analytical solution to the dynamical system $\dot{V} = a$. The exponentially decaying function $V(t) = E_L + (V_0 - E_L)e^{-g_L t/C}$ depicted in Fig.3.7, a solid curve, is an explicit analytical solution to the linear equation (3.1). (Check by differentiating).

Finding explicit solutions is often impossible even for such simple systems as (3.5), so quantitative analysis is carried out mostly via numerical simulations. The simplest procedure to solve (3.6) numerically, known as the first-order *Euler method*, replaces (3.6) with the discretized system

$$[V(t + h) - V(t)]/h = F(V(t)) ,$$

where $t = 0, h, 2h, 3h, \ldots$, is the discrete time and $h$ is a small time step. Knowing the current state $V(t)$, we can find the next state point via

$$V(t + h) = V(t) + hF(V(t)) . \qquad (3.7)$$

Iterating this *difference* equation starting with $V(0) = V_0$, we can approximate the analytical solution of (3.6) (see the dots in Fig.3.7). The approximation has a noticeable error of order $h$, so scientific software packages, such as MATLAB, use more sophisticated high-precision numerical methods.

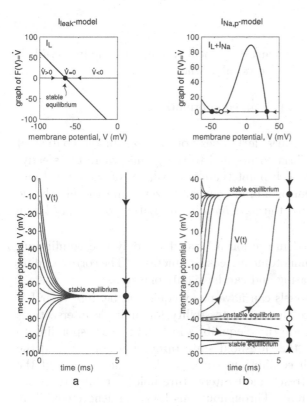

Figure 3.8: Graphs of the right-hand side functions of equations (3.1) and (3.5), and corresponding numerical solutions starting from various initial conditions.

In many cases, however, we do not need exact solutions, but qualitative understanding of the behavior of (3.6) and how it depends on parameters and the initial state $V_0$. For example, we might be interested in the number of equilibrium (rest) points the system could have, whether the equilibria are stable, their attraction domains, etc.

## 3.2.1 Geometrical Analysis

The first step in the qualitative geometrical analysis of any one-dimensional dynamical system is to plot the graph of the function $F$, as in Fig.3.8 (top). Since $F(V) = \dot{V}$, at every point $V$ where $F(V)$ is negative, the derivative $\dot{V}$ is negative, and hence the state variable $V$ decreases. In contrast, at every point where $F(V)$ is positive, $\dot{V}$ is positive, and the state variable $V$ increases; the greater the value of $F(V)$, the faster $V$ increases. Thus, the direction of movement of the state variable $V$, and hence the evolution of the dynamical system, is determined by the sign of the function $F(V)$.

The right-hand side of the $I_{leak}$-model (3.1) or the $I_{Na,p}$-model (3.5) in Fig.3.8 is the steady-state current-voltage (I-V) relation, $I_L(V)$ or $I_L(V)+I_{Na,p}(V)$ respectively, taken with the minus sign, see Fig.3.5. Positive values of the right-hand-side $F(V)$ mean negative I-V, corresponding to a net inward current that depolarizes the membrane. Conversely, negative values mean positive I-V, corresponding to a net outward current that hyperpolarizes the membrane.

### 3.2.2   Equilibria

The next step in the qualitative analysis of any dynamical system is to find its *equilibria* or *rest points*, that is, the values of the state variable where

$$F(V) = 0 \qquad (V \text{ is an equilibrium}).$$

At each such point $\dot{V} = 0$, the state variable $V$ does not change. In the context of membrane potential dynamics, equilibria correspond to the points where the steady-state I-V curve passes zero. At each such point there is a balance of the inward and outward currents so that the net transmembrane current is zero, and the membrane voltage does not change. (Incidentally, the part *libra* in the Latin word *aequilibrium* means balance).

The $I_K$- and $I_h$-models mentioned in section 3.1 can have only one equilibrium because their I-V relations $I(V)$ are monotonic increasing functions. The corresponding functions $F(V)$ are monotonic decreasing and can have only one zero.

In contrast, the $I_{Na,p}$- and $I_{Kir}$-models can have many equilibria because their I-V curves are not monotonic, and hence there is a possibility for multiple intersections with the $V$-axis. For example, there are three equilibria in Fig.3.8b corresponding to the resting state (around $-53$ mV), the threshold state (around $-40$ mV), and the excited state (around $30$ mV). Each equilibrium corresponds to the balance of the outward leak current and partially (rest), moderately (threshold), or fully (excited) activated persistent Na$^+$ inward current. Throughout this book we denote equilibria as small open or filled circles, depending on their stability, as in Fig.3.8.

### 3.2.3   Stability

If the initial value of the state variable is exactly at equilibrium, then $\dot{V} = 0$ and the variable will stay there forever. If the initial value is near the equilibrium, the state variable may approach the equilibrium or diverge from it. Both cases are depicted in Fig.3.8. We say that an equilibrium is *asymptotically stable* if all solutions starting sufficiently near the equilibrium will approach it as $t \to \infty$.

Stability of an equilibrium is determined by the signs of the function $F$ around it. The equilibrium is stable when $F(V)$ changes the sign from "plus" to "minus" as $V$ increases, as in Fig.3.8a. Obviously, all solutions starting near such an equilibrium converge to it. Such an equilibrium "attracts" all nearby solutions, so it is called an *attractor*. A stable equilibrium point is the only type of attractor that can exist in one-dimensional continuous dynamical systems defined on a state line $\mathbb{R}$. Multidimensional systems can have other attractors, e.g., limit cycles.

The differences between stable, asymptotically stable, and exponentially stable equilibria are discussed in exercise 18 at the end of the chapter. The reader is also encouraged to solve exercise 4 (piecewise continuous $F(V)$).

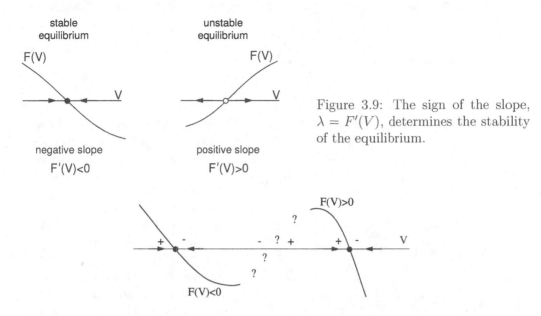

Figure 3.9: The sign of the slope, $\lambda = F'(V)$, determines the stability of the equilibrium.

Figure 3.10: Two stable equilibrium points must be separated by at least one unstable equilibrium point because $F(V)$ has to change the sign from "minus" to "plus".

### 3.2.4 Eigenvalues

A sufficient condition for an equilibrium to be stable is that the derivative of the function $F$ with respect to $V$ at the equilibrium is negative, provided the function is differentiable. We denote this derivative here by

$$\lambda = F'(V), \qquad (V \text{ is an equilibrium; that is, } F(V) = 0)$$

and note that it is the slope of the graph of $F$ at the point $V$ (see Fig.3.9). Obviously, when the slope, $\lambda$, is negative, the function changes the sign from "plus" to "minus", and the equilibrium is stable. Positive slope $\lambda$ implies instability. The parameter $\lambda$ defined above is the simplest example of an *eigenvalue* of an equilibrium. We introduce eigenvalues formally in chapter 4 and show that they play an important role in defining the types of equilibria of multidimensional systems.

### 3.2.5 Unstable Equilibria

If a one-dimensional system has two stable equilibrium points, then they must be separated by at least one unstable equilibrium point, as we illustrate in Fig.3.10. (This may not be true in multidimensional systems.) Indeed, a continuous function $F$ has to change the sign from "minus" to "plus" somewhere in between those equilibria; that is, it has to cross the $V$-axis at some point, as in Fig.3.8b. This point would be an unstable equilibrium, since all nearby solutions diverge from it. In the context

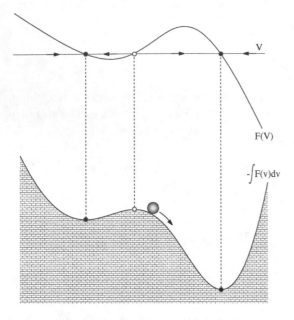

Figure 3.11: Mechanistic interpretation of stable and unstable equilibria. A massless (inertia-free) ball moves toward energy minima with the speed proportional to the slope. A one-dimensional system $\dot{V} = F(V)$ has the energy landscape $E(V) = -\int_{-\infty}^{V} F(v)\, dv$ (see exercise 17). Zeros of $F(V)$ with negative (positive) slope correspond to minima (maxima) of $E(V)$.

of neuronal models, unstable equilibria lie in the region of the steady-state I-V curve with negative conductance. (Please, check that this is in accordance with the fact that $F(V) = -I(V)/C$; see Fig.3.5.) An unstable equilibrium is sometimes called a *repeller*. Attractors and repellers have a simple mechanistic interpretation depicted in Fig.3.11.

If the initial condition $V_0$ is set to an unstable equilibrium point, then the solution will stay at this unstable equilibrium; that is, $V(t) = V_0$ for all $t$, at least in theory. In practice, the location of an equilibrium point is known only approximately. In addition, small noisy perturbations that are always present in biological systems can make $V(t)$ deviate slightly from the equilibrium point. Because of instability, such deviations will grow, and the state variable $V(t)$ will eventually diverge from the repelling equilibrium the same way that the ball set at the top of the hill in Fig.3.11 will eventually roll downhill. If the level of noise is low, it could take a long time to diverge from the repeller.

### 3.2.6 Attraction Domain

Even though unstable equilibria are hard to see experimentally, they still play an important role in dynamics, since they separate attraction domains. Indeed, the ball in Fig.3.11 could go left or right, depending on which side of the hilltop it is on initially. Similarly, the state variable of a one-dimensional system decreases or increases, depending on which side of the unstable equilibrium the initial condition is, as one can clearly see in Fig.3.8b.

In general, the *basin of attraction* or *attraction domain* of an attractor is the set

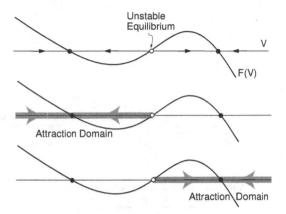

Figure 3.12: Two attraction domains in a one-dimensional system are separated by the unstable equilibrium.

of all initial conditions that lead to the attractor. For example, the attraction domain of the equilibrium in Fig.3.8a is the entire voltage range. Such an attractor is called *global*. In Fig.3.12 we plot attraction domains of two stable equilibria. The middle unstable equilibrium is always the boundary of the attraction domains.

### 3.2.7 Threshold and Action Potential

Unstable equilibria play the role of thresholds in one-dimensional bistable systems, i.e., in systems having two attractors. We illustrate this in Fig.3.13, which is believed to describe the essence of the mechanism of bistability in many neurons. Suppose the state variable is initially at the stable equilibrium point marked "state A" in the figure, and suppose that perturbations can kick it around the equilibrium. Small perturbations may not kick it over the unstable equilibrium so that the state variable continues to be in the attraction domain of "state A". We refer to such perturbations as *subthreshold*.

In contrast, we refer to perturbations as *superthreshold* (or *suprathreshold*) if they are large enough to push the state variable over the unstable equilibrium so that it becomes attracted to the "state B". We see that the unstable equilibrium acts as a threshold that separates two states.

The transition between two stable states separated by a threshold is relevant to the mechanism of excitability and generation of action potentials in many neurons, which is illustrated in Fig.3.14. In the $I_{Na,p}$-model (3.5) with the I-V relation in Fig.3.5 the existence of the resting state is largely due to the leak current $I_L$, while the existence of the excited state is largely due to the persistent inward Na$^+$ current $I_{Na,p}$. Small (subthreshold) perturbations leave the state variable in the attraction domain of the rest state, while large (superthreshold) perturbations initiate the regenerative process – the upstroke of an action potential – and the voltage variable becomes attracted to the excited state. Generation of the action potential must be completed via repolarization,

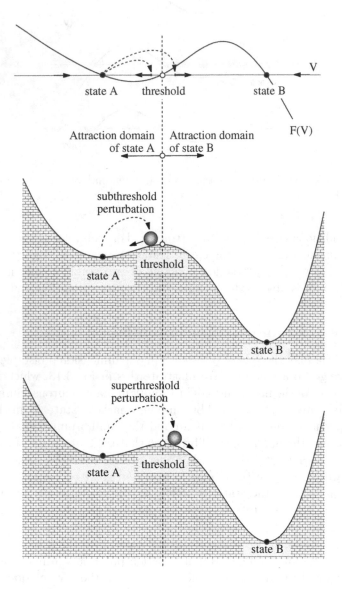

Figure 3.13: Unstable equilibrium plays the role of a threshold that separates two attraction domains.

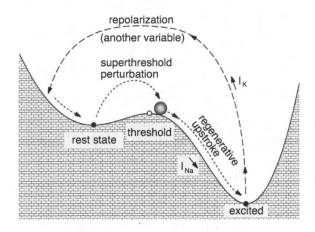

Figure 3.14: Mechanistic illustration of the mechanism of generation of an action potential.

which moves $V$ back to the resting state. Typically, repolarization occurs because of a relatively slow inactivation of Na$^+$ current and/or slow activation of an outward K$^+$ current, which are not taken into account in the one-dimensional system (3.5). To account for such processes, we consider two-dimensional systems in the next chapter.

Recall that the parameters of the $I_{Na,p}$-model (3.5) were obtained from a cortical pyramidal neuron. In Fig.3.15 (left), we stimulate (in vitro) the cortical neuron by short (0.1 ms) strong pulses of current to reset its membrane potential to various initial values, and interpret the results using the $I_{Na,p}$-model. Since activation of the Na$^+$ current is not instantaneous in real neurons, we allow variable $m$ to converge to $m_\infty(V)$, and ignore the 0.3-ms transient activity that follows each pulse. We also ignore

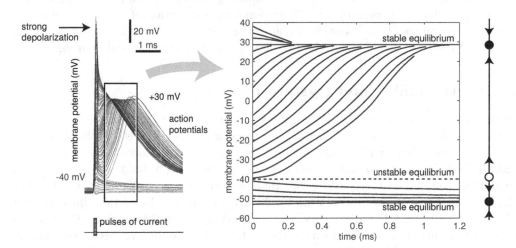

Figure 3.15: Upstroke dynamics of layer 5 pyramidal neuron in vitro (compare with the $I_{Na,p}$-model (3.5) in Fig.3.8b).

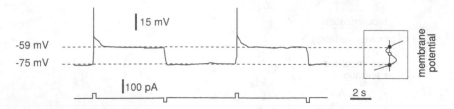

Figure 3.16: Membrane potential bistability in a cat TC neuron in the presence of ZD7288 (pharmacological blocker of $I_h$. (Modified from Fig. 6B of Hughes et al. 1999).

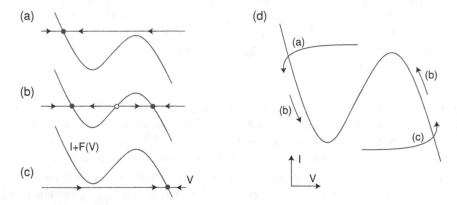

Figure 3.17: Bistability and hysteresis loop as $I$ changes.

the initial segment of the downstroke of the action potential, and plot the magnification of the voltage traces in Fig.3.15 (right). Comparing this figure with Fig.3.8b we see that the $I_{Na,p}$-model is a reasonable one-dimensional approximation of the action potential upstroke dynamics. It predicts the value of the resting ($-53$ mV), the instantaneous threshold ($-40$ mV), and the excited ($+30$ mV) states of the cortical neuron.

## 3.2.8 Bistability and Hysteresis

Systems having two (many) coexisting attractors are called *bistable* (*multistable*). Many neurons and neuronal models, such as the Hodgkin-Huxley model, exhibit bistability between resting (equilibrium) and spiking (limit cycle) attractors. Some neurons can exhibit bistability of two stable resting states in the subthreshold voltage range, for example, $-59$ mV and $-75$ mV in the thalamocortical neurons (Hughes et al. 1999) depicted in Fig.3.16, or $-50$ mV and $-60$ mV in mitral cells of the olfactory bulb (Heyward et al. 2001), or $-45$ mV and $-60$ mV in Purkinje neurons. Brief inputs can switch such neurons from one state to the other, as in Fig.3.16. Though the ionic mechanisms of bistability are different in the three neurons, the mathematical mechanism is the same.

Consider a one-dimensional system $\dot{V} = I + F(V)$ with function $F(V)$ having a cubic N-shape. Injection of a DC current $I$ shifts the function $I + F(V)$ up or down. When $I$ is negative, the system has only one equilibrium, depicted in Fig.3.17a. As we remove the injected current $I$, the system becomes bistable, as in Fig.3.17b, but its state is still at the left equilibrium. As we inject positive current, the left stable equilibrium disappears via another saddle-node bifurcation, and the state of the system jumps to the right equilibrium, as in Fig.3.17c. But as we slowly remove the injected current that caused the jump and go back to Fig.3.17b, the jump to the left equilibrium does not occur until a much lower value corresponding to Fig.3.17a is reached. The failure of the system to return to the original value when the injected current is removed is called *hysteresis*. If $I$ were a slow $V$-dependent variable, then the system could exhibit relaxation oscillations depicted in Fig.3.17d and described in the next chapter.

## 3.3  Phase Portraits

An important component in the qualitative analysis of any dynamical system is recon-struction of its *phase portrait*. It depicts all stable and unstable equilibria (as black and white circles, respectively), representative trajectories, and corresponding attrac-tion domains in the system's state/phase space, as we illustrate in Fig.3.18. The phase portrait is a geometrical representation of system dynamics. It depicts all possible evolutions of the state variable and how they depend on the initial state. Looking at the phase portrait, one immediately gets all important information about the system's qualitative behavior without even knowing the equation for $F$.

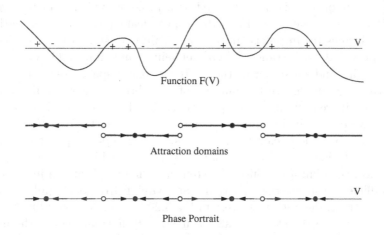

Figure 3.18: Phase portrait of a one-dimensional system $\dot{V} = F(V)$.

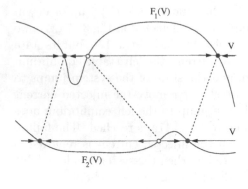

Figure 3.19: Two "seemingly different" dynamical systems, $\dot{V} = F_1(V)$ and $\dot{V} = F_2(V)$, are topologically equivalent. Hence they have qualitatively similar dynamics.

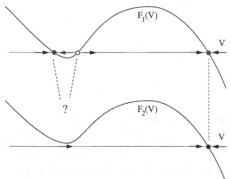

Figure 3.20: Two "seemingly alike" dynamical systems $\dot{V} = F_1(V)$ and $\dot{V} = F_2(V)$ are not topologically equivalent, hence they do not have qualitatively similar dynamics. (The first system has three equilibria, while the second system has only one.)

### 3.3.1 Topological Equivalence

Phase portraits can be used to determine qualitative similarity of dynamical systems. In particular, two one-dimensional systems are said to be *topologically equivalent* when the phase portrait of one of them, treated as a piece of rubber, can be stretched or shrunk to fit the other one, as in Fig.3.19. Topological equivalence is a mathematical concept that clarifies the imprecise notion of "qualitative similarity", and its rigorous definition is provided, for instance, by Guckenheimer and Holmes (1983).

The stretching and shrinking of the "rubber" phase space are topological transformations that do not change the number of equilibria or their stability. Thus, two systems having different numbers of equilibria cannot be topologically equivalent and, hence, they have qualitatively different dynamics, as we illustrate in Fig.3.20. Indeed, the top system is bistable because it has two stable equilibria separated by an unstable one. The evolution of the state variable depends on which attraction domain the initial condition is in initially. Such a system has "memory" of the initial condition. Moreover, sufficiently strong perturbations can switch it from one equilibrium state to another. In contrast, the bottom system in Fig.3.20 has only one equilibrium, which is a global attractor, and the state variable converges to it regardless of the initial condition. Such a system has quite primitive dynamics, and it is topologically equivalent to the linear system (3.1).

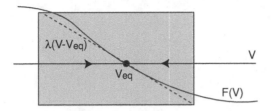

Figure 3.21: Hartman-Grobman theorem: The nonlinear system $\dot{V} = F(V)$ is topologically equivalent to the linear one $\dot{V} = \lambda(V - V_{eq})$ in the local (shaded) neighborhood of the hyperbolic equilibrium $V_{eq}$.

### 3.3.2 Local Equivalence and the Hartman-Grobman Theorem

In computational neuroscience, we usually face quite complicated systems describing neuronal dynamics. A useful strategy is to replace such systems with simpler ones having topologically equivalent phase portraits. For example, both systems in Fig.3.19 are topologically equivalent to $\dot{V} = V - V^3$ (readers should check this), which is easier to deal with analytically.

Quite often we cannot find a simpler system that is topologically equivalent to our neuronal model on the entire state line $\mathbb{R}$. In this case, we make a sacrifice: we restrict our analysis to a small neighborhood of the line $\mathbb{R}$ (e.g., a neighborhood of the resting state or of the threshold), and study behavior locally in this neighborhood.

An important tool in the local analysis of dynamical systems is the Hartman-Grobman theorem, which says that a nonlinear one-dimensional system

$$\dot{V} = F(V)$$

sufficiently near an equilibrium $V = V_{eq}$ is locally topologically equivalent to the linear system

$$\dot{V} = \lambda(V - V_{eq}) \,, \tag{3.8}$$

provided the eigenvalue

$$\lambda = F'(V_{eq})$$

at the equilibrium is nonzero, that is, the slope of $F(V)$ is nonzero. Such an equilibrium is called *hyperbolic*. Thus, nonlinear systems near hyperbolic equilibria behave as if they were linear, as in Fig.3.21.

It is easy to find the exact solution of the linearized system (3.8) with an initial condition $V(0) = V_0$. It is $V(t) = V_{eq} + e^{\lambda t}(V_0 - V_{eq})$ (readers should check by differentiating). If the eigenvalue $\lambda < 0$, then $e^{\lambda t} \to 0$ and $V(t) \to V_{eq}$ as $t \to \infty$, so that the equilibrium is stable. Conversely, if $\lambda > 0$, then $e^{\lambda t} \to \infty$ meaning that the initial displacement, $V_0 - V_{eq}$, grows with time and the equilibrium is unstable. Thus, the linearization predicts qualitative dynamics at the equilibrium, and the quantitative rate of convergence/divergence to/from the equilibrium.

If the eigenvalue $\lambda = 0$, then the equilibrium is non-hyperbolic, and analysis of the linearized system $\dot{V} = 0$ cannot describe the behavior of the nonlinear system. Typically, non-hyperbolic equilibria arise when the system undergoes a bifurcation, i.e., a qualitative change of behavior, which we consider next. To study stability, we need to consider higher-order terms of the Taylor series of $F(V)$ at $V_{eq}$.

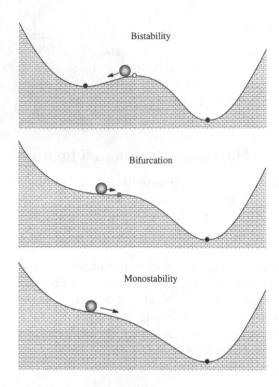

Figure 3.22: Mechanistic illustration of a bifurcation as a change of the landscape.

### 3.3.3   Bifurcations

The final and most advanced step in the qualitative analysis of any dynamical system is the bifurcation analysis. In general, a system is said to undergo a bifurcation when its phase portrait changes qualitatively. For example, the energy landscape in Fig.3.22 changes so that the system is no longer bistable. The precise mathematical definition of a bifurcation will be given later.

Qualitative change of the phase portrait may or may not necessarily reveal itself in a qualitative change of behavior, depending on the initial conditions. For example, there is a bifurcation in Fig.3.23 (left), but no change of behavior, because the ball remains in the attraction domain of the right equilibrium. To see the change, we need to drop the ball at different initial conditions and observe the disappearance of the left equilibrium. In the same veins, there is no bifurcation in Fig.3.23 (middle and right), – the phase portraits in each column are topologically equivalent, but the apparent change of behavior is caused by the expansion of the attraction domain of the left equilibrium or by the external input. Dropping the ball at different locations would result in the same qualitative picture – two stable equilibria whose attraction domains are separated by the unstable equilibrium. When mathematicians talk about bifurcations, they assume that all initial conditions could be sampled, in which case bifurcations do result in a qualitative change of behavior of the system as a whole.

To illustrate the importance of sampling all initial conditions, let us consider the in

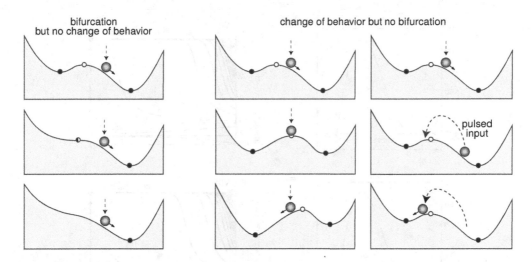

Figure 3.23: Bifurcations are not equivalent to qualitative change of behavior if the system is started with the same initial condition or subject to external input.

vitro recordings of a pyramidal neuron in Fig.3.24. We inject 0.1-ms strong pulses of current of various amplitudes to set the membrane potential to different initial values. Right after each pulse, we inject a 4-ms step of DC current of amplitude $I = 0$, $I = 16$, or $I = 60$ pA. The case of $I = 0$ pA is the same as in Fig.3.15, so some initial conditions result in upstroke of the action potential, while others do not. When $I = 60$ pA, all

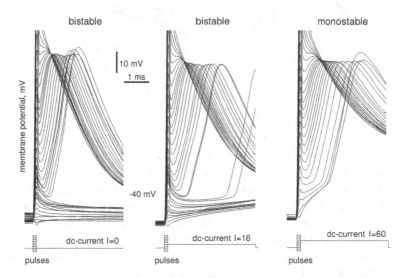

Figure 3.24: Qualitative change of the upstroke dynamics of a layer 5 pyramidal neuron from rat visual cortex (the same neuron as in Fig.3.15).

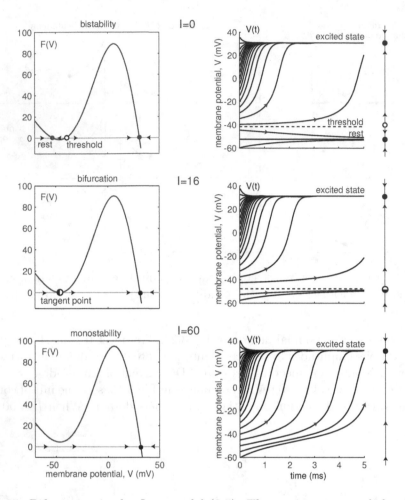

Figure 3.25: Bifurcation in the $I_{Na,p}$-model (3.5): The resting state and the threshold state coalesce and disappear when the parameter $I$ increases.

initial conditions result in the generation of an action potential. Clearly, a change of qualitative behavior occurs for some $I$ between 0 and 60.

To understand the qualitative dynamics in Fig.3.24, we consider the one-dimensional $I_{Na,p}$-model (3.5) having different values of the parameter $I$ and depict its trajectories in Fig.3.25. One can clearly see that the qualitative behavior of the model depends on whether $I$ is greater or less than 16. When $I = 0$ (top of Fig.3.25), the system is bistable. The resting and the excited states coexist. When $I$ is large (bottom of Fig.3.25) the resting state no longer exists because the leak outward current cannot balance the large injected DC current $I$ and the inward Na$^+$ current.

What happens when we change $I$ past 16? The answer lies in the details of the geometry of the right-hand-side function $F(V)$ of (3.5) and how it depends on the

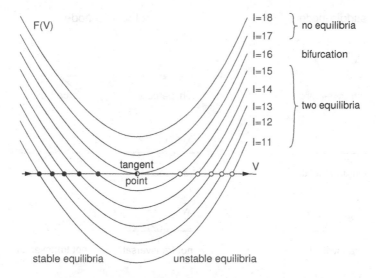

Figure 3.26: Saddle-node bifurcation: As the graph of the function $F(V)$ is lifted up, the stable and unstable equilibria approach each other, coalesce at the tangent point, and then disappear.

parameter $I$. Increasing $I$ elevates the graph of $F(V)$. The higher the graph of $F(V)$ is, the closer its intersections with the $V$-axis are, as we illustrate in Fig.3.26, which depicts only the low-voltage range of the system. When $I$ approaches 16, the distance between the stable and unstable equilibria vanishes; the equilibria coalesce and annihilate each other. The value $I = 16$, at which the equilibria coalesce, is called the *bifurcation value*. This value separates two qualitatively different regimes. When $I$ is near to but less than 16, the system has three equilibria and bistable dynamics. The quantitative features, such as the exact locations of the equilibria, depend on the particular values of $I$, but the qualitative behavior remains unchanged no matter how close $I$ is to the bifurcation value. In contrast, when $I$ is near to but greater than 16, the system has only one equilibrium and monostable dynamics.

In general, a dynamical system may depend on a vector of parameters, say $p$. A point in the parameter space, say $p = a$, is said to be a *regular* or non-bifurcation point, if the system's phase portrait at $p = a$ is topologically equivalent to the phase portrait at $p = c$ for any $c$ sufficiently close to $a$. For example, the value $I = 13$ in Fig.3.26 is regular, since the system has topologically equivalent phase portraits for all $I$ near 13. Similarly, the value $I = 18$ is also regular. Any point in the parameter space that is not regular is called a bifurcation point. Namely, a point $p = b$ is a bifurcation point if the system's phase portrait at $p = b$ is not topologically equivalent to the phase portrait at a point $p = c$ no matter how close $c$ is to $b$. The value $I = 16$ in Fig.3.26 is a bifurcation point. It corresponds to the *saddle-node* (also known as *fold* or *tangent*) bifurcation for reasons described later. It is one of the simplest bifurcations considered in this book.

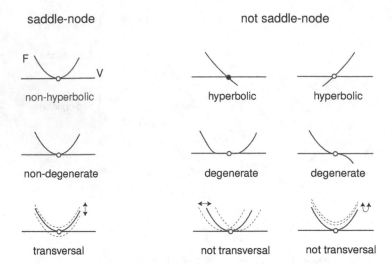

Figure 3.27: Geometrical illustration of the three conditions defining saddle-node bifurcations. Arrows denote the direction of displacement of the function $F(V, I)$ as the bifurcation parameter $I$ changes.

### 3.3.4   Saddle-Node (Fold) Bifurcation

In general, a one-dimensional system

$$\dot{V} = F(V, I),$$

having an equilibrium point $V = V_{\mathrm{sn}}$ for some value of the parameter $I = I_{\mathrm{sn}}$ (i.e., $F(V_{\mathrm{sn}}, I_{\mathrm{sn}}) = 0$), is said to be at a *saddle-node* bifurcation (sometimes called a *fold* bifurcation) if the following mathematical conditions, illustrated in Fig.3.27, are satisfied:

- *Non-hyperbolicity.* The eigenvalue $\lambda$ at $V_{\mathrm{sn}}$ is zero; that is,

$$\lambda = F_V(V, I_{\mathrm{sn}}) = 0 \qquad (\text{at } V = V_{\mathrm{sn}}),$$

where $F_V$ denotes the derivative of $F$ with respect to $V$, that is, $F_V = \partial F/\partial V$. Equilibria with zero or pure imaginary eigenvalues are called non-hyperbolic. Geometrically, this condition implies that the graph of $F$ has horizontal slope at the equilibrium.

- *Non-degeneracy.* The second-order derivative with respect to $V$ at $V_{\mathrm{sn}}$ is nonzero; that is,

$$F_{VV}(V, I_{\mathrm{sn}}) \neq 0 \qquad (\text{at } V = V_{\mathrm{sn}}).$$

Geometrically, this means that the graph of $F$ looks like the square parabola $V^2$ in Fig.3.27.

- *Transversality.* The function $F(V, I)$ is non-degenerate with respect to the bifurcation parameter $I$; that is,

$$F_I(V_{sn}, I) \neq 0 \qquad (\text{at } I = I_{sn}),$$

where $F_I$ denotes the derivative of $F$ with respect to $I$. Geometrically, this means that as $I$ changes past $I_{sn}$, the graph of $F$ approaches, touches, and then intersects the $V$-axis.

Saddle-node bifurcation results in appearance or disappearance of a pair of equilibria, as in Fig.3.26. None of the six examples on the right-hand side of Fig.3.27 can undergo a saddle-node bifurcation because at least one of the conditions above is violated.

The number of conditions involving strict equality ("=") is called the *codimension* of a bifurcation. The saddle-node bifurcation has *codimension-1* because there is only one condition involving "="; the other two conditions involve inequalities ("$\neq$"). Codimension-1 bifurcations can be reliably observed in systems with one parameter.

It is an easy exercise to check that the one-dimensional system

$$\dot{V} = I + V^2 \tag{3.9}$$

is at saddle-node bifurcation when $V = 0$ and $I = 0$ (readers should check all three conditions). This system is called the *topological normal form* for saddle-node bifurcation. The phase portraits of this system are topologically equivalent to those depicted in Fig.3.26, except that the bifurcation occurs at $I = 0$, and not at $I = 16$.

### 3.3.5 Slow Transition

All physical, chemical, and biological systems near saddle-node bifurcations possess certain universal features that do not depend on particulars of the systems. Consequently, all neural systems near such a bifurcation share common neurocomputational properties, which we will discuss in detail in chapter 7. Here we take a look at one such property – slow transition through the ruins (or ghost) of the resting state attractor, which is relevant to the dynamics of many neocortical neurons.

In Fig.3.28 we show the function $F(V)$ of the system (3.5) with $I = 30$ pA, which is greater than the bifurcation value 16 pA, and the corresponding behavior of a cortical neuron (compare with Fig.3.15). The system has only one attractor, the excited state, and any solution starting from an arbitrary initial condition should quickly approach this attractor. However, the solutions starting from the initial conditions around $-50$ mV do not seem to hurry. Instead, they slow down near $-46$ mV and spend a considerable amount of time in the voltage range corresponding to the resting state, as if the state were still present. The closer $I$ is to the bifurcation value, the more time the membrane potential spends in the neighborhood of the resting state. Obviously, such a slow transition cannot be explained by a slow activation of the inward $Na^+$ current, since $Na^+$ activation in a cortical neuron is practically instantaneous.

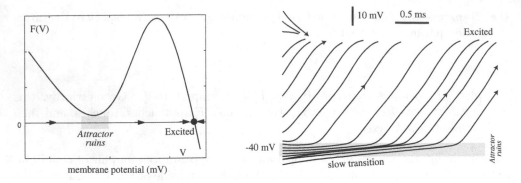

Figure 3.28: Slow transition through the ghost of the resting state attractor in a cortical pyramidal neuron with $I = 30$ pA (the same neuron as in Fig.3.15). Even though the resting state has already disappeared, the function $F(V)$, and hence the rate of change, $\dot{V}$, is still small when $V \approx -46$ mV.

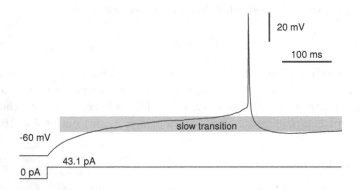

Figure 3.29: A 400-ms latency in a layer 5 pyramidal neuron of rat visual cortex.

The slow transition occurs because the neuron or the system (3.5) in Fig.3.28 is near a saddle-node bifurcation. Even though $I$ is greater than the bifurcation value, and the resting state attractor is already annihilated, the function $F(V)$ is barely above the $V$-axis at the "annihilation site". In other words, the resting state attractor has already been ruined, but its "ruins" (or its "ghost") can still be felt, because

$$\dot{V} = F(V) \approx 0 \qquad \text{(at attractor ruins, } V \approx -46 \text{ mV)},$$

as one can see in Fig.3.28. In chapter 7 we will show how this property explains the ability of many neocortical neurons, such as the one in Fig.3.29, to generate repetitive action potentials with small frequency, and how it predicts that all such neurons, considered as dynamical systems, reside near saddle-node bifurcations.

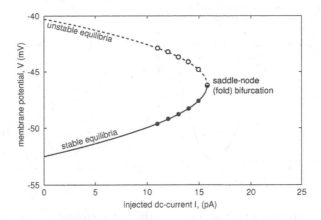

Figure 3.30: Bifurcation diagram of the system in Fig.3.26.

### 3.3.6 Bifurcation Diagram

The final step in the geometrical bifurcation analysis of one-dimensional systems is the analysis of bifurcation diagrams, which we do in Fig.3.30 for the saddle-node bifurcation shown in Fig.3.26. To draw the bifurcation diagram, we determine the locations of the stable and unstable equilibria for each value of the parameter $I$ and plot them as white or black circles in the $(I, V)$ plane in Fig.3.30. The equilibria form two branches that join at the fold point corresponding to the saddle-node bifurcation (hence the alternative name *fold* bifurcation). The branch corresponding to the unstable equilibria is dashed to stress its instability. As the bifurcation parameter $I$ varies from left to right, passing through the bifurcation point, the stable and unstable equilibria coalesce and annihilate each other. As the parameter varies from right to left, two equilibria – one stable and one unstable – appear from a single point. Thus, depending on the direction of movement of the bifurcation parameter, the saddle-node bifurcation explains disappearance or appearance of a new stable state. In any case, the qualitative behavior of the systems changes exactly at the bifurcation point.

### 3.3.7 Bifurcations and I-V Relations

In general, determining saddle-node bifurcation diagrams of neurons may be a daunting mathematical task. However, it is a trivial exercise when the bifurcation parameter is the injected DC current $I$. In this case, the bifurcation diagram, such as the one in Fig.3.30, is the steady-state I-V relation $I_\infty(V)$ plotted on the $(I, V)$-plane. Indeed, the equation

$$C\dot{V} = I - I_\infty(V) = 0$$

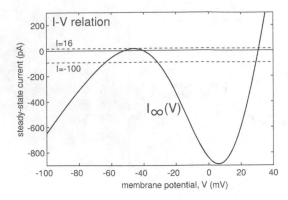

Figure 3.31: Equilibria are intersections of the steady-state I-V curve $I_\infty(V)$ and a horizontal line $I = $ const.

states that $V$ is an equilibrium if and only if the net membrane current, $I - I_\infty(V)$, is zero. For example, equilibria of the $I_{\mathrm{Na,p}}$-model are solutions of the equation

$$0 = I - \overbrace{(g_\mathrm{L}(V - E_\mathrm{L}) + g_\mathrm{Na}m_\infty(V)(V - E_\mathrm{Na}))}^{I_\infty(V)},$$

which follows directly from (3.5). In Fig.3.31 we illustrate how to find the equilibria geometrically: We plot the steady-state I-V curve $I_\infty(V)$ and draw a horizontal line with altitude $I$. Any intersection satisfies the equation $I = I_\infty(V)$, and hence is an equilibrium (stable or unstable). Obviously, when $I$ increases past 16, the saddle-node bifurcation occurs.

Note that the equilibria are points on the curve $I_\infty(V)$, so flipping and rotating the curve by 90°, as we do in Fig.3.32 (left), results in a complete saddle-node bifurcation diagram. The diagram conveys all important information about the qualitative behavior of the $I_{\mathrm{Na,p}}$-model in a very condensed manner. The three branches of the S-shaped

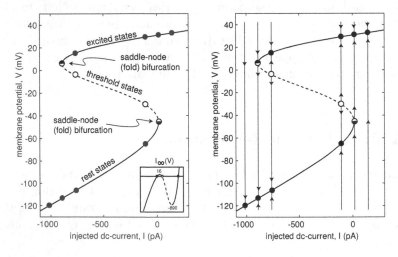

Figure 3.32: Bifurcation diagram of the $I_{\mathrm{Na,p}}$-model (3.5).

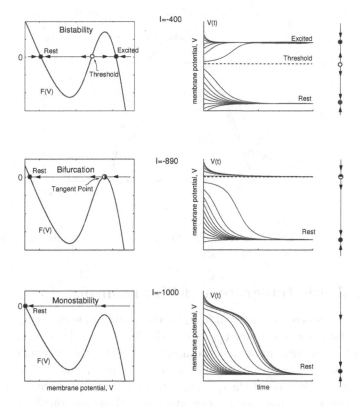

Figure 3.33: Bifurcation in the $I_{\text{Na,p}}$-model (3.5). The excited state and the threshold state coalesce and disappear when the parameter $I$ is sufficiently small.

curve, which is the 90°-rotated and flipped copy of the N-shaped I-V curve, correspond to the resting, threshold, and excited states of the model. Each slice $I = $ const represents the phase portrait of the system, as we illustrate in Fig.3.32 (right). Each point where the branches fold (max or min of $I_\infty(V)$) corresponds to a saddle-node bifurcation. Since there are two such folds, at $I = 16$ pA and at $I = -890$ pA, there are two saddle-node bifurcations in the system. The first one, studied in Fig.3.25, corresponds to the disappearance of the resting state. The other one, illustrated in Fig.3.33, corresponds to the disappearance of the excited state. It occurs because $I$ becomes so negative that the Na$^+$ inward current is no longer strong enough to balance the leak outward current and the negative injected DC current to keep the membrane in the depolarized (excited) state.

Below, the reader can find more examples of bifurcation analysis of the $I_{\text{Na,p}}$- and $I_{\text{Kir}}$-models, which have nonmonotonic I-V relations and can exhibit multistability of states. The $I_{\text{K}}$- and $I_{\text{h}}$-models have monotonic I-V relations, and hence only one equilibrium state. These models cannot have saddle-node bifurcations, as the reader is asked to prove in exercise 13 and 14.

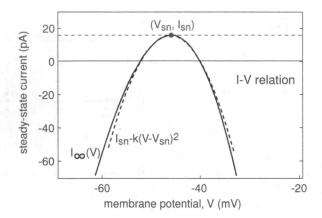

Figure 3.34: Magnification of the I-V curve in Fig.3.31 at the left knee shows that it can be approximated by a square parabola.

### 3.3.8   Quadratic Integrate-and-Fire Neuron

Let us consider the topological normal form for the saddle-node bifurcation (3.9). From $0 = I + V^2$ we find that there are two equilibria, $V_{\text{rest}} = -\sqrt{|I|}$ and $V_{\text{thresh}} = +\sqrt{|I|}$ when $I < 0$. The equilibria approach and annihilate each other via saddle-node bifurcation when $I = 0$, so there are no equilibria when $I > 0$. In this case, $\dot{V} \geq I$ and $V(t)$ increases to infinity. Because of the quadratic term, the rate of increase also increases, resulting in a positive feedback loop corresponding to the regenerative activation of the $\text{Na}^+$ current. In exercise 15 we show that $V(t)$ escapes to infinity in a finite time, which corresponds to the upstroke of the action potential. The same upstroke is generated when $I < 0$, if the voltage variable is pushed beyond the threshold value $V_{\text{thresh}}$.

Considering infinite values of the membrane potential may be convenient from a purely mathematical point of view, but this has no physical meaning and there is no way to simulate it on a digital computer. Instead, we fix a sufficiently large constant $V_{\text{peak}}$ and say that (3.9) generated a spike when $V(t)$ reached $V_{\text{peak}}$. After the peak of the spike is reached, we reset $V(t)$ to a new value $V_{\text{reset}}$. The topological normal form for the saddle-node bifurcation with the after-spike resetting,

$$\dot{V} = I + V^2 \, , \qquad \text{if } V \geq V_{\text{peak}}, \quad \text{then } V \leftarrow V_{\text{reset}} \tag{3.10}$$

is called the *quadratic integrate-and-fire neuron*. It is the simplest model of a spiking neuron. The name stems from its resemblance to the *leaky* integrate-and-fire neuron $\dot{V} = I - V$ considered in chapter 8. In contrast to the common folklore, the leaky neuron is not a *spiking model* because it does not have a spike generation mechanism, i.e., a regenerative upstroke of the membrane potential, whereas the quadratic neuron does. We discuss this and other issues in detail in chapter 8.

In general, the quadratic integrate-and-fire model could be derived directly from the equation $C\dot{V} = I - I_\infty(V)$ through approximating the steady-state I-V curve near

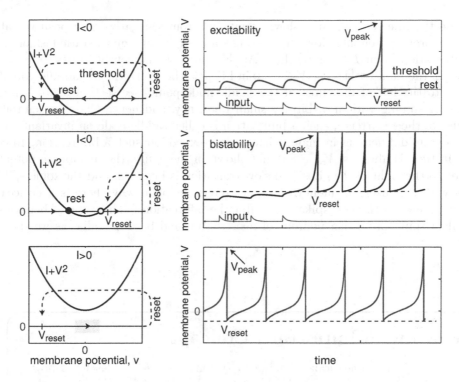

Figure 3.35: Quadratic integrate-and-fire neuron (3.10) with time-dependent input.

the resting state by the square parabola $I_\infty(V) \approx I_{sn} - k(V - V_{sn})^2$, where $k > 0$ and the peak of the curve $(V_{sn}, I_{sn})$ could easily be found experimentally (see Fig.3.34). Approximating the I-V curve by other functions – for example $I_\infty(V) = g_{leak}(V - V_{rest}) - ke^{pV}$, results in other forms of the model, such as the exponential integrate-and-fire model (Fourcaud-Trocme et al. 2003), which has certain advantages over the quadratic form. Unfortunately, the model is not solvable analytically, and it is expensive to simulate. The form $I_\infty(V) = g_{leak}(V - V_{leak}) - k(V - V_{th})_+^2$, where $x_+ = x$ when $x > 0$ and $x_+ = 0$ otherwise, combines the advantages of both models. The parameters $V_{peak}$ and $V_{reset}$ are derived from the shape of the spike. Normalization of variables and parameters results in the form (3.10) with $V_{peak} = 1$.

In Fig.3.35 we simulate the quadratic integrate-and-fire neuron to illustrate a number of its features, which will be described in detail in subsequent chapters using conductance-based models. First, the neuron is an integrator; each input pulse in Fig.3.35 (top), pushes $V$ closer to the threshold value; the higher the frequency of the input, the sooner $V$ reaches the threshold and starts the upstroke of a spike. The neuron is monostable when $V_{reset} \leq 0$ and can be bistable otherwise. Indeed, the first spike in Fig.3.35 (middle) is evoked by the input, but the subsequent spikes occur because the reset value is superthreshold.

The neuron can be Class 1 or Class 2 excitable, depending on the sign of $V_{reset}$.

Suppose the injected current $I$ slowly ramps up from a negative to a positive value. The membrane potential follows the resting state $-\sqrt{|I|}$ in a quasi-static fashion until the bifurcation point $I = 0$ is reached. At this moment, the neuron starts to fire tonic spikes. In the monostable case $V_{\text{reset}} < 0$ in Fig.3.35 (bottom), the membrane potential is reset to the left of the ghost of the saddle-node point (see section 3.3.5), thereby producing spiking with an arbitrary small frequency, and hence Class 1 excitability. Because of the recurrence, such a bifurcation is called saddle-node on invariant circle. Many pyramidal neurons in mammalian neocortex exhibit such a bifurcation. In contrast, in the bistable case $V_{\text{reset}} > 0$, not shown in the figure, the membrane potential is reset to the right of the ghost, no slow transition is involved, and the tonic spiking starts with a nonzero frequency. (As an exercise, explain why there is a noticeable latency [delay] to the first spike right after the bifurcation.) This type of behavior is typical in spiny projection neurons of neostriatum and basal ganglia, as we show in chapter 8.

## Review of Important Concepts

- The one-dimensional dynamical system $\dot{V} = F(V)$ describes how the rate of change of $V$ depends on $V$. Positive $F(V)$ means $V$ increases; negative $F(V)$ means $V$ decreases.

- In the context of neuronal dynamics, $V$ is often the membrane potential, and $F(V)$ is the steady-state I-V curve taken with the minus sign.

- A zero of $F(V)$ corresponds to an equilibrium of the system. (Indeed, if $F(V) = 0$, then the state of the system, $V$, neither increases nor decreases.)

- An equilibrium is stable when $F(V)$ changes the sign from "plus" to "minus". A sufficient condition for stability is that the eigenvalue $\lambda = F'(V)$ at the equilibrium be negative.

- A phase portrait is a geometrical representation of the system's dynamics. It depicts all equilibria, their stability, representative trajectories, and attraction domains.

- A bifurcation is a qualitative change of the system's phase portrait.

- The saddle-node (fold) is a typical bifurcation in one-dimensional systems. As a parameter changes, a stable and an unstable equilibrium approach, coalesce, and then annihilate each other.

# Bibliographical Notes

There is no standard textbook on dynamical systems theory. The classic book *Nonlinear Oscillations, Dynamical Systems, and Bifurcations of Vector Fields* by Guckenheimer and Holmes (1983) plays the same role in the dynamical systems community as the book *Ion Channels of Excitable Membranes* by Hille (2001) plays in the neuroscience community. A common feature of these books is that they are not suitable for beginners.

Most textbooks on differential equations, such as *Differential Equations and Dynamical Systems* by Perko (1996), develop the theory starting with a comprehensive analysis of linear systems, then applying it to local analysis of nonlinear systems, and then discussing global behavior. To get to bifurcations, the reader has to go through a lot of daunting math, which is fun only for mathematicians. Here we follow an approach similar to that in *Nonlinear Dynamics and Chaos* by Strogatz (1994). Instead of going from linear to nonlinear systems, we go from one-dimensional nonlinear systems (this chapter) to two-dimensional nonlinear systems (next chapter). Rather than burdening the theory with a lot of mathematics, we use the geometrical approach to stimulate the reader's intuition. (There is plenty of fun math in exercises and in later chapters.)

# Exercises

1. Consider a neuron having a $Na^+$ current with fast activation kinetics. Assume that inactivation of this current, as well as (in)activations of the other currents in the neuron are much slower. Prove that the initial segment of action potential upstroke of this neuron can be approximated by the $I_{Na,p}$-model (3.5). Use Fig.3.15 to discuss the applicability of this approximation.

2. Draw phase portraits of the systems in Fig.3.36. Clearly mark all equilibria, their stability, attraction domains, and direction of trajectories. Determine the signs of eigenvalues at each equilibrium.

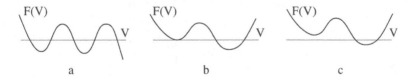

Figure 3.36: Draw a phase portrait of the system $\dot{V} = F(V)$ with shown $F(V)$.

3. Draw phase portraits of the following systems:

   (a) $\dot{x} = -1 + x^2$,

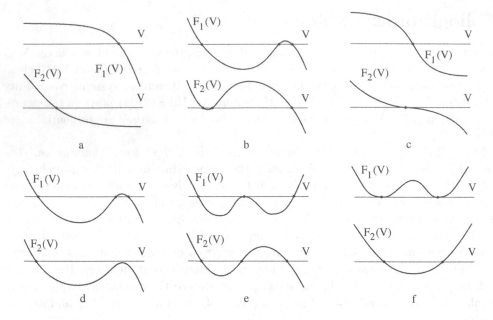

Figure 3.37: Which of the pairs correspond to topologically equivalent dynamical systems? (All intersections with the $V$-axis are marked as dots.)

(b) $\dot{x} = x - x^3$.

Determine the eigenvalues at each equilibrium.

4. Determine stability of the equilibrium $x = 0$ and draw phase portraits of the following piecewise continuous systems:

$$(a) \quad \dot{x} = \begin{cases} 2x, & \text{if } x < 0 \\ x, & \text{if } x \geq 0 \end{cases}$$

$$(b) \quad \dot{x} = \begin{cases} -1, & \text{if } x < 0 \\ 0, & \text{if } x = 0 \\ 1, & \text{if } x > 0 \end{cases}$$

$$(c) \quad \dot{x} = \begin{cases} -2/x, & \text{if } x \neq 0 \\ 0, & \text{if } x = 0 \end{cases}$$

5. Draw phase portraits of the systems in Fig.3.37. Which of the pairs in the figure correspond to topologically equivalent dynamical systems?

6. (Saddle-node bifurcation) Draw the bifurcation diagram and representative phase portraits of the system $\dot{x} = a + x^2$, where $a$ is a bifurcation parameter. Find the eigenvalues at each equilibrium.

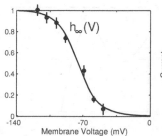 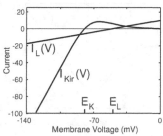 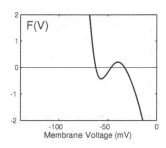

Figure 3.38: The $I_{\mathrm{Kir}}$-model having injected current ($I$), leak current ($I_{\mathrm{L}}$), and instantaneous K$^+$ inward rectifier current ($I_{\mathrm{Kir}}$) and described by (3.11). Inactivation curve $h_\infty(V)$ is modified from Wessel et al. (1999). Parameters: $C = 1$, $I = 6$, $g_{\mathrm{L}} = 0.2$, $E_{\mathrm{L}} = -50$, $g_{\mathrm{Kir}} = 2$, $E_{\mathrm{K}} = -80$, $V_{1/2} = -76$, $k = -12$ (see Fig.2.20).

7. (Saddle-node bifurcation) Use definition in section 3.3.4 to find saddle-node bifurcation points in the following systems:

   (a) $\dot{x} = a + 2x + x^2$,

   (b) $\dot{x} = a + x + x^2$,

   (c) $\dot{x} = a - x + x^2$,

   (d) $\dot{x} = a - x + x^3$ (Hint: Verify the non-hyperbolicity condition first.),

   (e) $\dot{x} = 1 + ax + x^2$,

   (f) $\dot{x} = 1 + 2x + ax^2$,

   where $a$ is the bifurcation parameter.

8. (Pitchfork bifurcation) Draw the bifurcation diagram and representative phase portraits of the system $\dot{x} = bx - x^3$, where $b$ is a bifurcation parameter. Find the eigenvalues at each equilibrium.

9. Draw the bifurcation diagram of the $I_{\mathrm{Kir}}$-model

$$C\dot{V} = I - g_{\mathrm{L}}(V - E_{\mathrm{L}}) - \overbrace{g_{\mathrm{Kir}}h_\infty(V)(V - E_{\mathrm{K}})}^{\text{instantaneous } I_{\mathrm{Kir}}}, \tag{3.11}$$

   using parameters from Fig.3.38 and treating $I$ as a bifurcation parameter.

10. Derive an explicit formula that relates the position of the equilibrium in the Hodgkin-Huxley model to the magnitude of the injected DC current $I$. Are there any saddle-node bifurcations?

11. Draw the bifurcation diagram of the $I_{\mathrm{Na,p}}$-model (3.5), using parameters from Fig.3.39 and treating

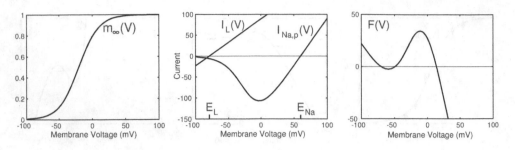

Figure 3.39: The $I_{\mathrm{Na,p}}$-model with leak current ($I_{\mathrm{L}}$) and persistent Na$^+$ current ($I_{\mathrm{Na,p}}$), described by (3.5) with the right-hand-side function $F(V)$. Parameters: $C = 1$, $I = 0$, $g_{\mathrm{L}} = 1$, $E_{\mathrm{L}} = -80$, $g_{\mathrm{Na}} = 2.25$, $E_{\mathrm{Na}} = 60$, $V_{1/2} = -20$, $k = 15$ (see Fig.2.20).

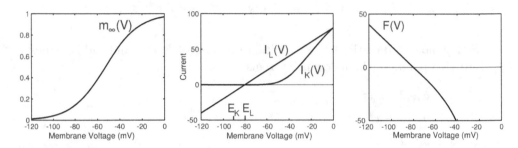

Figure 3.40: The $I_{\mathrm{K}}$-model with leak current ($I_{\mathrm{L}}$) and persistent K$^+$ current ($I_{\mathrm{K}}$), described by (3.12). Parameters: $C = 1$, $g_{\mathrm{L}} = 1$, $E_{\mathrm{L}} = -80$, $g_{\mathrm{K}} = 1$, $E_{\mathrm{K}} = -90$, $V_{1/2} = -53$, $k = 15$ (see Fig.2.20).

    (a) $g_{\mathrm{L}}$ as a bifurcation parameter, or

    (b) $E_{\mathrm{L}}$ as a bifurcation parameter.

12. Draw the bifurcation diagram of the $I_{\mathrm{Kir}}$-model (3.11), using parameters from Fig.3.38 and treating

    (a) $g_{\mathrm{L}}$ as a bifurcation parameter, or

    (b) $g_{\mathrm{Kir}}$ as a bifurcation parameter.

13. Show that the $I_{\mathrm{K}}$-model in Fig.3.40

$$C\dot{V} = -g_{\mathrm{L}}(V - E_{\mathrm{L}}) - \overbrace{g_{\mathrm{K}}m_\infty^4(V)(V - E_{\mathrm{K}})}^{\text{instantaneous } I_{\mathrm{K}}} . \tag{3.12}$$

cannot exhibit saddle-node bifurcation for $V > E_{\mathrm{K}}$. (Hint: Show that $F'(V) \neq 0$ for all $V > E_{\mathrm{K}}$.)

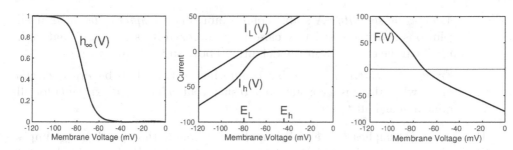

Figure 3.41: The $I_h$-model with leak current ($I_L$) and "hyperpolarization-activated" inward current $I_h$, described by (3.13). Parameters: $C = 1$, $g_L = 1$, $E_L = -80$, $g_h = 1$, $E_h = -43$, $V_{1/2} = -75$, $k = -5.5$ (Huguenard and McCormick 1992).

14. Show that the $I_h$-model in Fig.3.41,

$$C\dot{V} = -g_L(V - E_L) - \overbrace{g_h h_\infty(V)(V - E_h)}^{\text{instantaneous } I_h}\,, \tag{3.13}$$

cannot exhibit saddle-node bifurcation for any $V < E_h$.

15. Prove that the upstroke of the spike in the quadratic integrate-and-fire neuron (3.9) has the asymptote $1/(c - t)$ for some $c > 0$.

16. (Cusp bifurcation) Draw the bifurcation diagram and representative phase portraits of the system $\dot{x} = a + bx - x^3$, where $a$ and $b$ are bifurcation parameters. Plot the bifurcation diagram in the $(a, b, x)$-space and on the $(a, b)$-plane.

17. (Gradient systems) An $n$-dimensional dynamical system $\dot{x} = f(x)$, with $x = (x_1, \ldots, x_n) \in \mathbb{R}^n$ is said to be *gradient* when there is a potential (energy) function $E(x)$ such that

$$\dot{x} = -\text{ grad } E(x)\,,$$

where

$$\text{grad } E(x) = (E_{x_1}, \ldots, E_{x_n})$$

is the gradient of $E(x)$. Show that all one-dimensional systems are gradient. (Hint: See Fig.3.11.) Find potential (energy) functions for the following one-dimensional systems

(a) $\dot{V} = 0$,          (b) $\dot{V} = 1$,          (c) $\dot{V} = -V$,
(d) $\dot{V} = -1 + V^2$,    (e) $\dot{V} = V - V^3$,    (f) $\dot{V} = -\sin V$.

18. Consider a dynamical system $\dot{x} = f(x)$, $x(0) = x_0$.

(a) *Stability.* An equilibrium $y$ is *stable* if any solution $x(t)$ with $x_0$ sufficiently close to $y$ remains near $y$ for all time. That is, for all $\varepsilon > 0$ there exists $\delta > 0$ such that if $|x_0 - y| < \delta$ then $|x(t) - y| < \varepsilon$ for all $t \geq 0$.

(b) *Asymptotic stability.* A stable equilibrium $y$ is *asymptotically stable* if all solutions starting sufficiently close to $y$ approach it as $t \to \infty$. That is, if $\delta > 0$ can be chosen from the definition above so that $\lim_{t \to \infty} x(t) = y$.

(c) *Exponential stability.* A stable equilibrium $y$ is said to be *exponentially stable* when there is a constant $a > 0$ such that $|x(t) - y| < \exp(-at)$ for all $x_0$ near $y$ and all $t \geq 0$.

Prove that (c) implies (b), and (b) implies (a). Show that (a) does not imply (b) and (b) does not imply (c). That is, present a system having stable but not asymptotically stable equilibrium, and a system having asymptotically but not exponentially stable equilibrium.

19. ($I_{NMDA}$-model) Show that voltage-dependent activation of NMDA synaptic receptors in a passive dendritic tree with a constant concentration of glutamate is mathematically equivalent to the $I_{Na,p}$-model.

# Chapter 4

# Two-Dimensional Systems

In this chapter we introduce methods of phase plane analysis of two-dimensional systems. Most concepts will be illustrated using the $I_{\text{Na,p}}+I_{\text{K}}$-model in Fig.4.1:

$$
C\dot{V} = I - \overbrace{g_{\text{L}}(V-E_{\text{L}})}^{\text{leak } I_{\text{L}}} - \overbrace{g_{\text{Na}}\, m_{\infty}(V)\,(V-E_{\text{Na}})}^{\text{instantaneous } I_{\text{Na,p}}} - \overbrace{g_{\text{K}}\, n\,(V-E_{\text{K}})}^{I_{\text{K}}} \,, \tag{4.1}
$$

$$
\dot{n} = (n_{\infty}(V) - n)/\tau(V) \,, \tag{4.2}
$$

having leak current $I_{\text{L}}$, persistent Na$^+$ current $I_{\text{Na,p}}$ with instantaneous activation kinetic and a relatively slower persistent K$^+$ current $I_{\text{K}}$ with either high (Fig.4.1a) or low (Fig.4.1b) threshold (the two choices result in fundamentally different dynamics). The state of the $I_{\text{Na,p}}+I_{\text{K}}$-model is a two-dimensional vector $(V, n) \in \mathbb{R}^2$ on the *phase plane* $\mathbb{R}^2$. New types of equilibria, orbits, and bifurcations can exist on the phase plane that cannot exist on the phase line $\mathbb{R}$. Many interesting features of single neuron dynamics can be illustrated or explained using two-dimensional systems. Even neuronal bursting, which occurs in multidimensional systems, can be understood via bifurcation analysis of two-dimensional systems.

This model is equivalent in many respects to the well-known and widely used $I_{\text{Ca}}+I_{\text{K}}$-model proposed by Morris and Lecar (1981) to describe voltage oscillations in the barnacle giant muscle fiber.

## 4.1   Planar Vector Fields

Two-dimensional dynamical systems, also called *planar* systems, are often written in the form

$$
\begin{aligned}
\dot{x} &= f(x,y) \,, \\
\dot{y} &= g(x,y) \,,
\end{aligned}
$$

where the functions $f$ and $g$ describe the evolution of the two-dimensional state variable $(x(t), y(t))$. For any point $(x_0, y_0)$ on the phase plane, the vector $(f(x_0, y_0), g(x_0, y_0))$

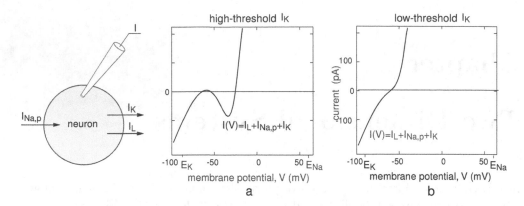

Figure 4.1: The $I_{\text{Na,p}}+I_{\text{K}}$-model (4.1, 4.2). Parameters in (a): $C = 1$, $I = 0$, $E_{\text{L}} = -80$ mV, $g_{\text{L}} = 8$, $g_{\text{Na}} = 20$, $g_{\text{K}} = 10$, $m_{\infty}(V)$ has $V_{1/2} = -20$ and $k = 15$, $n_{\infty}(V)$ has $V_{1/2} = -25$ and $k = 5$, and $\tau(V) = 1$, $E_{\text{Na}} = 60$ mV and $E_{\text{K}} = -90$ mV. Parameters in (b) as in (a) except $E_{\text{L}} = -78$ mV and $n_{\infty}(V)$ has $V_{1/2} = -45$; see section 2.3.5.

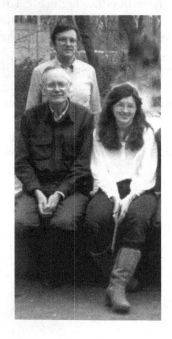

Figure 4.2: Harold Lecar (back), Richard FitzHugh (front), and Cathy Morris at NIH Biophysics Lab, summer of 1983.

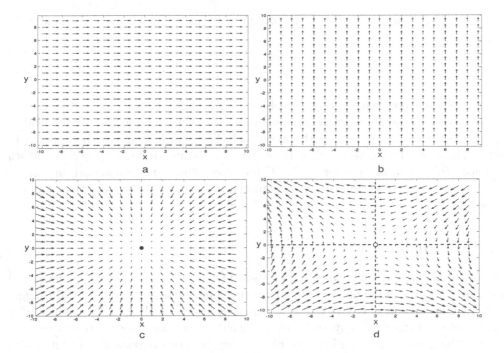

Figure 4.3: Examples of vector fields.

indicates the direction of change of the state variable. For example, negative $f(x_0, y_0)$ and positive $g(x_0, y_0)$ imply that $x(t)$ decreases and $y(t)$ increases at this particular point. Since each point on the phase plane $(x, y)$ has its own vector $(f, g)$, the system above is said to define a *vector field* on the plane, also known as a direction field or a velocity field, see Fig.4.3. Thus, the vector field defines the direction of motion; depending on where you are, it tells you *where you are going*.

Let us consider a few examples. The two-dimensional system

$$\dot{x} = 1\,,$$
$$\dot{y} = 0$$

defines a constant horizontal vector field in Fig.4.3a because each point has a horizontal vector $(1, 0)$ attached to it. (Of course, we depict only a small sample of vectors.) Similarly, the system

$$\dot{x} = 0\,,$$
$$\dot{y} = 1$$

defines a constant vertical vector field depicted in Fig.4.3b. The system

$$\dot{x} = -x\,,$$
$$\dot{y} = -y$$

defines a vector field that points to the origin $(0,0)$, as in Fig.4.3c, and the system

$$\dot{x} = -y \,, \tag{4.3}$$
$$\dot{y} = -x \tag{4.4}$$

defines a saddle vector field, as in Fig.4.3d. Vector fields provide geometrical information about the joint evolution of state variables. For example, the vector field in Fig.4.3d is directed rightward in the lower half-plane and leftward in the upper half-plane. Therefore the variable $x(t)$ increases when $y < 0$ and decreases otherwise, which obviously follows from equation (4.3). Quite often, however, geometrical analysis of vector fields can provide information about the behavior of the system that may not be obvious from the form of the functions $f$ and $g$.

### 4.1.1    Nullclines

The vector field in Fig.4.3d is directed rightward ($x$ increases) or leftward ($x$ decreases) in different regions of the phase plane. The set of points where the vector field changes its horizontal direction is called the *x-nullcline*, and it is defined by the equation $f(x, y) = 0$. Indeed, at any such point $x$ neither increases nor decreases because $\dot{x} = 0$. The $x$-nullcline partitions the phase plane into two regions where $x$ moves in opposite directions. Similarly, the *y-nullcline* is defined by the equation $g(x, y) = 0$, and it denotes the set of points where the vector field changes its vertical direction. This nullcline partitions the phase plane into two regions where $y$ either increases or decreases. The $x$- and $y$-nullclines partition the phase plane into four different regions: (a) $x$ and $y$ increase, (b) $x$ decreases and $y$ increases, (c) $x$ and $y$ decrease, and (d) $x$ increases and $y$ decreases, as we illustrate in Fig.4.4.

Each point of intersection of the nullclines is an *equilibrium point*, since $f(x, y) = g(x, y) = 0$, and hence $\dot{x} = \dot{y} = 0$. Conversely, every equilibrium of a two-dimensional system is the point of intersection of its nullclines. Because nullclines are so important, we consider two examples in detail below (the reader is urged to solve exercise 1 at the end of this chapter).

Let us determine nullclines of the system (4.3, 4.4) with the vector field shown in Fig.4.3d. From (4.3) it follows that the $x$-nullcline is the horizontal line $y = 0$, and from (4.4) it follows that the $y$-nullcline is the vertical line $x = 0$. These nullclines (dashed lines in Fig.4.3d) partition the phase plane into four quadrants, in each of which the vector field has a different direction. The intersection of the nullclines is the equilibrium $(0,0)$. Later in this chapter we will study how to determine stability of equilibria in two-dimensional systems, though in this particular case one can easily guess that the equilibrium is not stable.

As another example, let us determine the nullclines of the $I_{\mathrm{Na,p}}+I_{\mathrm{K}}$-model (4.1, 4.2). The $V$-nullcline is given by the equation

$$I - g_{\mathrm{L}}(V - E_{\mathrm{L}}) - g_{\mathrm{Na}}\, m_{\infty}(V)\,(V - E_{\mathrm{Na}}) - g_{\mathrm{K}}\, n\,(V - E_{\mathrm{K}}) = 0 \,,$$

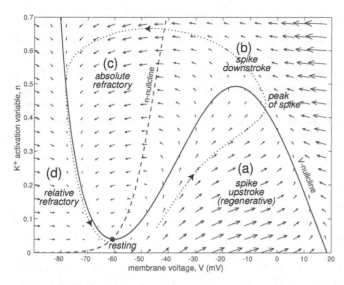

Figure 4.4: Nullclines of the $I_{\text{Na,p}}+I_{\text{K}}$-model (4.1, 4.2) with low-threshold K$^+$ current in Fig.4.1b. (The vector field is slightly distorted for the sake of clarity of illustration).

which has the solution

$$n = \frac{I - g_{\text{L}}(V - E_{\text{L}}) - g_{\text{Na}}\, m_\infty(V)\, (V - E_{\text{Na}})}{g_{\text{K}}\, (V - E_{\text{K}})} \qquad (V\text{-nullcline}) ,$$

depicted in Fig.4.4. It typically has the form of a cubic parabola. The equation

$$n_\infty(V) - n = 0$$

defines the $n$-nullcline

$$n = n_\infty(V) \qquad (n\text{-nullcline}),$$

which coincides with the K$^+$ steady-state activation function $n_\infty(V)$, though only an initial segment of this curve fits in Fig.4.4. It is easy to see how the $V$- and $n$-nullclines partition the phase plane into four regions, in each of which the vector field has a different direction:

(a) Both $V$ and $n$ increase. Both Na$^+$ and K$^+$ currents activate and lead to the upstroke of the action potential.

(b) $V$ decreases but $n$ still increases. The Na$^+$ current deactivates, but the slower K$^+$ current still activates and leads to the downstroke of the action potential.

(c) Both $V$ and $n$ decrease. Both Na$^+$ and K$^+$ currents deactivate while $V$ is small, leading to a refractory period.

(d) $V$ increases but $n$ still decreases. Partial activation of the Na$^+$ current combined with further deactivation of the residual K$^+$ current leads to a relative refractory period, then to an excitable period, and possibly to another action potential.

The intersection of the $V$- and $n$-nullclines in Fig.4.4 is an equilibrium corresponding to the resting state. The number and location of equilibria may be difficult to infer via analysis of equations (4.1, 4.2), but it is a trivial geometrical exercise once the nullclines are determined. Because nullclines are so useful and important in geometrical analysis of dynamical systems, few scientists bother to plot vector fields. Following this tradition, we will not show vector fields in the rest of the book (except for this chapter). Instead, we plot nullclines and representative trajectories, which we discuss next.

### 4.1.2   Trajectories

A vector function $(x(t), y(t))$ is a solution of the two-dimensional system

$$\dot{x} = f(x, y) ,$$
$$\dot{y} = g(x, y) ,$$

starting with an initial condition $(x(0), y(0)) = (x_0, y_0)$ when $dx(t)/dt = f(x(t), y(t))$ and $dy(t)/dt = g(x(t), y(t))$ at each $t \geq 0$. This requirement has a simple geometrical interpretation: a solution is a curve $(x(t), y(t))$ on the phase plane $\mathbb{R}^2$ which is tangent to the vector field, as we illustrate in Fig 4.5. Such a curve is often called a *trajectory* or an *orbit*.

One can think of the vector field as a stationary flow of a fluid. Then a solution is just a trajectory of a small particle dropped at a certain (initial) point and carried by the flow. To study the flow, it is useful to drop a few particles and see where they are going. Thus, to understand the geometry of a vector field, it is always useful to plot a few representative trajectories starting from various initial points, as we do in Fig.4.6. Due to the uniqueness of the solutions, the trajectories cannot cross, so they partition or foliate the phase space. This is an important step toward determining the phase portrait of a two-dimensional system.

Let us return to the $I_{\text{Na,p}} + I_{\text{K}}$-model (4.1, 4.2) with low-threshold K$^+$ current and explain two odd phenomena discussed in chapter 1: Failure to generate all-or-none action potentials (Fig.1.5b) and inability to have a fixed value of the threshold voltage.

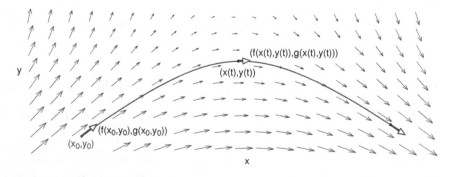

Figure 4.5: Solutions are trajectories tangent to the vector field.

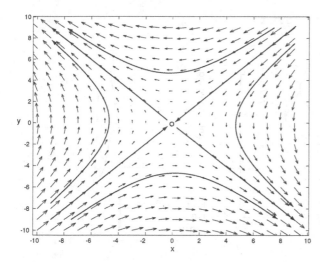

Figure 4.6: Representative trajectories of the two-dimensional system (4.3, 4.4).

Brief and strong current pulses in Fig.4.7 reset the value of the voltage variable $V$ but do not change the value of the K$^+$ activation variable $n$. Thus, each voltage trace after the pulse corresponds to a trajectory starting with different values of $V_0$ but the same value $n_0$. We see that each trajectory makes a counterclockwise excursion and returns to the resting state. However, the size of the excursion depends on the initial value of the voltage variable and can be small (subthreshold response), intermediate, or large (action potential). This phenomenon was considered theoretically by FitzHugh in the early 1960s (see bibliography) and demonstrated experimentally by Cole et al. (1970), using the squid giant axon at higher than normal temperatures.

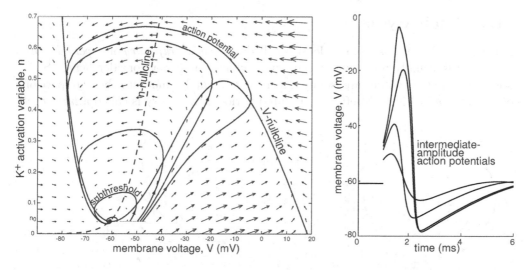

Figure 4.7: Failure to generate all-or-none action potentials in the $I_{\mathrm{Na,p}}+I_{\mathrm{K}}$-model.

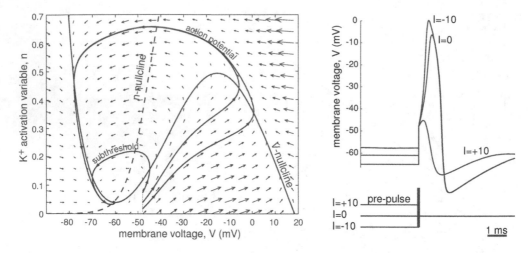

Figure 4.8: Failure to have a fixed value of threshold voltage in the $I_{Na,p}+I_K$-model.

In Fig.4.8 we apply a long pre-pulse current of various amplitudes to reset the $K^+$ activation variable $n$ to various values, and then a brief strong pulse to reset $V$ to exactly $-48$ mV. Each voltage trace after the pulse corresponds to a trajectory starting with the same $V_0 = -48$ mV, but different values of $n_0$. We see that some trajectories return immediately to the resting state, while others do so after generating a transient action potential. Therefore, $V = -48$ mV is a subthreshold value when $n_0$ is large, and a superthreshold value otherwise. In particular, the system does not have a clear-cut voltage threshold – a ubiquitous property of many neurons.

### 4.1.3   Limit Cycles

A trajectory that forms a closed loop is called a *periodic trajectory* or a *periodic orbit* (the latter is usually reserved for mappings, which we do not consider here). Sometimes periodic trajectories are isolated, as in Fig.4.9, and sometimes they are part of a continuum, as in Fig.4.13 (left). An isolated periodic trajectory is called a *limit cycle*.

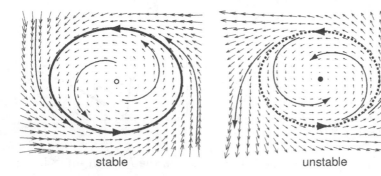

Figure 4.9: Limit cycles (periodic orbits).

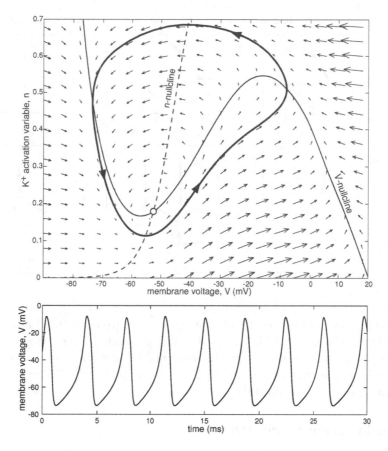

Figure 4.10: Stable limit cycle in the $I_{\text{Na,p}}+I_{\text{K}}$-model (4.1, 4.2) with low-threshold K$^+$ current and $I = 40$.

The existence of limit cycles is a major feature of two-dimensional systems that cannot exist in $\mathbb{R}^1$. If the initial point is on a limit cycle, then the solution $(x(t), y(t))$ stays on the cycle forever, and the system exhibits periodic behavior; that is,

$$x(t) = x(t + T) \qquad \text{and} \qquad y(t) = y(t + T) \qquad \text{(for all } t)$$

for some $T > 0$. The minimal $T$ for which this equality holds is called the *period* of the limit cycle. A limit cycle is said to be *asymptotically stable* if any trajectory with the initial point sufficiently near the cycle approaches the cycle as $t \to \infty$. Such asymptotically stable limit cycles are often called *limit cycle attractors*, since they "attract" all nearby trajectories. The stable limit cycle in Fig.4.9 is an attractor. The limit cycle in Fig.4.10 is also an attractor; it corresponds to the periodic (tonic) spiking of the $I_{\text{Na,p}}+I_{\text{K}}$-model (4.1, 4.2). The unstable limit cycle in Fig.4.9 is often called a *repeller*, since it repels all nearby trajectories. Notice that there is always at least one equilibrium inside any limit cycle on a plane.

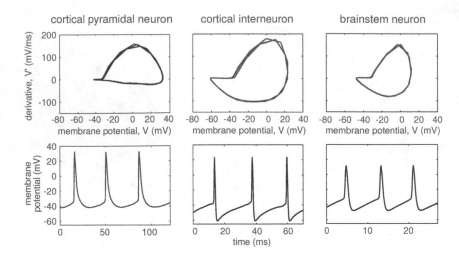

Figure 4.11: Limit cycles corresponding to tonic spiking of three types of neurons recorded in vitro.

In Fig.4.11 we depict limit cycles of three types of neurons recorded in vitro. Since we do not know the state of the internal variables, such as the magnitude of the activation and inactivation of $Na^+$ and $K^+$ currents, we plot the cycles on the $(V, V')$-plane, where $V'$ is the time derivative of $V$. The cycles look jerky because of the poor data sampling rate during each spike.

## 4.1.4    Relaxation Oscillators

Many models in science and engineering can be reduced to two-dimensional fast/slow systems of the form

$$\begin{aligned} \dot{x} &= f(x,y) \qquad \text{(fast variable)} \\ \dot{y} &= \mu g(x,y) \qquad \text{(slow variable)} , \end{aligned}$$

where the small parameter $\mu$ describes the ratio of time scales of variables $x$ and $y$. Typically, the fast variable $x$ has a cubic like nullcline that intersects the $y$-nullcline somewhere in the middle branch, as in Fig.4.12a, resulting in *relaxation oscillations*. The periodic trajectory of the system slides down along the left (stable) branch of the cubic nullcline until it reaches the left knee, A. At this moment, it quickly jumps to point B and then slowly slides up along the right (also stable) branch of the cubic nullcline. Upon reaching the right knee, C, the system jumps to the left branch and starts to slide down again, thereby completing one oscillation. Relaxation oscillations are easy to grasp conceptually, but some of their features are quite difficult to study mathematically. (We consider relaxation oscillations in detail in section 6.3.4).

Note that the jumps in Fig.4.12a are nearly horizontal – a distinctive signature of relaxation oscillations that is due to the disparately different time scales in the system.

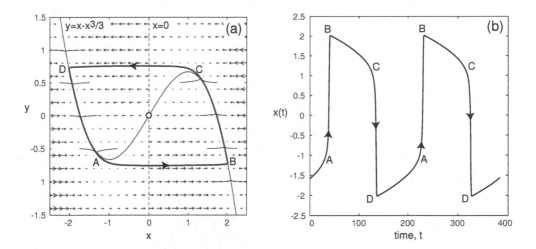

Figure 4.12: Relaxation oscillations in the van der Pol model $\dot{x} = x - x^3/3 - y$, $\dot{y} = \mu x$ with $\mu = 0.01$.

Although many neuronal models have fast and slow time scales and could be reduced to the fast/slow form above, they do not exhibit relaxation oscillations because the parameter $\mu$ is not small enough. Anybody who records from neurons would probably notice the weird square shape of "spikes" in Fig.4.12b, something that most biological neurons do not exhibit. Nevertheless, relaxation oscillations in fast/slow systems are important when we consider neuronal bursting in chapter 9; the fast variable $x$ is two-dimensional there.

## 4.2 Equilibria

An important step in the analysis of any dynamical system is to find its equilibria, that is, points where

$$
\begin{aligned}
f(x, y) &= 0 \,, \\
g(x, y) &= 0
\end{aligned}
\qquad \text{(point } (x, y) \text{ is an equilibrium).}
$$

As mentioned before, equilibria are intersections of nullclines. If the initial point $(x_0, y_0)$ is an equilibrium, then $\dot{x} = 0$ and $\dot{y} = 0$, and the trajectory stays at equilibrium; that is, $x(t) = x_0$ and $y(t) = y_0$ for all $t \geq 0$. If the initial point is near the equilibrium, then the trajectory may converge to or diverge from the equilibrium, depending on its stability.

From the electrophysiological point of view, any equilibrium of a neuronal model is the zero crossing of its steady-state I-V relation $I_\infty(V)$. For example, the $I_{\text{Na,p}} + I_{\text{K}}$-model (4.1, 4.2) with high-threshold K$^+$ current has an I-V curve with three zeroes

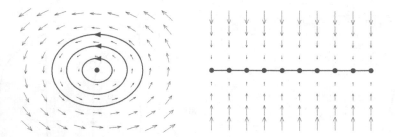

Figure 4.13: Neutrally stable equilibria. Some trajectories neither converge to nor diverge from the equilibria.

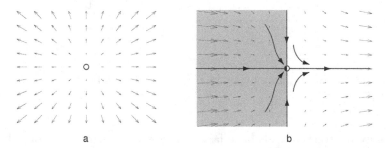

a                                                                    b

Figure 4.14: Unstable equilibria.

(Fig.4.1a); hence it has three equilibria: around $-66$ mV, $-56$ mV, and $-28$ mV. In contrast, the same model with low-threshold K$^+$ current has a monotonic I-V curve with only one zero (Fig.4.1b); hence it has a unique equilibrium, which is around $-61$ mV.

## 4.2.1    Stability

In chapter 3, exercise 18, we provide rigorous definitions of stability of equilibria in one-dimensional systems. The same definitions apply to higher-dimensional systems. Briefly, an equilibrium is *stable* if any trajectory starting sufficiently close to the equilibrium remains near it for all $t \geq 0$. If, in addition, all such trajectories converge to the equilibrium as $t \to \infty$, the equilibrium is *asymptotically stable*, as in Fig.4.3c. When the convergence rate is exponential or faster, then the equilibrium is said to be *exponentially stable*. Note that stability does not imply asymptotic stability. For example, all equilibria in Fig.4.13 are stable but not asymptotically stable. They are often referred to as *neutrally stable*.

An equilibrium is called *unstable*, if it is not stable. Obviously, if all nearby trajectories diverge from the equilibrium, as in Fig.4.14a, then it is unstable. This, however, is an exceptional case. For instability it suffices to have at least one trajectory that diverges from the equilibrium no matter how close the initial condition is to the equilibrium, as in Fig.4.14b. Indeed, any trajectory starting in the shaded area (attraction domain) converges to the equilibrium, but any trajectory starting in the white area diverges from it, regardless of how close the initial point is to the equilibrium.

In contrast to the one-dimensional case, the stability of a two-dimensional equilibrium cannot be inferred from the slope of the steady-state I-V curve. For example, the equilibrium around $-28$ mV in Fig.4.1a is unstable even though the I-V curve has positive slope.

To determine the stability of an equilibrium, we need to look at the behavior of the two-dimensional vector field in a small neighborhood of the equilibrium. Quite often visual inspection of the vector field does not give conclusive information about stability. For example, is the equilibrium in Fig.4.4 stable? What about the equilibrium in Fig.4.10? The vector fields in the neighborhoods of the two equilibria exhibit subtle differences that are difficult to spot without the help of analytical tools, which we discuss next.

### 4.2.2 Local Linear Analysis

Below we remind the reader of some basic concepts of linear algebra, assuming that he or she has some familiarity with matrices, eigenvectors, and eigenvalues. Consider a two-dimensional dynamical system

$$\dot{x} = f(x, y) \tag{4.5}$$
$$\dot{y} = g(x, y) \tag{4.6}$$

having an equilibrium point $(x_0, y_0)$. The nonlinear functions $f$ and $g$ can be linearized near the equilibrium; that is, written in the form

$$f(x, y) = a(x - x_0) + b(y - y_0) + \text{higher-order terms},$$
$$g(x, y) = c(x - x_0) + d(y - y_0) + \text{higher-order terms},$$

where higher-order terms include $(x - x_0)^2$, $(x - x_0)(y - y_0)$, $(x - x_0)^3$, and so on, and

$$a = \frac{\partial f}{\partial x}(x_0, y_0), \qquad b = \frac{\partial f}{\partial y}(x_0, y_0),$$
$$c = \frac{\partial g}{\partial x}(x_0, y_0), \qquad d = \frac{\partial g}{\partial y}(x_0, y_0)$$

are the partial derivatives of $f$ and $g$ with respect to the state variables $x$ and $y$ evaluated at the equilibrium $(x_0, y_0)$. (First, evaluate the derivatives, then substitute $x = x_0$ and $y = y_0$; if you do in the opposite order, you will always get zero). Many questions regarding the stability of the equilibrium can be answered by considering the corresponding linear system

$$\dot{u} = au + bw, \tag{4.7}$$
$$\dot{w} = cu + dw, \tag{4.8}$$

where $u = x - x_0$ and $w = y - y_0$ are the deviations from the equilibrium, and the higher-order terms $u^2$, $uw$, $w^3$, and so on, are neglected. We can write this system in the vector form

$$\begin{pmatrix} \dot{u} \\ \dot{w} \end{pmatrix} = \begin{pmatrix} a & b \\ c & d \end{pmatrix} \begin{pmatrix} u \\ w \end{pmatrix} .$$

The linearization matrix

$$L = \begin{pmatrix} a & b \\ c & d \end{pmatrix}$$

is called the *Jacobian matrix* of the system (4.5, 4.6) at the equilibrium $(x_0, y_0)$. For example, the Jacobian matrix of the system (4.3, 4.4) at the origin is

$$\begin{pmatrix} 0 & -1 \\ -1 & 0 \end{pmatrix} . \tag{4.9}$$

It is important to remember that Jacobian matrices are defined for equilibria, and that a nonlinear system can have many equilibria, and hence many different Jacobian matrices.

### 4.2.3    Eigenvalues and Eigenvectors

A nonzero vector $v \in \mathbb{R}^2$ is said to be an *eigenvector* of the matrix $L$ corresponding to the *eigenvalue* $\lambda$ if

$$Lv = \lambda v \qquad \text{(matrix notation)} .$$

For example, the matrix (4.9) has two eigenvectors,

$$v_1 = \begin{pmatrix} 1 \\ 1 \end{pmatrix} \qquad \text{and} \qquad v_2 = \begin{pmatrix} 1 \\ -1 \end{pmatrix},$$

corresponding to the eigenvalues $\lambda_1 = -1$ and $\lambda_2 = 1$, respectively. Any textbook on linear algebra explains how to find eigenvectors and eigenvalues of an arbitrary matrix. It is important for the reader to get comfortable with these notions, since they are used extensively in the rest of the book.

Eigenvalues play an important role in the analysis of stability of equilibria. To find the eigenvalues of a $2 \times 2$-matrix $L$, one solves the *characteristic equation*

$$\det \begin{pmatrix} a - \lambda & b \\ c & d - \lambda \end{pmatrix} = 0 .$$

This equation can be written in the polynomial form $(a - \lambda)(d - \lambda) - bc = 0$ or

$$\lambda^2 - \tau\lambda + \Delta = 0 ,$$

where

$$\tau = \operatorname{tr} L = a + d \qquad \text{and} \qquad \Delta = \det L = ad - bc$$

are the *trace* and the *determinant* of the matrix $L$, respectively. Such a quadratic polynomial has two solutions of the form

$$\lambda_1 = \frac{\tau + \sqrt{\tau^2 - 4\Delta}}{2} \quad \text{and} \quad \lambda_2 = \frac{\tau - \sqrt{\tau^2 - 4\Delta}}{2} , \tag{4.10}$$

and they are either real (when $\tau^2 - 4\Delta \geq 0$) or complex-conjugate (when $\tau^2 - 4\Delta < 0$). What can you say about the case $\tau^2 = 4\Delta$?

In general, $2 \times 2$ matrices have two eigenvalues with distinct (independent) eigenvectors. In this case a general solution of the linear system has the form

$$\left( \begin{array}{c} u(t) \\ w(t) \end{array} \right) = c_1 e^{\lambda_1 t} v_1 + c_2 e^{\lambda_2 t} v_2 ,$$

where $c_1$ and $c_2$ are constants that depend on the initial condition. This formula is valid for real and complex-conjugate eigenvalues. When both eigenvalues are negative (or have negative real parts), $u(t) \to 0$ and $w(t) \to 0$, meaning $x(t) \to x_0$ and $y(t) \to y_0$, so that the equilibrium $(x_0, y_0)$ is exponentially (and hence asymptotically) stable. It is unstable when at least one eigenvalue is positive or has a positive real part. We denote stable equilibria by filled circles • and unstable equilibria by open circles ∘ throughout the book.

### 4.2.4 Local Equivalence

An equilibrium whose Jacobian matrix does not have zero eigenvalues or eigenvalues with zero real parts is called *hyperbolic*. Such an equilibrium can be stable or unstable. The Hartman-Grobman theorem states that the vector field, and hence the dynamics of a nonlinear system, such as (4.5, 4.6), near such a hyperbolic equilibrium is topologically equivalent to that of its linearization (4.7, 4.8). That is, the higher-order terms that are neglected when (4.5, 4.6) is replaced by (4.7, 4.8) do not play any qualitative role. Thus, understanding and classifying the geometry of vector fields of linear systems provides an exhaustive description of all possible behaviors of nonlinear systems near hyperbolic equilibria.

A zero eigenvalue (or eigenvalues with zero real parts) arises when the equilibrium undergoes a bifurcation, as in Fig.4.14b; such equilibria are called non-hyperbolic. Linear analysis cannot answer the question of stability of a nonlinear system in this case, since small nonlinear (high-order) terms play a crucial role here. We denote equilibria undergoing a bifurcation by half-filled circles, ◐.

### 4.2.5 Classification of Equilibria

Besides defining the stability of an equilibrium, the eigenvalues also define the geometry of the vector field near the equilibrium, as we illustrate in Fig.4.15, and as the reader is asked to prove in exercise 4. (The proof is a straightforward consequence of (4.10).) There are three major types of equilibria.

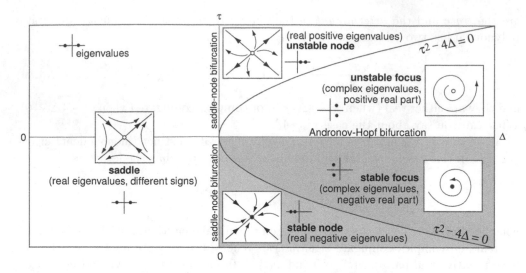

Figure 4.15: Classification of equilibria according to the trace ($\tau$) and the determinant ($\Delta$) of the Jacobian matrix $L$. The shaded region corresponds to stable equilibria.

**Node (Fig.4.16).** The eigenvalues are real and of the same sign. The node is stable when the eigenvalues are negative, and unstable when they are positive. The trajectories tend to converge to or diverge from the node along the eigenvector corresponding to the eigenvalue having the smallest absolute value.

**Saddle (Fig.4.17).** The eigenvalues are real and of opposite signs. Saddles are always unstable, since one of the eigenvalues is always positive. Most trajectories approach the saddle equilibrium along the eigenvector corresponding to the negative (stable) eigenvalue and then diverge from it along the eigenvector corresponding to the positive (unstable) eigenvalue.

**Focus (Fig.4.18).** The eigenvalues are complex-conjugate. Foci are stable when the eigenvalues have negative real parts, and unstable when the eigenvalues have positive real parts. The imaginary part of the eigenvalues determines the frequency of rotation of trajectories around the focus equilibrium.

When the system undergoes a saddle-node bifurcation, one of the eigenvalues becomes zero and a mixed type of equilibrium occurs – saddle-node equilibrium, illustrated in Fig.4.14b. There could be other types of mixed equilibria, such as saddle-focus or focus-node, and so on, in dynamical systems having dimension 3 and higher.

Depending upon the value of the injected current $I$, the $I_{Na,p}+I_K$-model (4.1, 4.2) with a low-threshold K$^+$ current has a stable focus (Fig.4.8) or an unstable focus (Fig.4.10) surrounded by a stable limit cycle. In Fig.4.19 we depict the vector field and nullclines of the same model with a high-threshold K$^+$ current. As one expects from the shape of the steady-state I-V curve in Fig.4.1a, the model has three equilibria:

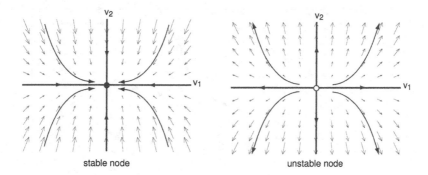

Figure 4.16: Node equilibrium occurs when both eigenvalues are real and have the same sign, for example, $\lambda_1 = -1$ and $\lambda_2 = -3$ (stable) or $\lambda_1 = +1$ and $\lambda_2 = +3$ (unstable). Most trajectories converge to or diverge from the node along the eigenvector $v_1$ corresponding to the eigenvalue having the smallest absolute value.

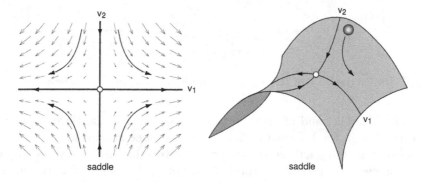

Figure 4.17: Saddle equilibrium occurs when two real eigenvalues have opposite signs, such as $\lambda_1 = +1$ and $\lambda_2 = -1$. Most trajectories diverge from the equilibrium along the eigenvector corresponding to the positive eigenvalue (in this case, $v_1$).

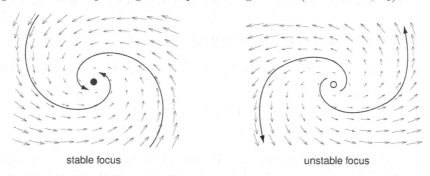

Figure 4.18: Focus equilibrium occurs when the eigenvalues are complex-conjugate, for instance, $\lambda = -3 \pm i$ (stable) or $\lambda = +3 \pm i$ (unstable). The imaginary part (here, 1) determines the frequency of rotation around the focus.

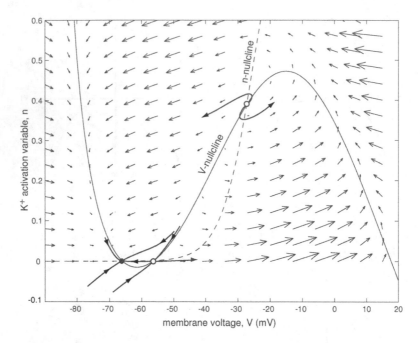

Figure 4.19: Phase portrait of the $I_{\mathrm{Na,p}}+I_{\mathrm{K}}$-model having high-threshold $\mathrm{K}^+$ current.

a stable node, a saddle, and an unstable focus. Notice that the third equilibrium is unstable even though the I-V relation has a positive slope around it.

Also notice that the $y$-axis starts at the negative value -0.1. However, the gating variable $n$ represents the proportion (probability) of the $\mathrm{K}^+$ channels in the open state; hence a value less than zero has no physical meaning. So while we can happily calculate the nullclines for the negative $n$, and even start the trajectory with the initial condition $n < 0$, we cannot interpret the result. (As an exercise, prove that if all gating variables of a model are initially in the range $[0,1]$, then they stay in the range for all $t \geq 0$.)

## 4.2.6    Example: FitzHugh-Nagumo Model

The FitzHugh-Nagumo model (FitzHugh 1961; Nagumo et al. 1962; Izhikevich and FitzHugh 2006)

$$\dot{V} = V(a - V)(V - 1) - w + I \,, \qquad (4.11)$$
$$\dot{w} = bV - cw \,, \qquad\qquad\qquad (4.12)$$

imitates generation of action potentials by Hodgkin-Huxley-type models having cubic (N-shaped) nullclines, as in Fig.4.4. Here $V$ mimics the membrane voltage and the "recovery" variable $w$ mimics activation of an outward current. Parameter $I$ mimics the injected current, and for the sake of simplicity we set $I = 0$ in our analysis below. Parameter $a$ describes the shape of the cubic parabola $V(a - V)(V - 1)$, and parameters

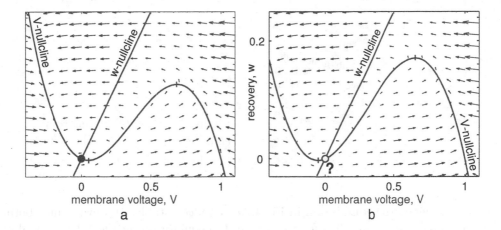

Figure 4.20: Nullclines in the FitzHugh-Nagumo model (4.11, 4.12). Parameters: $I = 0, b = 0.01, c = 0.02, a = 0.1$ (left) and $a = -0.1$ (right).

$b > 0$ and $c \geq 0$ describe the kinetics of the recovery variable $w$. When $b$ and $c$ are small, the model may exhibit relaxation oscillations.

The nullclines of the FitzHugh-Nagumo model have the cubic and linear form

$$w = V(a - V)(V - 1) + I \qquad (V\text{-nullcline}),$$
$$w = b/c\,V \qquad\qquad\qquad (w\text{-nullcline}),$$

and they can intersect in one, two, or three points, resulting in one, two, or three equilibria, all of which may be unstable. Below, we consider the simple case $I = 0$, so that the origin, $(0, 0)$, is an equilibrium. Indeed, the nullclines of the model, depicted in Fig.4.20, always intersect at $(0, 0)$ in this case. The intersection may occur on the left (Fig.4.20a) or middle (Fig.4.20b) branch of the cubic $V$-nullcline, depending on the sign of the parameter $a$. Let us determine how the stability of the equilibrium $(0, 0)$ depends on the parameters $a$, $b$, and $c$.

There is a common dogma that the equilibrium in Fig.4.20a corresponding to $a > 0$ is always stable, the equilibrium in Fig.4.20b corresponding to $a < 0$ is always unstable, and the loss of stability occurs "exactly" at $a = 0$, that is, at the bottom of the left knee. Let us check that this is not necessarily true, at least when $c \neq 0$. The Jacobian matrix of the FitzHugh-Nagumo model (4.11,4.12) at the equilibrium $(0, 0)$ has the form

$$L = \begin{pmatrix} -a & -1 \\ b & -c \end{pmatrix}.$$

It is easy to check that

$$\tau = \operatorname{tr} L = -a - c \qquad \text{and} \qquad \Delta = \det L = ac + b\,.$$

Using Fig.4.15, we conclude that the equilibrium is stable when $\operatorname{tr} L < 0$ and $\det L > 0$, which corresponds to the shaded region in Fig.4.21. Both conditions are always satisfied

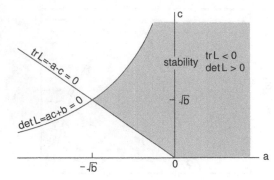

Figure 4.21: Stability diagram of the equilibrium $(0,0)$ in the FitzHugh-Nagumo model (4.11,4.12).

when $a > 0$; hence the equilibrium in Fig.4.20a is indeed stable. However, since both conditions may also be satisfied for negative $a$, the equilibrium in Fig.4.20b may also be stable. Thus, the equilibrium loses stability not at the left knee, but slightly to the right of it, so that a part of the "unstable branch" of the cubic nullcline is actually stable. The part is small when $b$ and $c$ are small, i.e., when (4.11,4.12) is in a relaxation regime.

## 4.3   Phase Portraits

An important step in geometrical analysis of dynamical systems is sketching their phase portraits. The *phase portrait* of a two-dimensional system is a partitioning of the phase plane into orbits or trajectories. Instead of depicting all possible trajectories, it usually suffices to depict some representative trajectories. The phase portrait contains all important information about qualitative behavior of the dynamical system, such as relative location and stability of equilibria, their attraction domains, separatrices, limit cycles, and other special trajectories that are discussed in this section.

### 4.3.1   Bistability and Attraction Domains

Nonlinear two-dimensional systems can have many coexisting attractors. For example, the FitzHugh-Nagumo model (4.11,4.12) with nullclines depicted in Fig.4.22 has two stable equilibria separated by an unstable equilibrium. Such a system is called *bistable* (*multi-stable* when there are more than two attractors). Depending on the initial conditions, the trajectory may approach the left or the right equilibrium. The shaded area denotes the *attraction domain* of the right equilibrium; that is, the set of all initial conditions that lead to this equilibrium. Since there are only two attractors, the complementary white area denotes the attraction domain of the other equilibrium. The domains are separated not by equilibria, as in the one-dimensional case, but by special trajectories called separatrices, which we discuss in section 4.3.2.

Many neural models are bistable or can be made bistable when the parameters have appropriate values. Often bistability results from the coexistence of an equilibrium

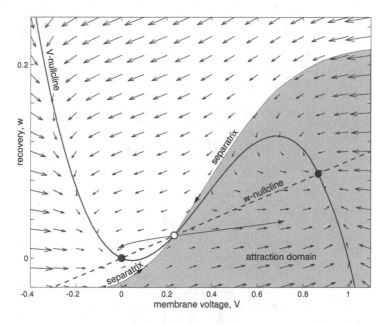

Figure 4.22: Bistability of two equilibrium attractors (black circles) in the FitzHugh-Nagumo model (4.11,4.12). The shaded area – attraction domain of the right equilibrium. Parameters: $I = 0$, $b = 0.01$, $a = c = 0.1$.

attractor corresponding to the resting state and a limit cycle attractor corresponding to the repetitive firing state. Figure 4.23 depicts one of many possible cases. Here we use the $I_{Na,p}+I_K$-model with a high-threshold fast K$^+$ current. The resting state exists due to the balance of partially activated Na$^+$ and leak currents. The repetitive spiking state persists because the K$^+$ current deactivates too fast and cannot bring the membrane potential into the subthreshold voltage range. If the initial state is in the shaded area, which is the attraction domain of the limit cycle attractor, the trajectory approaches the limit cycle attractor and the neuron fires an infinite train of action potentials.

## 4.3.2 Stable/Unstable Manifolds

In contrast with one-dimensional systems, in two-dimensional systems unstable equilibria do not necessarily separate attraction domains. Nevertheless, they play an important role in defining the boundary of attraction domains, as in Fig.4.22 and Fig.4.23. In both cases the attraction domains are separated by a pair of trajectories, called *separatrices*, which converge to the saddle equilibrium. Such trajectories form the *stable manifold* of a saddle point. Locally, the manifold is parallel to the eigenvector corresponding to the negative (stable) eigenvalue; see Fig.4.24. Similarly, the *unstable manifold* of a saddle is formed by the two trajectories that originate exactly from the

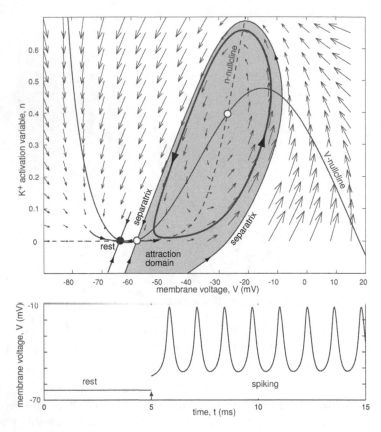

Figure 4.23: Bistability of rest and spiking states in the $I_{Na,p}+I_K$-model (4.1, 4.2) with high-threshold fast ($\tau(V) = 0.152$) K$^+$ current and $I = 3$. A brief strong pulse of current (arrow at $t = 5$ ms) brings the state vector of the system into the attraction domain of the stable limit cycle.

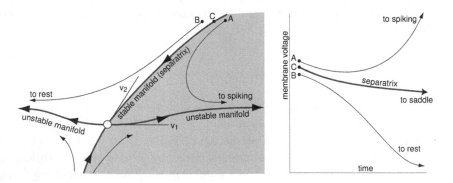

Figure 4.24: Stable and unstable manifolds to a saddle. The eigenvectors $v_1$ and $v_2$ correspond to positive and negative eigenvalues, respectively.

saddle (or approach the saddle if the time is reversed). Locally, the unstable manifold is parallel to the eigenvector corresponding to the positive (unstable) eigenvalue.

The stable manifold of the saddle in Fig.4.23 plays the role of a threshold, since it separates resting and spiking states. We illustrate this concept in Fig.4.24: if the initial state of the system, denoted as A, is in the shaded area, the trajectory will converge to the spiking attractor (right) no matter how close the initial condition is to the stable manifold. In contrast, if the initial condition, denoted as B, is in the white area, the trajectory will converge to the resting attractor (left). If the initial condition is precisely on the stable manifold (point C), the trajectory converges neither to resting nor to spiking, but to the saddle equilibrium. Of course, this case is highly unstable, and small perturbations will certainly push the trajectory to one side or the other. The important message in Fig.4.24 is that a threshold is not a point, i.e., a single voltage value, but a trajectory on the phase plane. (Find an exceptional case where the threshold looks like a single voltage value. Hint: See Fig.4.17.)

### 4.3.3   Homoclinic/Heteroclinic Trajectories

Figure 4.24 shows that trajectories forming the unstable manifold originate from the saddle. Where do they go? Similarly, the trajectories forming the stable manifold terminate at the saddle. Where do they come from? We say that a trajectory is *heteroclinic* if it originates at one equilibrium and terminates at another equilibrium, as in Fig.4.25. A trajectory is *homoclinic* if it originates and terminates at the same equilibrium. These types of trajectories play an important role in geometrical analysis of dynamical systems.

Heteroclinic trajectories connect unstable and stable equilibria, as in Fig.4.26, and they are ubiquitous in dynamical systems having two or more equilibrium points. In fact, there are infinitely many heteroclinic trajectories in Fig.4.26, since all trajectories inside the bold loop originate at the unstable focus and terminate at the stable node. (Find the exceptional trajectory that ends elsewhere.)

In contrast, homoclinic trajectories are rare. First, a homoclinic trajectory diverges from an equilibrium, so the equilibrium must be unstable. Next, the trajectory makes a loop and returns to the same equilibrium, as in Fig.4.27. It needs to hit the unstable equilibrium precisely, since a small error would make it deviate from the unstable equilibrium. Though uncommon, homoclinic trajectories indicate that the system undergoes a bifurcation – appearance or disappearance of a limit cycle. The homoclinic trajectory in Fig.4.27 indicates that the limit cycle in Fig.4.23 is about to (dis)appear

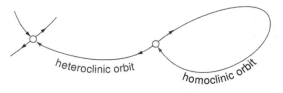

Figure 4.25: A heteroclinic orbit starts and ends at different equilibria. A homoclinic orbit starts and ends at the same equilibrium.

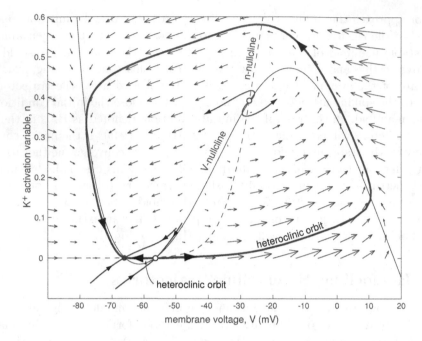

Figure 4.26: Two heteroclinic orbits (bold curves connecting stable and unstable equilibria) in the $I_{\mathrm{Na,p}}+I_{\mathrm{K}}$-model with high-threshold $\mathrm{K}^+$ current.

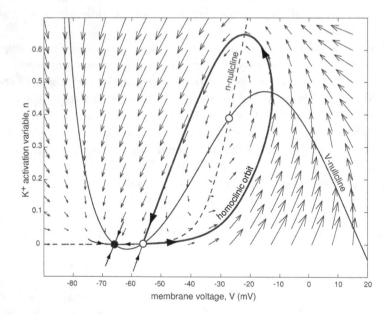

Figure 4.27: Homoclinic orbit (bold) in the $I_{\mathrm{Na,p}}+I_{\mathrm{K}}$-model with high-threshold fast $(\tau(V) = 0.152)$ $\mathrm{K}^+$ current.

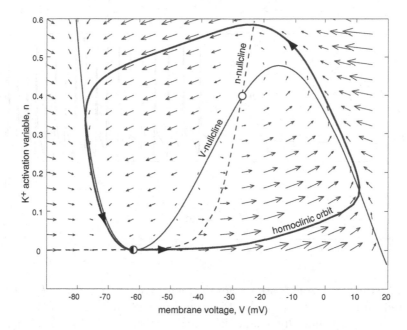

Figure 4.28: Homoclinic orbit (bold) to saddle-node equilibrium in the $I_{Na,p}+I_K$-model with high-threshold K$^+$ current and $I = 4.51$.

via *saddle homoclinic orbit* bifurcation. The homoclinic trajectory in Fig.4.28 indicates that a limit cycle is about to (dis)appear via *saddle-node on invariant circle* bifurcation. We study these bifurcations in detail in chapter 6.

### 4.3.4  Saddle-Node Bifurcation

In Fig.4.29 we simulate the injection of a ramp current $I$ into the $I_{Na,p}+I_K$-model having high-threshold K$^+$ current. Our goal is to understand the transition from the resting state to repetitive spiking. When $I$ is small, the phase portrait of the model is similar to the one depicted in Fig.4.26 for $I = 0$. There are two equilibria in the low-voltage range – a stable node corresponding to the resting state and a saddle. The equilibria are the intersections of the cubic $V$-nullcline and the $n$-nullcline. Increasing the parameter $I$ changes the shape of the cubic nullcline and shifts it upward, but does not change the $n$-nullcline. As a result, the distance between the equilibria decreases, until they coalesce as in Fig.4.28 so that the nullclines touch each other only in the low-voltage range. Further increase of $I$ results in the disappearance of the saddle and node equilibrium, and hence in the disappearance of the resting state. The new phase portrait is depicted in Fig.4.30; it has only a limit cycle attractor corresponding to repetitive firing. We see that increasing $I$ past the value $I = 4.51$ results in transition from resting to periodic spiking dynamics. What kind of bifurcation occurs when $I = 4.51$?

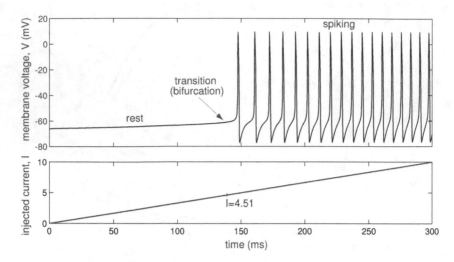

Figure 4.29: Transition from resting state to repetitive spiking in the $I_{\text{Na,p}}+I_{\text{K}}$-model with injected ramp current $I$ (see also Fig.4.26, Fig.4.28, and Fig.4.30). Note that the frequency of spiking is initially small, then increases as the amplitude of the injected current increases.

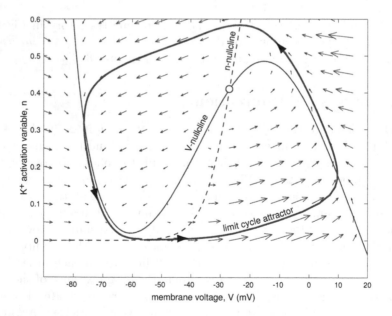

Figure 4.30: Limit cycle attractor (bold) in the $I_{\text{Na,p}}+I_{\text{K}}$-model when $I = 10$ (compare with Fig.4.26 and 4.28).

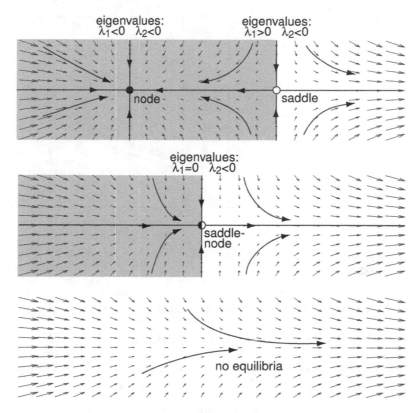

Figure 4.31: Saddle-node bifurcation: The saddle and node equilibria approach each other, coalesce, and annihilate each other (shaded area is the basin of attraction of the stable node).

Those readers who did not skip section 3.3.3 in chapter 3 will immediately recognize the saddle-node bifurcation, whose major stages are summarized in Fig.4.31. As a bifurcation parameter changes, the saddle and the node equilibrium approach each other, coalesce, and then annihilate each other so there are no equilibria left. When they coalesce, the joint equilibrium is neither a saddle nor a node, but a *saddle-node*. Its major feature is that it has precisely one zero eigenvalue, and it is stable on one side of the neighborhood and unstable on the other side. In chapter 6 we will provide an exact definition of a saddle-node bifurcation in a multi-dimensional system, and will show that there are two important subtypes of this bifurcation, resulting in slightly different neurocomputational properties.

It is a relatively simple exercise to determine bifurcation diagrams for saddle-node bifurcations in neuronal models. For this, we just need to determine all equilibria of the model and how they depend on the injected current $I$. Any equilibrium of the

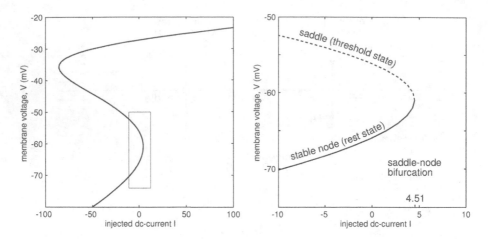

Figure 4.32: Saddle-node bifurcation diagram of the $I_{\mathrm{Na,p}}+I_{\mathrm{K}}$-model. The curve is given by the equation (4.13).

$I_{\mathrm{Na,p}}+I_{\mathrm{K}}$-model satisfies the one-dimensional equation

$$0 = I - g_{\mathrm{L}}(V-E_{\mathrm{L}}) - g_{\mathrm{Na}}\, m_{\infty}(V)\,(V-E_{\mathrm{Na}}) - g_{\mathrm{K}}\, n_{\infty}(V)\,(V-E_{\mathrm{K}})\ ,$$

where $n = n_{\infty}(V)$. Instead of solving this equation for $V$, we use $V$ as a free parameter and solve it for $I$,

$$I = \overbrace{g_{\mathrm{L}}(V-E_{\mathrm{L}}) + g_{\mathrm{Na}}\, m_{\infty}(V)\,(V-E_{\mathrm{Na}}) + g_{\mathrm{K}}\, n_{\infty}(V)\,(V-E_{\mathrm{K}})}^{\text{steady-state } I_{\infty}(V)}\ , \qquad (4.13)$$

and then depict the solution as a curve in the $(I, V)$ plane in Fig.4.32. In the magnification (Fig.4.32, right) one can clearly see how two branches of equilibria approach and annihilate each other as $I$ approaches the bifurcation value 4.51. (Is there any other saddle-node bifurcation in the figure?)

### 4.3.5   Andronov-Hopf Bifurcation

In Fig.4.33 we repeat the current ramp experiment, using the $I_{\mathrm{Na,p}}+I_{\mathrm{K}}$-model with a low-threshold K$^{+}$ current. The phase portrait of such a model is simple – it has a unique equilibrium, as we illustrate in Fig.4.34. When $I$ is small, the equilibrium is a stable focus corresponding to the resting state. When $I$ increases past $I = 12$, the focus loses stability and gives birth to a small-amplitude limit cycle attractor. The amplitude of the limit cycle grows as $I$ increases. We see that increasing $I$ beyond $I = 12$ results in the transition from resting to spiking behavior. What kind of bifurcation occurs there?

Recall that stable foci have a pair of complex-conjugate eigenvalues with negative real part. When $I$ increases, the real part of the eigenvalues also increases until it

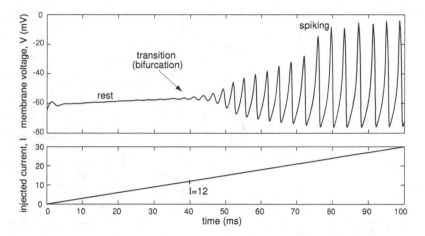

Figure 4.33: Transition from resting state to repetitive spiking in the $I_{Na,p}+I_K$-model with ramp injected current $I$; see also Fig.4.34 (small-amplitude noise is added to the model to mask the slow passage effect). Note that the frequency of spiking is relatively constant for a wide range of injected current.

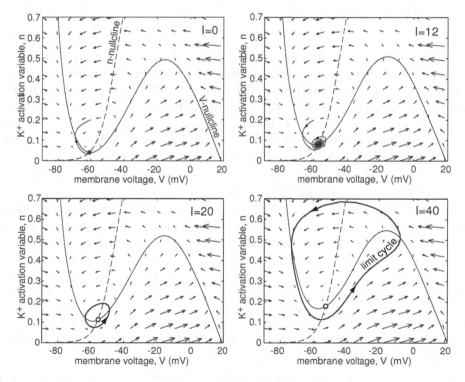

Figure 4.34: Supercritical Andronov-Hopf bifurcation in the $I_{Na,p}+I_K$-model (4.1, 4.2) with low-threshold K$^+$ current when $I = 12$ (see also Fig.4.33).

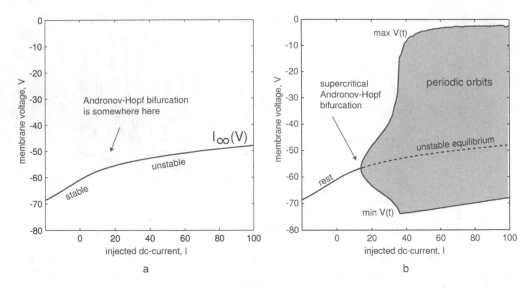

Figure 4.35: Andronov-Hopf bifurcation diagram in the $I_{Na,p}+I_K$-model with low-threshold $K^+$ current. a. Equilibria of the model (solution of (4.13)). b. Equilibria and limit cycles of the model.

becomes zero (at $I = 12$) and then positive (when $I > 12$), meaning that the focus is no longer stable. The transition from stable to unstable focus described above is called the *Andronov-Hopf* bifurcation. It occurs when the eigenvalues become purely imaginary, as happens when $I = 12$. We will study Andronov-Hopf bifurcations in detail in chapter 6, where we will show that they can be *supercritical* or *subcritical*. The former correspond to birth of a small-amplitude limit cycle attractor, as in Fig.4.34. The latter correspond to the death of an unstable limit cycle.

In Fig.4.35a we plot the solution of (4.13) as an attempt to determine the bifurcation diagram for the Andronov-Hopf bifurcation in the $I_{Na,p}+I_K$-model. However, all we can see is that the equilibrium persists as $I$ increases, but there is no information on its stability or on the existence of a limit cycle attractor. To study the limit cycle attractor, we need to simulate the model with various values of parameter $I$. For each $I$, we disregard the transient period and plot min $V(t)$ and max $V(t)$ on the $(I, V)$-plane, as in Fig.4.35b. When $I$ is small, the solutions converge to the stable equilibrium, and both min $V(t)$ and max $V(t)$ are equal to the resting voltage. When $I$ increases past $I = 12$, the min $V(t)$ and max $V(t)$ values start to diverge, meaning that there is a limit cycle attractor whose amplitude increases as $I$ does. This method is appropriate for analysis of supercritical Andronov-Hopf bifurcations, but it fails for subcritical Andronov-Hopf bifurcations. (Why?)

Figure 4.36 depicts an interesting phenomenon observed in many biological neurons, *excitation block*. Spiking activity of the layer 5 pyramidal neuron of rat's visual cortex is blocked by strong excitation (i.e., injection of strong depolarizing current). The

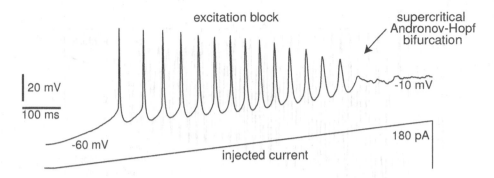

Figure 4.36: Excitation block in layer 5 pyramidal neuron of rat's visual cortex as the amplitude of the injected current ramps up.

geometry of this phenomenon is illustrated in Fig.4.37 (bottom). As the magnitude of the injected current increases, the unstable equilibrium, which is the intersection point of the nullclines, moves to the right branch of the cubic $V$-nullcline and becomes stable. The limit cycle shrinks and the spiking activity disappears, typically but not necessarily via the supercritical Andronov-Hopf bifurcation. Thus, the $I_{Na,p}+I_K$-model with low-threshold K$^+$ current can exhibit two such bifurcations in response to ramping up of the injected current, one leading to the appearance of periodic spiking activity (Fig.4.34), and then one leading to its disappearance (Fig.4.37).

Supercritical and subcritical Andronov-Hopf bifurcations in neurons result in slightly different neurocomputational properties. In contrast, the saddle-node and Andronov-Hopf bifurcations result in *dramatically* different neurocomputational properties. In particular, neurons near a saddle-node bifurcation act as *integrators* – they prefer high-frequency input. The higher the frequency of the input, the sooner they fire. In contrast, neural systems near Andronov-Hopf bifurcations have damped oscillatory potentials and act as *resonators* – they prefer oscillatory input with the same frequency as that of damped oscillations. Increasing the frequency may delay or even terminate their response. We discuss this and other neurocomputational properties in chapter 7.

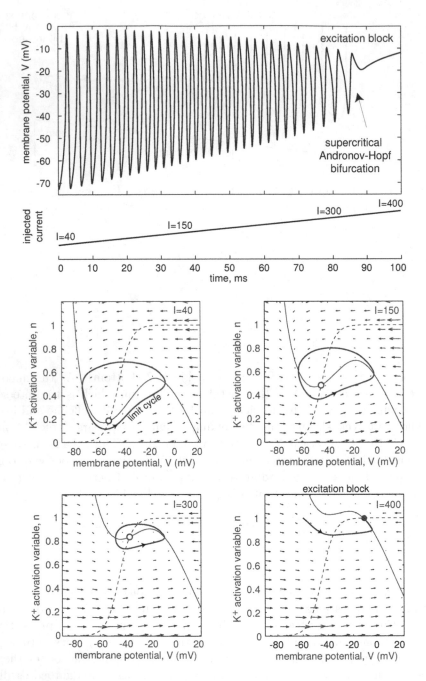

Figure 4.37: Excitation block in the $I_{\text{Na,p}}+I_{\text{K}}$-model. As the magnitude of the injected current $I$ ramps up, the spiking stops.

# Review of Important Concepts

- A two-dimensional system of differential equations

$$
\begin{aligned}
\dot{x} &= f(x, y) \\
\dot{y} &= g(x, y) \,,
\end{aligned}
$$

  describes joint evolution of state variables $x$ and $y$, which often are the membrane voltage and a "recovery" variable.

- Solutions of the system are trajectories on the phase plane $\mathbb{R}^2$ that are tangent to the vector field $(f, g)$.

- The sets given by the equations $f(x, y) = 0$ and $g(x, y) = 0$ are the $x$- and $y$-nullclines, respectively, where trajectories change their $x$ and $y$ directions.

- Intersections of the nullclines are equilibria of the system.

- Periodic dynamics correspond to closed loop trajectories.

- Some special trajectories (e.g., separatrices) define thresholds and separate attraction domains.

- An equilibrium or a periodic trajectory is stable if all nearby trajectories are attracted to it.

- To determine the stability of an equilibrium, one needs to consider the Jacobian matrix of partial derivatives

$$
L = \begin{pmatrix} f_x & f_y \\ g_x & g_y \end{pmatrix} \,.
$$

- The equilibrium is stable when both eigenvalues of $L$ are negative or have negative real parts.

- The equilibrium is a saddle, a node, or a focus when $L$ has real eigenvalues of opposite signs, of the same signs, or complex-conjugate eigenvalues, respectively.

- When the equilibrium undergoes a saddle-node bifurcation, one of the eigenvalues becomes zero.

- When the equilibrium undergoes an Andronov-Hopf bifurcation (birth or death of a small periodic trajectory), the complex-conjugate eigenvalues become purely imaginary.

- The saddle-node and Andronov-Hopf bifurcations are ubiquitous in neural models, and they result in different neurocomputational properties.

# Bibliographical Notes

Among many textbooks on the mathematical theory of dynamical systems we recommend the following three.

- *Nonlinear Dynamics and Chaos* by Strogatz (1994) is suitable as an introductory book for undergraduate math or physics majors or graduate students in life sciences. It contains many exercises and worked-out examples.

- *Differential Equations and Dynamical Systems* by Perko (1996, 3rd ed., 2000) is suitable for math and physics graduate students, but may be too technical for life scientists. Nevertheless, it should be a standard textbook for computational neuroscientists.

- *Elements of Applied Bifurcation Theory* by Kuznetsov (1995, 3rd ed., 2004) is suitable for advanced graduate students in mathematics or physics and for computational neuroscientists who want to pursue bifurcation analysis of neural models.

The second edition of *The Geometry of Biological Time* by Winfree (2001) is a good introduction to oscillations, limit cycles, and synchronization in biology. It requires little background in mathematics and can be suitable even for undergraduate life science majors. *Mathematical Biology* by Murray (2nd ed., corr., 1993, 3rd ed., 2003) is an excellent example of how dynamical system theory can solve many problems in population biology and shed light on pattern formation in biological systems. Most of this book is suitable for advanced undergraduate or graduate students in mathematics and physics. *Mathematical Physiology* by Keener and Sneyd (1998) is similar to Murray's book, but is more focused on neural systems. *Spikes, Decisions, and Actions* by H. R. Wilson (1999) is a short introduction to dynamical systems with many neuroscience examples.

# Exercises

1. Use a pencil (as in Fig.4.39) to sketch the nullclines of the vector fields depicted in figures 4.40 through 4.44.

2. Assume that the continuous curve is the $x$-nullcline and the dashed curve is the $y$-nullcline in Fig.4.38, and that $\dot{x}$ or $\dot{y}$ changes sign when $(x, y)$ passes through the corresponding nullcline. The arrow indicates the direction of the vector field in one region. Determine the approximate directions of the vector field in the other regions of the phase plane.

3. Use a pencil (as in Fig.4.39) to sketch phase portraits of the vector fields depicted in figures 4.40 through 4.44. Clearly mark all equilibria, their stability, and their attraction domains. Show directions of all homoclinic, heteroclinic, and periodic

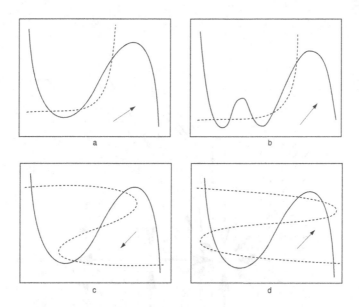

Figure 4.38: Determine the approximate direction of the vector field in each region between the nullclines. Continuous (dashed) curve is the $x$-nullcline ($y$-nullcline), and the direction of the vector field in one region is indicated by the arrow.

trajectories, as well as other representative trajectories. Estimate the signs of eigenvalues at each equilibrium.

4. Prove the classification diagram in Fig.4.15.

5. (van der Pol oscillator) Determine nullclines and draw the phase portrait of the van der Pol oscillator given in the Liénard (1928) form

$$\dot{x} = x - x^3/3 - y ,$$
$$\dot{y} = bx ,$$

where $b > 0$ is a parameter.

6. (Bonhoeffer–van der Pol oscillator) Determine the nullclines and sketch representative phase portraits of the Bonhoeffer–van der Pol oscillator

$$\dot{x} = x - x^3/3 - y ,$$
$$\dot{y} = b(x - a) - cy ,$$

in the case of $c = 0$. Treat $a$ and $b > 0$ as parameters.

7. (Hindmarsh-Rose spiking neuron) The following system is a generalization of the FitzHugh-Nagumo model (Hindmarsh and Rose 1982):

$$\dot{x} = f(x) - y + I ,$$
$$\dot{y} = g(x) - y ,$$

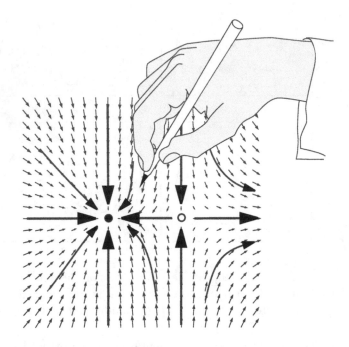

Figure 4.39: Phase portrait of a vector field. Use pencil to draw phase portraits in figures 4.40 through 4.44.

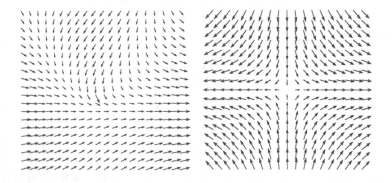

Figure 4.40: Use a pencil to draw a phase portrait, as in Fig.4.39.

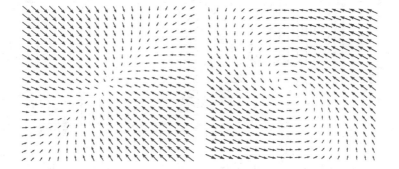

Figure 4.41: Use a pencil to draw a phase portrait, as in Fig.4.39.

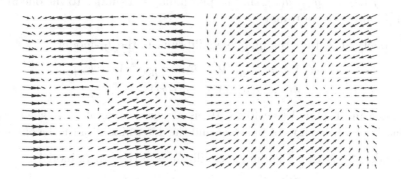

Figure 4.42: Use a pencil to draw a phase portrait, as in Fig.4.39.

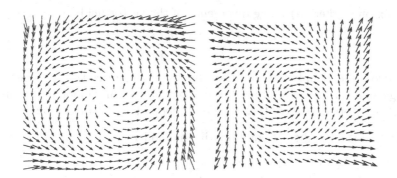

Figure 4.43: Use a pencil to draw a phase portrait, as in Fig.4.39.

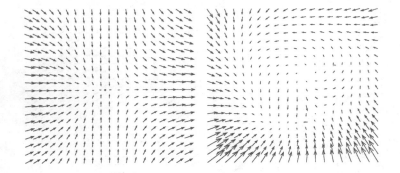

Figure 4.44: Use a pencil to draw a phase portrait, as in Fig.4.39.

where $f(x) = -ax^3 + bx^2$, $g(x) = -c + dx^2$, and $a, b, c, d$, and $I$ are parameters. Suppose $(\bar{x}, \bar{y})$ is an equilibrium. Determine its type and stability as a function of $f' = f'(\bar{x})$ and $g' = g(\bar{x})$; that is, plot a diagram similar to the one in Fig.4.15, with $f'$ and $g'$ as coordinates.

8. ($I_{\mathrm{K}}$-model) Show that the unique equilibrium in the $I_{\mathrm{K}}$-model

$$C\dot{V} = -g_{\mathrm{L}}(V - E_{\mathrm{L}}) - g_{\mathrm{K}}m^4(V - E_{\mathrm{K}}) \,, \qquad (4.14)$$
$$\dot{m} = (m_\infty(V) - m)/\tau(V) \,. \qquad (4.15)$$

discussed in chapter 3 (see Fig.3.40), is always stable, at least when $E_{\mathrm{L}} > E_{\mathrm{K}}$. (Hint: Look at the signs of the trace and the determinant of the Jacobian matrix).

9. ($I_{\mathrm{h}}$-model) Show that the unique equilibrium in the full $I_{\mathrm{h}}$-model

$$C\dot{V} = -g_{\mathrm{L}}(V - E_{\mathrm{L}}) - g_{\mathrm{h}}h(V - E_{\mathrm{h}}) \,,$$
$$\dot{h} = (h_\infty(V) - h)/\tau(V) \,,$$

discussed in chapter 3 is always stable.

10. (Bendixson's criterion) If the divergence of the vector field

$$\frac{\partial f(x,y)}{\partial x} + \frac{\partial g(x,y)}{\partial y}$$

of a two-dimensional dynamical system is not identically zero, and does not change sign on the plane, then the dynamical system cannot have limit cycles. Use this criterion to show that the $I_{\mathrm{K}}$-model and the $I_{\mathrm{h}}$-model cannot oscillate.

11. Determine the stability of equilibria in the model

$$\dot{x} = a + x^2 - y \,,$$
$$\dot{y} = bx - cy \,,$$

where $a \in \mathbb{R}$, $b \geq 0$, and $c > 0$ are some parameters.

# Chapter 5

# Conductance-Based Models and Their Reductions

In this chapter we present examples of geometrical phase plane analysis of various two-dimensional neural models. In particular, we consider minimal models, i.e., those having minimal sets of currents that enable the models to generate action potentials. The remarkable fact is that all these models can be reduced to planar systems having N-shaped $V$-nullclines. We will see that the behavior of the models depends not so much on the ionic currents as on the relationship between (in)activation curves and the time constants. That is, models involving completely different currents can have identical dynamics and, conversely, models involving similar currents can have completely different dynamics.

## 5.1   Minimal Models

There are a few dozen known voltage- and $Ca^{2+}$-gated currents having diverse activation and inactivation dynamics, and this number grows every year. Some of them are summarized in section 2.3.5. Almost any combination of the currents would result in interesting nonlinear behavior, such as excitability. Therefore, there are billions (more than $2^{30}$) of different electrophysiological models of neurons. Here we say that two models are "different" if, for example, one has the h-current $I_h$ and the other does not, without even considering how much of the $I_h$ there is. How can we classify all such models?

Let us do the following thought experiment. Consider a conductance-based model capable of exhibiting periodic spiking, that is, having a limit cycle attractor. Let us completely remove a current or one of its gating variables, then ask the question "Does the reduced model have a limit cycle attractor, at least for some values of parameters?" If it does, we remove one more gating variable or current, and proceed until we arrive at a model that satisfies the following two properties:

- It has a limit cycle attractor, at least for some values of parameters.

- If one removes any current or gating variable, the model has only equilibrium attractors for any values of parameters.

We refer to such a model as being *minimal* or *irreducible* for spiking. Thus, minimal models can exhibit periodic activity, even if it is of small amplitude, but their reductions cannot. According to this definition, any space-clamped conductance-based model of a neuron either is a minimal model or could be reduced to a minimal model or models by removing gating variables. This will be the basis for our classification of electrophysiological mechanisms in neurons.

For example, the Hodgkin-Huxley model considered in section 2.3 is not minimal for spiking. Recall that the model consists of three currents: leakage $I_L$, transient sodium $I_{Na,t}$ (gating variables $m$ and $h$), and persistent potassium $I_K$ (gating variable $n$); see Fig.5.1. Which of these currents are responsible for excitability and spiking?

We can remove the leakage current and the gating variable, $h$, for the inactivation of the sodium current: The resulting $I_{Na,p}+I_K$-model

$$
C\dot{V} = I - \overbrace{g_K n^4 (V - E_K)}^{I_K} - \overbrace{g_{Na} m^3 (V - E_{Na})}^{I_{Na,p}} ,
$$
$$
\dot{n} = (n_\infty(V) - n)/\tau_n(V) ,
$$
$$
\dot{m} = (m_\infty(V) - m)/\tau_m(V) ,
$$

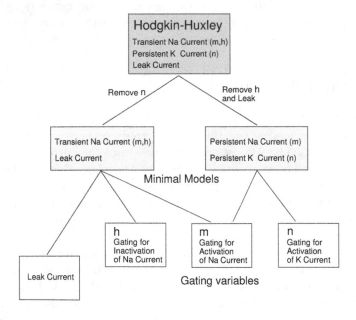

Figure 5.1: The Hodgkin-Huxley model (top box) is a combination of minimal models (shaded boxes on second level). Each minimal model can oscillate for at least some values of its parameters.

was considered in the previous chapter where we have shown that it could oscillate due to the interplay between the activation of persistent sodium and potassium currents. Alternatively, we can remove the K$^+$ current from the Hodgkin-Huxley model, yet the new $I_{\text{Na,t}}$-model

$$
\begin{aligned}
C\dot{V} &= I - \overbrace{g_{\text{Na}}m^3 h(V - E_{\text{Na}})}^{I_{\text{Na,t}}} - \overbrace{g_{\text{L}}(V - E_{\text{L}})}^{I_{\text{L}}}\,, \\
\dot{m} &= (m_\infty(V) - m)/\tau_m(V)\,, \\
\dot{h} &= (h_\infty(V) - h)/\tau_h(V)\,,
\end{aligned}
$$

can still oscillate via the interplay between activation and inactivation of the Na$^+$ current, as we will see later in this chapter. Both models are minimal, because removal of any other gating variable results in the $I_{\text{Na,p}}$-, $I_{\text{K}}$-, or $I_{\text{h}}$-models, none of which can have a limit cycle attractor, as the reader is asked to prove at the end of chapter 4.

We see that the Hodgkin-Huxley model is not minimal by itself, but is a combination of two minimal models. Minimal models are appealing because they are relatively simple; each individual variable has an established electrophysiological meaning, and its role in dynamics can be easily identified. As we show below, many minimal models can be reduced to planar systems, which are amenable to analysis using geometrical phase plane methods. In section 5.2 we discuss other methods of reducing multidimensional models, e.g., the Hodgkin-Huxley model, to planar systems.

There are only few minimal models, and understanding their dynamics can shed light on dynamics of more complicated electrophysiological models. However, the reader should be aware of the limitations of such an approach: Understanding minimal models cannot provide exhaustive information about all electrophysiological models (just as understanding the zeros of the equations $y = x$ and $y = x^2$ does not provide complete information about the zeros of the equation $y = x + x^2$).

## 5.1.1 Amplifying and Resonant Gating Variables

The definition of the minimal models involves a top-down approach: take a complicated model and strip it down to minimal ones. It is unlikely that this could be done for all $2^{30}$ or so electrophysiological models. Instead, we employ here a bottom-up approach, which is based on the following rule of thumb: a mixture of one amplifying and one resonant (recovery) gating variable (plus an Ohmic leak current) results in a minimal model. Indeed, neither of the variables alone can produce oscillation, but together they can (as we will see below).

The *amplifying* gating variable is the activation variable $m$ for voltage-gated inward current or the inactivation variable $h$ for voltage-gated outward current, as in Fig.5.2. These variables amplify voltage changes via a positive feedback loop. Indeed,

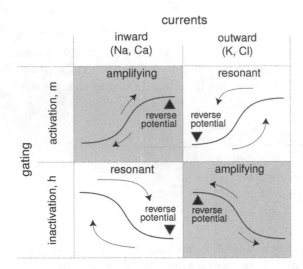

Figure 5.2: Gating variables may be amplifying or resonant depending on whether they represent activation/inactivation of inward/outward currents (see also Fig.3.3 and 3.4).

a small depolarization increases $m$ and decreases $h$, which in turn increases inward and decreases outward currents and increases depolarization. Similarly, a small hyperpolarization decreases $m$ and increases $h$, resulting in less inward and more outward current, and hence in more hyperpolarization.

The *resonant* gating variable is the inactivation variable $h$ for an inward current or the activation variable $n$ for an outward current. These variables resist voltage changes via a negative feedback loop. A small depolarization decreases $h$ and increases $n$, which in turn decreases inward and increases outward currents and produces a net outward current that resists the depolarization. Similarly, a small hyperpolarization produces inward current and, possibly, rebound depolarization.

Currents with amplifying gating variables can result in bistability, and they behave essentially like the $I_{\text{Na,p}}$-model or $I_{\text{Kir}}$-model considered in chapter 3. Currents with resonant gating variables have one stable equilibrium with possibly damped oscillation, and they behave essentially like the $I_{\text{K}}$-model or the $I_{\text{h}}$-model (compare Fig.5.2 with Fig.3.3). A typical neuronal model consists of at least one amplifying and at least one resonant gating variable. (Amplifying and resonant gating variables for $Ca^{2+}$-sensitive currents are discussed later in this chapter).

To get spikes in a minimal model, we need a fast positive feedback and a slower negative feedback. Indeed, if an amplifying gating variable has a slow time constant, it would act more as a low-pass filter, hardly affecting fast fluctuations and amplifying only slow fluctuations. If a resonant gating variable has a fast time constant, it will act to damp input fluctuations (faster than they can be amplified by the amplifying variable), resulting in stability of the resting state. Instead, the resonant variable acts as a band-pass filter; it has no effect on oscillations with a period much smaller than its time constant; it damps oscillations having a period much larger than its time constant, because the variable oscillates in phase with the voltage fluctuations; it amplifies oscillations with a period that is about the same as its time constant because

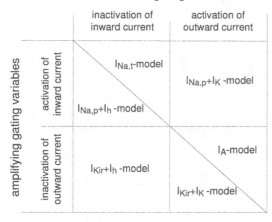

Figure 5.3: Any combination of one amplifying variable and one resonant gating variable results in a spiking model.

the variable lags the voltage fluctuations.

Since the amplifying gating variable, say $m$, has relatively fast kinetics, it can be replaced by its equilibrium (steady-state) value $m_\infty(V)$. This allows us to reduce the dimension of the minimal models from 3 (say $V$, $m$, $n$) to 2 ($V$ and $n$).

Two amplifying and two resonant gating variables produce four different combinations, depicted in Fig.5.3. However, the number of minimal models is not four, but six. The additional models arise due to the fact that a pair of gating variables may describe activation/inactivation properties of the same current or of two different currents. For example, the activation and inactivation gating variables $m$ and $h$ may describe the dynamics of a transient inward current, such as $I_{\mathrm{Na,t}}$, or the dynamics of a combination of one persistent inward current, such as $I_{\mathrm{Na,p}}$, and one "hyperpolarization-activated" inward current, such as $I_{\mathrm{h}}$. Hence this pair results in two models, $I_{\mathrm{Na,t}}$ and $I_{\mathrm{Na,p}}+I_{\mathrm{h}}$. Similarly, the pair of activation and inactivation variables of an outward current may describe the dynamics of the same transient current, such as $I_{\mathrm{A}}$, or the dynamics of two different outward currents; hence the two models, $I_{\mathrm{A}}$ and $I_{\mathrm{Kir}}+I_{\mathrm{K}}$.

Below we present the geometrical analysis of the six minimal voltage-gated models shown in Fig.5.3. Though they are based on different ionic currents, the models have many similarities from the dynamical systems point of view. In particular, all can exhibit saddle-node and Andronov-Hopf bifurcations. For each model we first provide a word description of the mechanism of generation of sustained oscillations, and then use phase plane analysis to provide a geometrical description. The first two, the $I_{\mathrm{Na,p}}+I_{\mathrm{K}}$-model and the $I_{\mathrm{Na,t}}$-model, are common; they describe the mechanism of generation of action potentials or subthreshold oscillations by many cells. The other four models are rare; they might even be classified as weird or bizarre by biologists, since they reveal rather unexpected mechanisms for voltage oscillations. Nevertheless, it is educational to consider all six models to see how the theory of dynamical systems works where intuition and common sense fail.

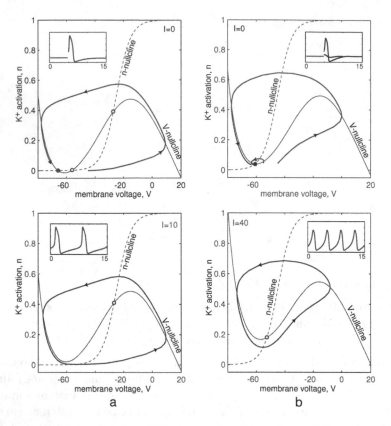

Figure 5.4: Possible forms of nullclines in the $I_{\mathrm{Na,p}}+I_{\mathrm{K}}$-model (parameters as in Fig.4.1).

## 5.1.2   $I_{\mathrm{Na,p}}+I_{\mathrm{K}}$-Model

One of the most fundamental models in computational neuroscience is the $I_{\mathrm{Na,p}}+I_{\mathrm{K}}$-model (pronounced *persistent sodium plus potassium model*), which consists of a fast $\mathrm{Na}^+$ current and a relatively slower $\mathrm{K}^+$ current:

$$C\dot{V} = I - \overbrace{g_{\mathrm{L}}(V-E_{\mathrm{L}})}^{\text{leak } I_{\mathrm{L}}} - \overbrace{g_{\mathrm{Na}}m(V-E_{\mathrm{Na}})}^{I_{\mathrm{Na,p}}} - \overbrace{g_{\mathrm{K}}n(V-E_{\mathrm{K}})}^{I_{\mathrm{K}}},$$
$$\dot{m} = (m_{\infty}(V)-m)/\tau_m(V),$$
$$\dot{n} = (n_{\infty}(V)-n)/\tau_n(V).$$

This model is in many respects equivalent to the $I_{\mathrm{Ca}}+I_{\mathrm{K}}$-model proposed by Morris and Lecar (1981) to describe voltage oscillations in the barnacle giant muscle fiber. A reasonable assumption based on experimental observations is that the $\mathrm{Na}^+$ gating variable $m(t)$ is much faster than the voltage variable $V(t)$, so that $m$ approaches the asymptotic value $m_\infty(V)$ practically instantaneously. In this case we can substitute $m = m_\infty(V)$ into the voltage equation and reduce the three-dimensional system above to a planar system,

$$C\dot{V} = I - \overbrace{g_L(V-E_L)}^{\text{leak } I_L} - \overbrace{g_{Na}\,m_\infty(V)\,(V-E_{Na})}^{\text{instantaneous } I_{Na,p}} - \overbrace{g_K\,n\,(V-E_K)}^{I_K} \qquad (5.1)$$
$$\dot{n} = (n_\infty(V)-n)/\tau(V)\,, \qquad (5.2)$$

which was considered in detail in chapter 4. In Fig.5.4 we summarize the dynamic repertoire of the model. A striking observation is that the other minimal models can have similar nullclines and similar dynamic repertoire, even though they consist of quite different ionic currents.

## 5.1.3 $I_{Na,t}$-model

An interesting example of a spiking mechanism, implicitly present in practically every biological neuron, is given by the $I_{Na,t}$-model (pronounced *transient sodium model*),

$$C\dot{V} = I - \overbrace{g_L(V-E_L)}^{\text{leak } I_L} - \overbrace{g_{Na}m^3h(V-E_{Na})}^{I_{Na,t}}\,,$$
$$\dot{m} = (m_\infty(V)-m)/\tau_m(V)\,,$$
$$\dot{h} = (h_\infty(V)-h)/\tau_h(V)\,,$$

consisting only of an Ohmic leak current and a transient voltage-gated inward $Na^+$ current. How could such a model generate action potentials? The upstroke of an action potential is generated because of the regenerative process involving the activation gate $m$. This mechanism is similar to that in the Hodgkin-Huxley model and the $I_{Na,p}+I_K$-model: increase of $m$ results in an increase of the inward current; hence more depolarization and further increase of $m$ until the excited state is achieved. At the excited state there is a balance of the $Na^+$ inward current and the leak outward current.

Since there is no $I_K$, the downstroke from the excited state occurs via a different mechanism. While in the excited state, the $Na^+$ current inactivates (turns off) and the Ohmic leak current slowly repolarizes the membrane potential toward the leak reverse potential $E_L$, which determines the resting state. While at rest, the $Na^+$ current deinactivates (i.e., becomes available), and the neuron is ready to generate another action potential. This mechanism is summarized in Fig.5.5.

To study the dynamics of the $I_{Na,t}$-model, we first reduce it to a planar system. Assuming that activation dynamics is instantaneous, we use $m = m_\infty(V)$ in the voltage equation and obtain

$$C\dot{V} = I - \overbrace{g_L(V-E_L)}^{\text{leak } I_L} - \overbrace{g_{Na}m_\infty^3(V)h(V-E_{Na})}^{I_{Na,t},\text{ inst. activation}}\,,$$

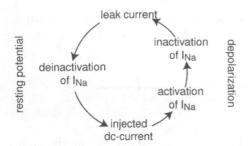

Figure 5.5: Mechanism of generation of sustained oscillations in the $I_{\text{Na,t}}$-model.

$$\dot{h} = (h_\infty(V) - h)/\tau_h(V) .$$

One can easily find the nullclines

$$h = \frac{I - g_{\text{L}}(V - E_{\text{L}})}{g_{\text{Na}}m_\infty^3(V)(V - E_{\text{Na}})} \qquad (V\text{-nullcline})$$

and

$$h = h_\infty(V) \qquad (h\text{-nullcline}) .$$

The $V$-nullcline looks like a cubic parabola (flipped N-shape), and the $h$-nullcline has a sigmoid shape. In Fig.5.6 we depict two typical cases (we invert the $h$-axis so that the vector field is directed counterclockwise, and this phase portrait is consistent with the other phase portraits in this book).

When the inactivation curve $h_\infty(V)$ has a high threshold (i.e., $I_{\text{Na,t}}$ is a window current), there are three intersections of the nullclines, and hence three equilibria, as in Fig.5.6a. A stable node (filled circle) corresponds to the resting state, and a nearby saddle corresponds to the threshold state. Another equilibrium, an unstable focus denoted by a white circle at the top of the figure, determines the shape of the action potential since all "spiking" trajectories have to go around it. Because of the high threshold of inactivation, the $I_{\text{Na,t}}$ current is deinactivated at rest. Moreover, small fluctuations of $V$ do not produce significant changes of the inactivation variable $h$ because the $h$-nullcline is nearly horizontal at rest. Such a system does not perform damped oscillations, and the nonlinear dynamics of the $V$ *near resting state* can be described by the one-dimensional system (where $h = h_\infty(V)$)

$$C\,\dot{V} = I - g_{\text{L}}(V - E_{\text{L}}) - g_{\text{Na}}m_\infty^3(V)h_\infty(V)(V - E_{\text{Na}})$$

studied in chapter 3. When $I$ increases, the stable node and the saddle approach, coalesce, and annihilate each other via saddle-node bifurcation. When $I = 0.5$, there is a periodic trajectory with a long period (compare the time scales in the bottom insets in Fig.5.6a and 5.6b).

When the Na$^+$ inactivation curve $h_\infty(V)$ has a low threshold, the nullclines have only one intersection; hence there is only one equilibrium, as in Fig.5.6b. When $I = 0$, the equilibrium (filled circle) is stable, and all trajectories converge to it. There

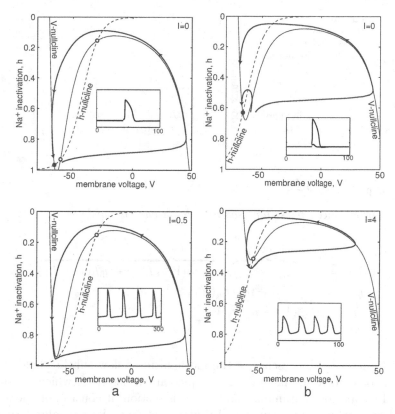

Figure 5.6: Possible forms of nullclines in the $I_{\mathrm{Na,t}}$-model. Notice that the $h$-axis is inverted. Parameters for $I_{\mathrm{Na,t}}$ are as in the Hodgkin-Huxley model, except that $\tau_h(V) = 5$ ms. $E_{\mathrm{Na}} = 60$ mV, $E_{\mathrm{L}} = -70$ mV, $g_{\mathrm{L}} = 1$, $g_{\mathrm{Na}} = 15$ (in b) and $g_{\mathrm{Na}} = 10$ and $V_{1/2} = -42$ mV (in a).

are damped oscillations near the equilibrium, though they can hardly be seen in the figure. The oscillations occur because the $I_{\mathrm{Na,t}}$ current is partially inactivated at rest. An increase of $V$ leads to more inactivation, less inward current, and hence rebound decrease of $V$, which in turn leads to partial deinactivation, more inward current, and to rebound increase of $V$. When the applied DC current $I$ increases, the equilibrium loses stability via Andronov-Hopf bifurcation. When $I = 4$, the equilibrium is an unstable focus (white circle in the figure), and there is a stable limit cycle attractor around it corresponding to periodic spiking.

We see that the $I_{\mathrm{Na,t}}$-model exhibits essentially the same dynamic repertoire as the $I_{\mathrm{Na,p}}+I_{\mathrm{K}}$-model, even though the models are quite different from the electrophysiological point of view.

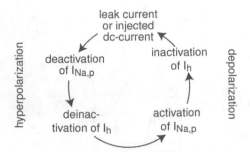

Figure 5.7: Mechanism of generation of sustained voltage oscillations in the $I_{\text{Na,p}}{+}I_{\text{h}}$-model.

### 5.1.4  $I_{\text{Na,p}}{+}I_{\text{h}}$-Model

The system (pronounced *persistent sodium plus h-current model*)

$$C\dot{V} = I - \overbrace{g_{\text{L}}(V-E_{\text{L}})}^{\text{leak } I_{\text{L}}} - \overbrace{g_{\text{Na}}m(V-E_{\text{Na}})}^{I_{\text{Na,p}}} - \overbrace{g_{\text{h}}h(V-E_{\text{h}})}^{I_{\text{h}}},$$
$$\dot{m} = (m_\infty(V)-m)/\tau_m(V),$$
$$\dot{h} = (h_\infty(V)-h)/\tau_h(V),$$

is believed to describe the essence of the mechanism of slow subthreshold voltage oscillations in some cortical, thalamic, and hippocampal neurons, which we summarize in Fig.5.7. Like any other minimal model in this section, it consists of one amplifying ($I_{\text{Na,p}}$) and one resonant ($I_{\text{h}}$) current. Both currents may be partially active at resting voltage. Recall that we treat the h-current as an inward current that is always activated (its activation variable $m=1$ all the time), but can be inactivated (turned off) by depolarization and deinactivated (turned on) by hyperpolarization. At resting voltage this current is usually inactivated (turned off). A sufficient hyperpolarization of $V$ deinactivates (turns on) the h-current, resulting in rebound depolarization. While depolarized, the h-current inactivates (turns off), and the leak current repolarizes the membrane potential toward the resting state. Without the persistent Na$^+$ current, or some other amplifying current, these oscillations always subside, as the reader was asked to prove in chapter 4, exercise 10. However, they may become sustained when $I_{\text{Na,p}}$ is involved.

To study dynamics of the $I_{\text{Na,p}}{+}I_{\text{h}}$-model, we assume that the activation kinetics of the Na$^+$ current is instantaneous, and use $m=m_\infty(V)$ in the voltage equation to obtain a two-dimensional system

$$C\dot{V} = I - \overbrace{g_{\text{L}}(V-E_{\text{L}})}^{\text{leak } I_{\text{L}}} - \overbrace{g_{\text{Na}}m_\infty(V)(V-E_{\text{Na}})}^{\text{instantaneous } I_{\text{Na,p}}} - \overbrace{g_{\text{h}}h(V-E_{\text{h}})}^{I_{\text{h}}},$$
$$\dot{h} = (h_\infty(V)-h)/\tau_h(V).$$

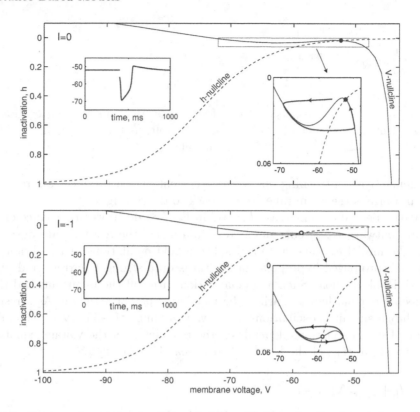

Figure 5.8: Rest and sustained subthreshold oscillations in the $I_{\text{Na,p}}+I_{\text{h}}$-model. Parameters for currents are as in thalamocortical neurons, $E_{\text{Na}} = 20$ mV, $E_{\text{h}} = -43$ mV, $E_{\text{L}} = -80$ mV, $g_{\text{L}} = 1.3$, $g_{\text{Na}} = 0.9$, and $g_{\text{h}} = 3$.

The nullclines of this system,

$$h = \frac{I - g_{\text{L}}(V - E_{\text{L}}) - g_{\text{Na}}m_\infty(V)(V - E_{\text{Na}})}{g_{\text{h}}(V - E_{\text{h}})} \qquad (V\text{-nullcline})$$

and

$$h = h_\infty(V) \qquad (h\text{-nullcline}),$$

have the familiar N- and sigmoid shapes depicted in Fig.5.8. We take the parameters for both currents from the experimental studies of thalamic relay neurons (see section 2.3.5). This choice results in one intersection of the nullclines in the relevant voltage range, which corresponds to only one equilibrium. This equilibrium is a stable resting state when no current is injected, i.e., when $I = 0$. In Fig.5.8 (top), one can clearly see that $h \approx 0$; that is, the h-current is inactivated (turned off). The resting state is due to the balance of the inward persistent Na$^+$ current and the Ohmic leak current. A small hyperpolarization deactivates the fast Na$^+$ current and shifts the balance toward the leak current, which brings $V$ closer to $E_{\text{leak}}$. This, in turn, results

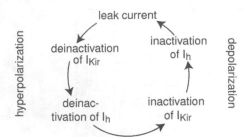

Figure 5.9: Mechanism of generation of sustained voltage oscillations in the $I_h+I_{Kir}$-model.

in slow deinactivation (turning on) of the h-current, which produces a strong inward current and brings the membrane voltage back to the resting state.

Negative injected current (case $I = -1$ in Fig.5.8) destroys the balance of inward ($I_{Na,p}$) and outward ($I_{leak}$) currents at rest, and makes the resting state unstable. As a result, the model exhibits sustained subthreshold oscillations of membrane potential. Indeed, prolonged hyperpolarization turns on a strong h-current and produces prolonged depolarization. Such a depolarization turns off the h-current, and the negative injected current hyperpolarizes the membrane potential again. As a result, the model exhibits sustained oscillations in the voltage range of $-55$ mV to $-65$ mV. The frequency of such oscillations depends on the parameters of the voltage equation and the time constant $\tau(V)$ of the h-current; it is near 4 Hz in Fig.5.8.

### 5.1.5  $I_h+I_{Kir}$-Model

The persistent Na$^+$ current, which amplifies the damped oscillations in the $I_{Na,p}+I_h$-model, can be replaced by the K$^+$ inwardly rectifying current $I_{Kir}$ to achieve the same amplifying effect. The resulting $I_h+I_{Kir}$-model (pronounced *h-current plus inwardly rectifying potassium model*)

$$
\begin{aligned}
C\dot{V} &= I - \overbrace{g_L(V-E_L)}^{\text{leak } I_L} - \overbrace{g_{Kir}h_{Kir}(V-E_K)}^{I_{Kir}} - \overbrace{g_h h(V-E_h)}^{I_h} , \\
\dot{h}_{Kir} &= (h_{Kir,\infty}(V) - h_{Kir})/\tau_{Kir}(V) , \\
\dot{h} &= (h_\infty(V) - h)/\tau_h(V) ,
\end{aligned}
$$

can exhibit sustained subthreshold oscillations of membrane voltage via a rather weird mechanism illustrated in Fig.5.9. The inwardly rectifying K$^+$ current $I_{Kir}$ behaves like $I_h$, except that the former is an outward current. A brief hyperpolarization deinactivates (turns on) the fast outward current $I_{Kir}$ and produces more hyperpolarization via a positive feedback loop. Such a regenerative process results in a prolonged hyperpolarization that deinactivates (turns on) the slower inward current $I_h$ and produces a rebound depolarization. This depolarization is enhanced by inactivation (turning off) of the fast $I_{Kir}$. However, the membrane potential cannot hold long in the depolarized state because of the slow depolarization-triggered decrease of $I_h$, and the leak

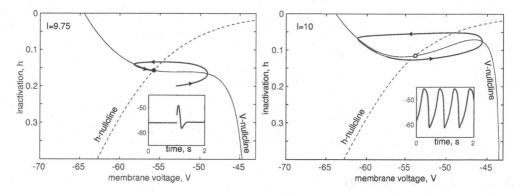

Figure 5.10: Resting and sustained subthreshold oscillations in the $I_h+I_{Kir}$-model. Parameters: $E_K = -80$ mV, $E_h = -43$ mV, $E_L = -50$ mV, $g_{Kir} = 4$, $g_h = 0.5$, $g_L = 0.44$. The h-current is the same as in section 5.1.4, except $V_{1/2} = -65$ mV. Instantaneous $I_{Kir}$ has $V_{1/2} = -76$ mV and $k = -11$.

current repolarizes the membrane potential. The repolarization is enhanced by the deinactivation of $I_{Kir}$ and becomes a hyperpolarization again, leading to the oscillations summarized in Fig.5.9.

Since the kinetics of $I_{Kir}$ is practically instantaneous, one can use $h_{Kir} = h_{Kir,\infty}(V)$ in the voltage equation above and consider the two-dimensional system

$$C\dot{V} = I - \overbrace{g_L(V-E_L)}^{\text{leak } I_L} - \overbrace{g_{Kir}h_{Kir,\infty}(V)(V-E_K)}^{\text{instantaneous } I_{Kir}} - \overbrace{g_h h(V-E_h)}^{I_h},$$
$$\dot{h} = (h_\infty(V) - h)/\tau_h(V).$$

One can easily find the nullclines of this system,

$$h = \frac{I - g_L(V-E_L) - g_{Kir}h_{Kir,\infty}(V)(V-E_K)}{g_h(V-E_h)} \qquad (V\text{-nullcline})$$

and

$$h = h_\infty(V) \qquad (h\text{-nullcline}),$$

which have the familiar form depicted in Fig.5.10. Most values of the parameters result in a phase portrait similar to the one depicted in Fig.5.10 (left). The $V$-nullcline is a monotonic curve that intersects the $h$-nullcline in one point corresponding to a stable resting state. An injected DC current $I$ shifts the resting state, but does not change its stability: Voltage perturbations always subside, resulting only in damped oscillations. There is, however, a narrow region in parameter space (it took the author a few hours to find that region) that produces just the right relationship between inactivation curves and conductances so that the $V$-nullcline becomes N-shaped and the subthreshold oscillations become sustained, as in Fig.5.10 (right).

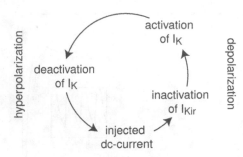

Figure 5.11: Mechanism of generation of sustained voltage oscillations in the $I_K+I_{Kir}$-model.

### 5.1.6   $I_K+I_{Kir}$-Model

The last two minimal models consist exclusively of outward K$^+$ currents, yet they can exhibit sustained oscillations of membrane voltage. The models defy the imagination of many biologists: How can a neuron with only outward K$^+$ currents and no inward Na$^+$ or Ca$^{2+}$ currents fire action potentials?

In the $I_K+I_{Kir}$-model (pronounced *persistent plus inwardly rectifying potassium model*)

$$C\dot{V} = I - \overbrace{g_{Kir}h(V - E_K)}^{I_{Kir}} - \overbrace{g_K n(V - E_K)}^{I_K},$$
$$\dot{n} = (n_\infty(V) - n)/\tau_n(V),$$
$$\dot{h} = (h_\infty(V) - h)/\tau_h(V),$$

the amplifying current is $I_{Kir}$ with inactivation gating variable $h$, and the resonant current is $I_K$ with activation variable $n$. The mechanism of generation of action potentials is summarized in Fig.5.11. A strong injected current depolarizes the membrane potential and inactivates (turns off) $I_{Kir}$, which amplifies the depolarization. While depolarized, the slower K$^+$ current $I_K$ activates and brings the potential down with possible hyperpolarization, which is amplified by the deinactivation of $I_{Kir}$. While the membrane potential is hyperpolarized, $I_K$ deactivates and the strong injected current brings the potential up again. Thus, the upstroke of the action potential is due exclusively to the injected DC current $I$, while the downstroke is due to the persistent outward K$^+$ current.

To perform the geometrical phase plane analysis of the model, we take advantage of the same observation as before: the kinetics of the amplifying current $I_{Kir}$ is relatively fast, so that $h = h_\infty(V)$ can be used in the voltage equation to reduce the three-dimensional system above to the two-dimensional system

$$C\dot{V} = I - \overbrace{g_{Kir}h_\infty(V)(V - E_K)}^{\text{instantaneous } I_{Kir}} - \overbrace{g_K n(V - E_K)}^{I_K},$$
$$\dot{n} = (n_\infty(V) - n)/\tau_n(V).$$

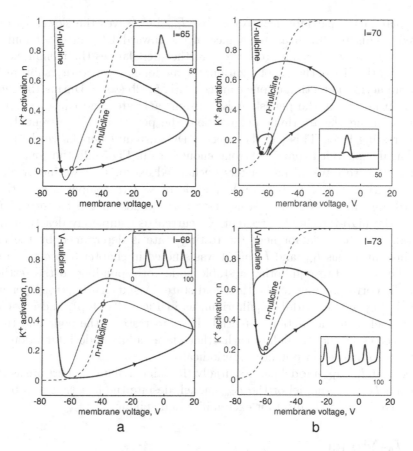

Figure 5.12: Possible intersections of nullclines in the $I_K+I_{Kir}$-model. Parameters: $E_K = -80$ mV, $g_{Kir} = 20$, $g_K = 2$. Instantaneous $I_{Kir}$ with $V_{1/2} = -80$ mV and $k = -12$. Slower $I_K$ with $k = 5$, $\tau(V) = 5$ ms, and $V_{1/2} = -40$ mV (in a) or $V_{1/2} = -55$ mV (in b).

It is an easy exercise to find the nullclines

$$n = I/\{g_K(V - E_K)\} - g_{Kir}h_\infty(V)/g_K \qquad (V\text{-nullcline})$$

and

$$n = n_\infty(V) \qquad (n\text{-nullcline}) ,$$

which we depict in Fig.5.12. There are two interesting cases corresponding to high-threshold (Fig.5.12a) and low-threshold (Fig.5.12b) $K^+$ current $I_K$.

When the $I_K$ has a low threshold, it is partially activated at resting potential. In this case, the resting state corresponds to the balance of partially activated $I_K$, partially inactivated $I_{Kir}$, and a strong injected DC current $I$. (Without the DC current the membrane voltage would converge to $E_K = -80$ mV and stay there forever.) A small depolarization partially inactivates fast $I_{\text{Kir}}$ but leaves the slower $I_{\text{K}}$ relatively unchanged. This results in an imbalance of the inward DC current $I$ and all outward currents, and the net inward current further depolarizes the membrane voltage. Depending on the size of the depolarization, the model may generate a subthreshold response or an action potential, as one can see in Fig.5.12b (top). During the generation of the action potential, the persistent K$^+$ current activates and causes afterhyperpolarization. During the afterhyperpolarization, the persistent K$^+$ current deactivates below the resting level. This lets the injected DC current $I$ depolarize the membrane potential again, provided that $I$ is strong enough, as in Fig.5.12b (bottom).

In Fig.5.12a we leave all parameters unchanged except that we increase the half-voltage activation $V_{1/2}$ of $I_{\text{K}}$ by 15 mV, and decrease $I$ to compensate for the deficit of outward current. Now, the resting state corresponds to the balance of $I_{\text{Kir}}$ and $I$, because the high-threshold persistent K$^+$ current is completely deactivated in this voltage range. The behavior near the resting state is determined by the interplay between instantaneous $I_{\text{Kir}}$ and $I$, and it was studied in chapter 3 (see exercises, $I_{\text{Kir}}$-model). There are two equilibria: a stable node corresponding to the resting state and a saddle corresponding to the threshold state. A sufficiently strong perturbation can push $V$ beyond the saddle equilibrium, as in Fig.5.12a (top), and can cause the minimal model to fire an action potential. If we increase $I$, the node and the saddle approach, coalesce, and annihilate each other via a saddle-node bifurcation, and the model starts to fire action potentials periodically.

We see that $I_{\text{K}}+I_{\text{Kir}}$-model has essentially the same dynamic repertoire as the more conventional $I_{\text{Na,p}}+I_{\text{K}}$-model or the $I_{\text{Na,t}}$-model, despite the fact that it is based on a rather bizarre ionic mechanism for excitability and spiking.

### 5.1.7  $I_{\text{A}}$-Model

The last minimal voltage-gated model has only one transient K$^+$ current, often referred to as the A-current $I_{\text{A}}$, yet it can also generate sustained oscillations. In some sense, the model is similar to the $I_{\text{Na,t}}$-model. Indeed, each consists of only one transient current and an Ohmic leak current. The only difference is that the A-current is outward, and as a result the action potentials are fired downward; see Fig.5.14 and Fig.5.15.

The A-current has activation and inactivation variables $m$ and $h$, respectively, and the $I_{\text{A}}$-model (pronounced *transient potassium model* or *A-current model*) has the form

$$C\dot{V} = I - \overbrace{g_{\text{L}}(V - E_{\text{L}})}^{\text{leak } I_{\text{L}}} - \overbrace{g_{\text{A}}mh(V - E_{\text{K}})}^{I_{\text{A}}}$$
$$\dot{m} = (m_\infty(V) - m)/\tau_m(V)$$
$$\dot{h} = (h_\infty(V) - h)/\tau_h(V) .$$

The mechanism of generation of downward action potentials is summarized in Fig.5.13. Due to a strong injected DC current, the resting state is in the depolarizing voltage

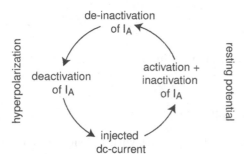

Figure 5.13: Mechanism of generation of sustained voltage oscillations in the $I_A$-model.

range, and it corresponds to the balance of the partially activated, partially inactivated A-current, the leak outward current, and the injected DC current. A small hyperpolarization can simultaneously deactivate and deinactivate the A-current, that is, decrease variable $m$ and increase variable $h$. Depending on the relationship between the activation and inactivation time constants, this may result in an increase of the A-current conductance, which is proportional to the product $mh$. More outward current produces more hyperpolarization and even more outward current. As a result of this regenerative process, the membrane voltage produces a sudden downstroke. While hyperpolarized, the A-current deactivates (variable $m \to 0$), and the injected DC current slowly brings the membrane potential toward the resting state, resulting in a slow upstroke. A fast downstroke and a slower upstroke from a depolarized resting state look like an action potential pointing downward.

If activation kinetics is much faster than inactivation kinetics, we can substitute $m = m_\infty(V)$ into the voltage equation above and reduce the $I_A$-model to a two-dimensional system, which hopefully would have the right kind of nullclines and a limit cycle attractor. After all, this is what we have done with previous minimal models, and it has always worked. As the reader is asked to prove in exercise 1, the $I_A$-model cannot have a limit cycle attractor when the A-current activation kinetics is instantaneous. Oscillations are possible only when the activation and inactivation kinetics have comparable time constants or inactivation is much faster than activation.

Even though none of the experimentally measured A-currents show fast inactivation and a relatively slower activation, this case is still interesting from the pure theoretical point of view, since it shows how a single K$^+$ current can give rise to oscillations. Assuming instantaneous inactivation and using $h = h_\infty(V)$ in the voltage equation, we obtain a two-dimensional system,

$$C\dot{V} = I - \overbrace{g_L(V - E_L)}^{\text{leak } I_L} - \overbrace{g_A m\, h_\infty(V)(V - E_K)}^{I_A, \text{ inst. inactivation}},$$
$$\dot{m} = (m_\infty(V) - m)/\tau_m(V),$$

whose nullclines can easily be found:

$$m = \frac{I - g_{\mathrm{L}}(V - E_{\mathrm{L}})}{g_{\mathrm{A}} h_\infty(V)(V - E_{\mathrm{K}})} \qquad (V\text{-nullcline})$$

and

$$m = m_\infty(V) \qquad (m\text{-nullcline}) \,.$$

Two typical cases are depicted in Fig.5.14a and 5.14b. We start with the simpler case in Fig.5.14b.

Figure 5.14b depicts nullclines when the A-current has a low activation threshold. There is only one intersection of the nullclines; hence there is only one equilibrium, which is a stable focus when the injected DC current $I$ is not strong enough (Fig.5.14b, top). Increasing $I$ makes the equilibrium lose stability via a supercritical Andronov-Hopf bifurcation that gives birth to a small amplitude limit cycle attractor (not shown in the figure). A further increase of $I$ increases the amplitude of oscillations (e.g., when $I = 10$ in the middle of Fig.5.14b), and the attractor corresponds to periodic firing of action potentials. When $I = 10.5$, the attractor disappears and the equilibrium becomes stable (via Andronov-Hopf bifurcation) again. The model, however, becomes excitable. A small hyperpolarization does not significantly change the A-current, and the voltage returns to resting state, resulting in a "subthreshold response". A sufficiently large hyperpolarization deinactivates enough $I_{\mathrm{A}}$ to open the $K^+$ current and hyperpolarize the membrane even further. This regenerative process produces the downstroke and brings $V$ close to $E_{\mathrm{K}}$. During the state of hyperpolarization, the A-current deactivates ($m \to 0$), and the DC current $I$ brings $V$ back to resting state. Notice that the action potential is directed downward.

In Fig.5.14a we consider the $I_{\mathrm{A}}$-model with exactly the same parameters except that we shift the half-voltage activation $V_{1/2}$ of $I_{\mathrm{A}}$ by 10 mV, so that the A-current has a higher activation threshold. This does not greatly affect the behavior of the system when $I$ is small. However, when $I \approx 10.7$, the spiking limit cycle attractor undergoes another kind of bifurcation – saddle-node bifurcation – resulting in the appearance of two new equilibria: a stable node and a saddle. If the reader looks at Fig.5.14a upside-down, he or she will notice that this figure resembles figure 5.4a, 5.6a, or 5.12a, with all the consequences: the node corresponds to a resting state, and the saddle corresponds to the threshold state. The large-amplitude trajectory that starts at the saddle and terminates at the node corresponds to an action potential, though a weird one. Thus, the behavior of this model is similar to the behavior of other models, with the exception that the $V$-axis is reversed.

The existence of "upside-down" $K^+$ spikes may (or, better say, *does*) look bizarre to many researchers, even though "inverted" $K^+$ and $Cl^-$ spikes were reported in many preparations, including frog and toad axons, squid axons, lobster muscle fibers, and dog cardiac muscle, as reviewed by Reuben et al. (1961) and Grundfest (1971). Two such cases are depicted in Fig.5.15. Interestingly, Reuben et al. (1961) postulated, albeit reluctantly, that the inverted spikes are caused by the inactivation of the $K^+$

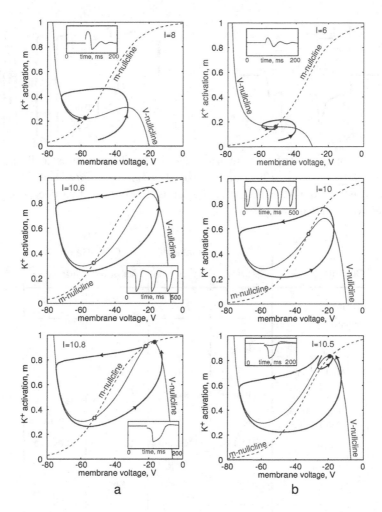

Figure 5.14: Possible intersections of nullclines in the $I_A$-model. Parameters: $E_K = -80$ mV, $E_L = -60$ mV, $g_A = 5$, $g_L = 0.2$. Instantaneous inactivation kinetics with $V_{1/2} = -66$ mV and $k = -10$. Activation of the A-current with $k = 10$, $\tau(V) = 20$ ms, and $V_{1/2} = -45$ mV (in a) or $V_{1/2} = -35$ mV (in b).

current. The reluctance was due to the fact that transient $K^+$ $I_A$ was not known at that time.

By now the reader must be convinced that quite different models can have practically identical dynamics. Conversely, the same model could have quite different behavior if only one parameter, e.g., $V_{1/2}$, is changed by as little as 10 mV. Such dramatic conclusions emphasize the importance of geometrical phase plane analysis of neuronal models, since the conclusions can hardly be drawn from mere word descriptions of the spiking mechanisms.

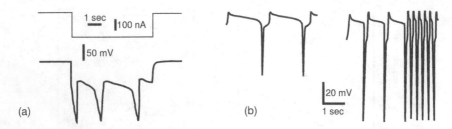

Figure 5.15: Anomalous (upside-down) spikes in (a) lobster muscle fibers (modified from Fig.2 of Reuben et al. 1961) and in (b) *Ascaris* esophageal cells (modified from Fig.16 of del Castillo and Morales 1967; the cell is depolarized by injected DC current). The voltage axis is not inverted.

| Currents | Voltage-Gated | | Ca$^{2+}$-Gated | |
|---|---|---|---|---|
| | Activation | Inactivation | Activation | Inactivation |
| $I_{leak}$ | | | | |
| **Inward** | | | | |
| $I_{Na,p}$  $I_{Ca}$ | fast | | | |
| $I_{Na,t}$  $I_{Ca(T)}$ | fast | fast | | |
| $I_{Ca(P)}$ | fast | slow | | |
| $I_{Ca(L)}$ | fast | | | slow |
| $I_{Ca(N)}$ | fast | medium | | medium |
| $I_h$ | | medium | | |
| $I_{CAN}$ | | | slow | |
| **Outward** | | | | |
| $I_K$ | fast | | | |
| $I_{K(M)}$ | slow | | | |
| $I_A$ | fast | fast | | |
| $I_{K(D)}$ | medium | slow | | |
| $I_{K(Ca)}$ | fast | | fast | |
| $I_{AHP}$ | | | slow | |
| $I_{Kir}$ | | fast | | |

Figure 5.16: Some representative voltage- and Ca$^{2+}$-gated ionic currents (Johnston and Wu 1995; Hille 2001; Shepherd 2004).

### 5.1.8 Ca$^{2+}$-Gated Minimal Models

So far, we have considered minimal models consisting of voltage-gated currents only. However, there are many ionic currents that depend not only on the membrane potential but also on the concentration of intracellular ions, mostly Ca$^{2+}$. Such currents are referred to as Ca$^{2+}$-gated, and they are summarized in Fig.5.16. In addition, there are Cl$^-$-gated, K$^+$-gated, and Na$^+$-gated currents, such as the SLO gene family of Cl$^-$-gated K$^+$ currents discovered in C. elegans, and the related "slack and slick" family of Na$^+$-gated K$^+$ currents (Yuan et al. 2000, 2003). Considering minimal models involving these currents lies outside the scope of this book, but it could be a good intellectual exercise for an expert reader (see also exercise 7 and 8).

Ca$^{2+}$-gated currents can also be divided into amplifying and resonant currents. Ca$^{2+}$-activated inward currents, such as the cation nonselective $I_{\mathrm{CAN}}$, act as amplifying currents. Indeed, activation of such a current leads to an influx of Ca$^{2+}$ ions and to more activation. Similarly, a hypothetical outward current inactivated by Ca$^{2+}$(not present in the figure) might also act as an amplifying current. Indeed, a depolarization due to the Ca$^{2+}$ influx inactivates such a hypothetical outward current, thereby producing a net shift toward inward currents and leading to more depolarization.

In contrast, Ca$^{2+}$-inactivating inward currents and Ca$^{2+}$-activating outward currents, such as $I_{\mathrm{Ca(L)}}$ and $I_{\mathrm{AHP}}$, respectively, act as resonant currents. Indeed, a depolarization due to the Ca$^{2+}$ influx inactivates the inward current and activates the outward current, and resists further depolarization.

Any combination of one voltage- or Ca$^{2+}$-gated amplifying current and one voltage- or Ca$^{2+}$-gated resonant current leads to a minimal model for spiking. All such combinations are depicted in Fig.5.17. Here, $I_1$ denotes a hypothetical Ca$^{2+}$-activated voltage-inactivated transient inward current. Though such a current is not presently known, one can easily write a conductance-gated model for it. A biologist would treat such a current as hyperpolarization- and Ca$^{2+}$-activated. $I_2$ is a hypothetical Ca$^{2+}$ current that is inactivated by Ca$^{2+}$. $I_3$ is a hypothetical voltage-inactivated Ca$^{2+}$ current. $I_4$ is an outward Ca$^{2+}$-inactivated current.

We see that there are many minimal models in Fig.5.17. Six of them are purely voltage-gated, and they have been investigated above. The others are mixed-mode or purely Ca$^{2+}$-gated models. An interested reader can work out the details of their phase portraits.

## 5.2 Reduction of Multidimensional Models

### 5.2.1 Hodgkin-Huxley model

Let us again consider the Hodgkin-Huxley model

$$C\dot{V} = I - \overbrace{g_{\mathrm{K}}n^4(V - E_{\mathrm{K}})}^{I_{\mathrm{K}}} - \overbrace{g_{\mathrm{Na}}m^3h(V - E_{\mathrm{Na}})}^{I_{\mathrm{Na}}} - \overbrace{g_{\mathrm{L}}(V - E_{\mathrm{L}})}^{I_{\mathrm{L}}},$$

|  |  | resonant gate | | | |
|  |  | voltage-gated | | Ca$^{2+}$-gated | |
|  |  | inactivation of inward current | activation of outward current | inactivation of inward current | activation of outward current |
|---|---|---|---|---|---|
| amplifying gate / voltage-gated | activation of inward current | I$_{Na,p}$+I$_h$  I$_{Na,t}$ | I$_{Na,p}$+I$_K$ | I$_{Ca}$+I$_2$  I$_{Ca(L)}$ | I$_{Ca}$+I$_{K(Ca)}$ |
|  | inactivation of outward current | I$_{Kir}$+I$_h$ | I$_{Kir}$+I$_K$  I$_A$ | I$_{Kir}$+I$_2$ |  |
| Ca$^{2+}$-gated | activation of inward current | I$_{CAN}$+I$_h$  I$_1$ | I$_{CAN}$+I$_K$ | I$_{CAN}$+I$_2$  I$_{CAN,t}$ | I$_{CAN}$+I$_{K(Ca)}$ |
|  | inactivation of outward current | I$_4$+I$_3$ |  | I$_4$+I$_2$ |  |

Figure 5.17: Voltage- and Ca$^{2+}$-gated minimal models. $I_1, \ldots, I_4$ are hypothetical currents that could exist theoretically, but have never been recorded experimentally (see text).

$$\dot{n} = (n_\infty(V) - n)/\tau_n(V) ,$$
$$\dot{m} = (m_\infty(V) - m)/\tau_m(V) ,$$
$$\dot{h} = (h_\infty(V) - h)/\tau_h(V) ,$$

with the original values of parameters presented in chapter 2. How can we understand the qualitative dynamics of this model? One way, discussed above, is to throw away the variable $h$ or $n$ and to reduce this model to the $I_{Na,p}+I_K$-model or $I_{Na,t}$-model, respectively. Although the reduced minimal models can tell a lot about the behavior of the original model, they are not equivalent to the Hodgkin-Huxley model from the electrophysiological or the dynamical systems point of view. Below we discuss another method of reduction of multidimensional electrophysiological models to planar systems.

The Hodgkin-Huxley model has four independent variables. Early computer simulations by Krinskii and Kokoz (1973) have shown that there is a relationship between the gating variables $n(t)$ and $h(t)$, namely,

$$n(t) + h(t) \approx 0.84 ,$$

as shown in Fig.5.18. In fact, plotting the variables on the $(n, h)$ plane, as we do in Fig.5.19, reveals that the orbit is near the straight line

$$h = 0.89 - 1.1n .$$

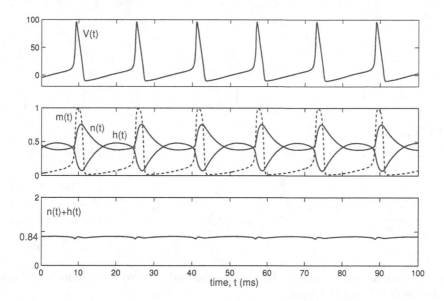

Figure 5.18: The sum $n(t) + h(t) \approx 0.84$ in the Hodgkin-Huxley model. Parameters are as in chapter 2 and $I = 8$.

We can use this relationship in the voltage equation to reduce the Hodgkin-Huxley model to a three-dimensional system. If, in addition, we assume that the activation kinetics of the Na$^+$ current is instantaneous, that is, $m = m_\infty(V)$, then the Hodgkin-Huxley model can be reduced to the two-dimensional system

$$C\dot{V} = I - \overbrace{g_K n^4 (V - E_K)}^{I_K} - \overbrace{g_{Na} m_\infty^3(V)(0.89 - 1.1n)(V - E_{Na})}^{\text{instantaneous } I_{Na}} - \overbrace{g_L(V - E_L)}^{I_L},$$
$$\dot{n} = (n_\infty(V) - n)/\tau_n(V),$$

whose solutions retain qualitative and some quantitative agreement with the original four-dimensional Hodgkin-Huxley system (see Fig.5.20). The first step in the analysis

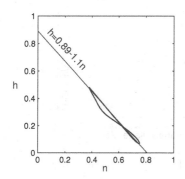

Figure 5.19: The relationship between $n(t)$ and $h(t)$ in the Hodgkin-Huxley model can be better described by $h = 0.89 - 1.1n$.

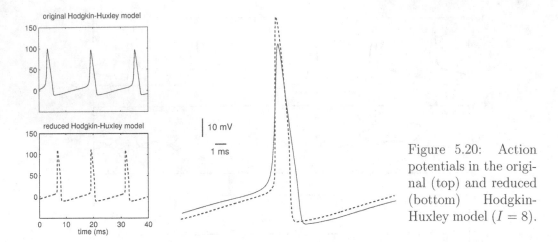

Figure 5.20: Action potentials in the original (top) and reduced (bottom) Hodgkin-Huxley model ($I = 8$).

of any two-dimensional system is to find its nullclines. The $V$-nullcline can be found by numerically solving the equation

$$I - g_K n^4(V - E_K) - g_{Na}m_\infty^3(V)(0.89 - 1.1n)(V - E_{Na}) - g_L(V - E_L) = 0$$

for $n$. The nullcline has the familiar N-shape depicted in Fig.5.21. Notice that it has only one intersection with the $n$-nullcline $n = n_\infty(V)$, hence there is only one equilibrium, which is stable when $I = 0$. When the parameter $I$ increases, the equilibrium loses stability via subcritical Andronov-Hopf bifurcation, as discussed in the next chapter. When $I$ is sufficiently large (e.g. $I = 12$ in Fig.5.21), there is a limit cycle attractor corresponding to periodic spiking. In exercise 2 we discuss what happens when $I$ becomes very large.

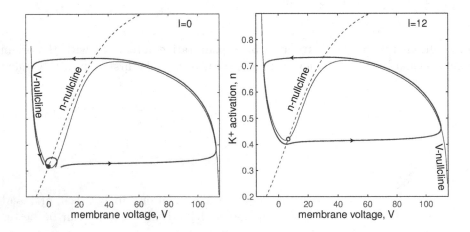

Figure 5.21: Reduction of the Hodgkin-Huxley model to the $(V, n)$ phase plane.

## 5.2.2 Equivalent Potentials

Inspired by the reduction idea of Krinskii and Kokoz (1973), Kepler et al. (1992) suggested a systematic method of reducing the complexity of conductance-based Hodgkin-Huxley-type models

$$\begin{aligned} C\dot{V} &= I - I(V, x_1, \ldots, x_n) \\ \dot{x}_i &= (m_{i,\infty}(V) - x_i)/\tau_i(V) , \qquad i = 1, \ldots, n , \end{aligned}$$

where $x_1, \ldots, x_n$ is a set of gating variables. The goal is to find certain patterns or combinations of the gating variables that can be lumped to reduce the dimension of the system. For example, we want to combine all resonant variables operating on a similar time scale into a "master" recovery variable, then do the same for amplifying variables.

Let us convert each variable $x_i(t)$ to the *equivalent potential* $v_i(t)$ that satisfies

$$x_i = m_{i,\infty}(v_i) .$$

In other words, the equivalent potential is the voltage which, in a voltage clamp, would give the value $x_i$ when the model is at an equilibrium. Applying the chain rule to $v_i = m_{i,\infty}^{-1}(x_i)$, we express the model above in terms of equivalent potentials:

$$\begin{aligned} C\dot{V} &= I - I(V, m_{1,\infty}(v_1), \ldots, m_{n,\infty}(v_n)) , \\ \dot{v}_i &= (m_{i,\infty}(V) - m_{i,\infty}(v_i))/(\tau_i(V)\, m'_{i,\infty}(v_i)) . \end{aligned}$$

Since the Boltzmann functions $m_{i,\infty}(V)$ are invertible, the denominators do not vanish. No approximations have been made yet; the new model is entirely equivalent to the original one – it is just expressed in a different coordinate system. The new coordinates, however, expose many patterns among the equivalent voltage variables that were not obvious in the original, gating coordinate system.

Kepler et al. (1992) developed an algorithm that replaces resonant and amplifying variables with their weighted averages. The weights are found using Lagrange multipliers and strictly local criteria aimed at preserving the bifurcation structure of the model. There is also a set of tests that informs the user when the method is likely to fail. The method results in a lower-dimensional system that is easier to simulate, visualize, and understand.

## 5.2.3 Nullclines and I-V Relations

We saw that the form and the position of nullclines provided important information about the neuron dynamics, that is, the number of equilibria, their stability, the existence of limit cycle attractors, and so on. The same information, in principle, can also be obtained from the analysis of the neuronal current-voltage (I-V) relations. This is not a coincidence, since there is a profound relationship between nullclines and experimentally measured I-V curves.

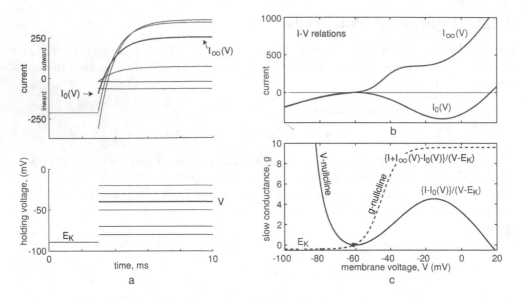

Figure 5.22: Voltage-clamp protocol to measure instantaneous (peak) and steady-state current-voltage (I-V) relations. (Shown are simulations of the $I_{Na,p}+I_K$-model from Fig.5.4b.)

Let us illustrate the relationship by using the $I_{Na,p}+I_K$-model, which we write in the form

$$C\dot{V} = I - I_0(V) - g(V - E_K) ,  \qquad (5.3)$$
$$\dot{g} = f(V,g) ,  \qquad (5.4)$$

where

$$I_0(V) = g_L(V - E_L) + g_{Na}m_\infty(V)(V - E_{Na})$$

is the instantaneous (peak) current, and $g = g_K n$ is the slow conductance. The function $f(V,g)$ describes the dynamics of $g$, and its form is not important here. The method described below is quite general, and it can be used in many circumstances when little is known about the neuron's electrophysiology.

In Fig.5.22 we describe a typical voltage-clamp experiment to measure the instantaneous (peak) and the steady-state I-V relations, denoted here as $I_0(V)$ and $I_\infty(V)$, respectively. The holding voltage (Fig.5.22a, bottom) is kept at $E_K$ and then stepped to various values $V$. The recorded current (Fig.5.22a, top) typically consists of a fast (peak) component $I_0(V)$ that is due to the instantaneous activation of Na$^+$ currents, leak current, and other fast currents, and then it relaxes to the asymptotic steady-state value $I_\infty(V)$. Repeating this experiment for various $V$, one can measure the I-V functions $I_0(V)$ and $I_\infty(V)$ depicted in Fig.5.22b. Note that $I_0(V)$ has the N-shape with a large region of negative slope. This region corresponds to the regenerative activation of the Na$^+$ current, and it is responsible for the excitability property of the neuron. It is also responsible for the N-shape of the $V$-nullcline, as we see next.

Once the I-V relations are found, we can find the nullclines of the system (5.3, 5.4). From the equation

$$I - I_0(V) - g(V - E_K) = 0$$

we can easily find the $V$-nullcline

$$g = \{I - I_0(V)\}/(V - E_K) \qquad (V\text{-nullcline}) ,$$

which has the inverted N-shape depicted in Fig.5.22c because $I_0(V)$ does. While measuring $I_\infty(V)$, we hold $V$ long enough so that all conductances reach their steady-state values. The steady-state value $g = g_\infty(V)$ can be obtained from the equation

$$I - I_0(V) - g(V - E_K) = -I_\infty(V) ,$$

which says that the asymptotic steady-state current is the sum of the steady-state fast current and steady-state slow current. Therefore,

$$g = \{I + I_\infty(V) - I_0(V)\}/(V - E_K) \qquad (g\text{-nullcline})$$

depicted in Fig.5.22c. Since we used the $I_{Na,p}+I_K$-model with parameters as in Fig.5.4b (top), we are not surprised that the $V$- and $g$-nullclines found here have the same shape and relative position as those in Fig.5.4b (top). In exercise 5 we further explore the relationship between the I-V curves and neuronal dynamics.

## 5.2.4   Reduction to Simple Model

All models discussed in this chapter can be reduced to two-dimensional systems having a fast voltage variable, $V$, and a slower "recovery" variable, $u$, with N-shaped and sigmoidal nullclines, respectively. The decision to fire or not to fire is made at the resting state, which is the intersection of the nullclines near the left knee, as we illustrate in Fig.5.23a. To model the subthreshold behavior of such neurons and the initial segment of the upstroke of an action potential, we need to consider only a small neighborhood of the left knee confined to the shaded square in Fig.5.23. The rest of the phase space is needed only to model the peak and the downstroke of the action potential. If the shape of the action potential is less important than the subthreshold dynamics leading to this action potential, then we can retain detailed information about the left knee and its neighborhood, and simplify the vector field outside the neighborhood. This approach results in a simple model capable of exhibiting quite realistic dynamics, as we will see in chapter 8.

### Derivation via Nullclines

The fast nullcline in Fig.5.23b can be approximated by the quadratic parabola

$$u = u_{min} + p(V - V_{min})^2,$$

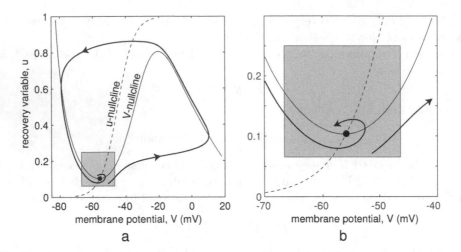

Figure 5.23: Phase portrait (a) and its magnification (b) of a typical neuronal model having voltage variable $V$ and a recovery variable $u$.

where $(V_{\min}, u_{\min})$ is the location of the minimum on the left knee, and $p \geq 0$ is a scaling coefficient. Similarly, the slow nullcline can be approximated by the straight line

$$u = s(V - V_0) \, ,$$

where $s$ is the slope and $V_0$ is the $V$-intercept. All these parameters can easily be determined geometrically or analytically.

Using these nullclines, we approximate the dynamics in the shaded region in Fig.5.23 by the system

$$\dot{V} = \tau_{\mathrm{f}} \left\{ p(V - V_{\min})^2 - (u - u_{\min}) \right\} \, ,$$
$$\dot{u} = \tau_{\mathrm{s}} \left\{ s(V - V_0) - u \right\} \, ,$$

where the parameters $\tau_{\mathrm{f}}$ and $\tau_{\mathrm{s}}$ describe the fast and slow time scales. Because of the term $(V - V_{\min})^2$, the variable $V$ can escape to infinity in a finite time. This corresponds to the firing of an action potential, more precisely, to its upstroke. To model the downstroke, we assume that $V_{\max}$ is the peak value of the action potential, and we reset the state of the system

$$(V, u) \leftarrow (V_{\mathrm{reset}}, u + u_{\mathrm{reset}}) \, , \qquad \text{when } V = V_{\max},$$

as if the spiking trajectory disappears at the right edge and appears at the left edge in Fig.5.23b. Here $V_{\mathrm{reset}}$ and $u_{\mathrm{reset}}$ are parameters. Appropriate rescaling of variables transforms the simple model into the equivalent form

$$\dot{v} = I + v^2 - u \qquad\qquad \text{if } v \geq 1, \text{ then} \qquad\qquad (5.5)$$
$$\dot{u} = a(bv - u) \qquad\qquad\qquad v \leftarrow c, \, u \leftarrow u + d \qquad\qquad (5.6)$$

having only four dimensionless parameters.

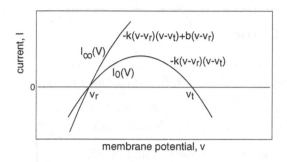

Figure 5.24: The relationship between the parameters of the simple model (5.7, 5.8) and the instantaneous and steady-state I-V relations, $I_0(V)$ and $I_\infty(V)$, respectively.

## Derivation via I-V Relations

The parameters of the simple model can be derived using instantaneous (peak) and steady-state I-V relations. Let us represent the model in the equivalent form

$$C\dot{v} = k(v - v_r)(v - v_t) - u + I \qquad \text{if } v \geq v_{\text{peak}}, \text{ then} \qquad (5.7)$$
$$\dot{u} = a\{b(v - v_r) - u\} \qquad \qquad v \leftarrow c, \ u \leftarrow u + d \qquad (5.8)$$

where $v$ is the membrane potential, $u$ is the recovery current, and $C$ is the membrane capacitance. The quadratic polynomial $-k(v - v_r)(v - v_t)$ approximates the subthreshold part of the instantaneous I-V relation $I_0(V)$. Here, $v_r$ is the resting membrane potential, and $v_t$ is the instantaneous threshold potential, as in Fig.5.24. That is, instantaneous depolarizations above $v_t$ result in spike response. The polynomial $-k(v - v_r)(v - v_t) + b(v - v_r)$ approximates the subthreshold part of the steady-state I-V relation $I_\infty(V)$. When $b < 0$, its maximum approximates the rheobase current of the neuron, i.e., the minimal amplitude of a DC current needed to fire a cell. Its derivative with respect to $v$ at $v = v_r$, that is, $b - k(v_r - v_t)$, corresponds to the resting input conductance, which is the inverse of the input resistance. Knowing both the rheobase and the input resistance of a neuron, one can use the two equations above to determine the parameters $k$ and $b$. We do that in chapter 8 using recordings of real neurons. This method does not work when $b > 0$.

The sum of all slow currents that modulate the spike generation mechanism is combined in the phenomenological variable $u$, with outward currents taken with the plus sign. The form of (5.8) ensures that $u = 0$ at rest (i.e., when $I = 0$ and $v = v_r$). The sign of $b$ determines whether $u$ is an amplifying ($b < 0$) or a resonant ($b > 0$) variable. In the latter case, the neuron sags in response to hyperpolarized pulses of current, peaks in response to depolarized subthreshold pulses, and produces rebound (postinhibitory) responses. The recovery time constant is $a$. The spike cutoff value is $v_{\text{peak}}$, and the voltage reset value is $c$. The parameter $d$ describes the total amount of outward minus inward currents activated during the spike and affecting the after-spike behavior. All these parameters can easily be fit to any particular neuron type, as we show in chapter 8.

## Review of Important Concepts

- Amplifying gating variables describe activation of an inward current or inactivation of an outward current. They amplify voltage changes.

- Resonant gating variables describe inactivation of an inward current or activation of an outward current. They resist voltage changes.

- To exhibit excitability, it is enough to have one amplifying and one resonant gating variable in a neuronal model.

- Many models can be reduced to two-dimensional systems with one equation for voltage and instantaneous amplifying currents, and one equation for a resonant gating variable.

- The behavior of a two-dimensional model depends on the position of its nullclines. Many models have an N-shaped $V$-nullcline and a sigmoid-shaped nullcline for the gating variable.

- There is a relationship between nullclines and I-V curves.

- Quite different electrophysiological models can have similar nullclines, and hence essentially the same dynamics.

- The spike generation mechanism of detailed electrophysiological models depends on the dynamics near the left knee of the fast $V$-nullcline, and it can be captured by a simple model (5.5, 5.6).

## Bibliographical Notes

Richard FitzHugh pioneered the use of phase planes and nullclines to study the Hodgkin-Huxley model (FitzHugh 1955). First, he used an analog computer, consisting of operational amplifiers, function generators, and vacuum tubes, to simulate the model. According to FitzHugh (see Izhikevich and FitzHugh 2006), the tubes were continually failing, and he had to find and replace several tubes a week. The heat from all these tubes overloaded the air conditioning, so that on hot summer days he had to take off his shirt and wear shorts to be comfortable. Not surprisingly, FitzHugh came up with a simple model with N-shaped cubic $V$-nullcline and a straight-line slow nullcline, known as the FitzHugh-Nagumo model, to illustrate the mechanism of excitability of the Hodgkin-Huxley system. However, it was Krinskii and Kokoz (1973) who first discovered the relationship $n(t) + h(t) \approx$ const, and thus were able to reduce the four-dimensional Hodgkin-Huxley model to a two-dimensional system. Since then, the phase plane analysis of neuronal models has become standard, at least in Russian-language literature.

Current awareness of the geometrical methods of phase plane analysis of neuronal models is mostly due to the seminal paper by John Rinzel and Bard Ermentrout *Analysis of Neural Excitability and Oscillations*, published as a chapter in Koch and Segev's book *Methods in Neuronal Modeling* (1989, 2nd ed., 1999). Not only did they introduce the geometrical methods to a wide computational neuroscience audience, but they also were able to explain a number of outstanding problems, such as the origin of Class 1 and 2 excitability observed by Hodgkin in 1948.

Rinzel and Ermentrout illustrated most of the concepts using the Morris-Lecar (1981) model, which is a $I_{Ca} + I_K$-minimal voltage-gated model equivalent of the $I_{Na,p}$ $+ I_K$-model considered above. Due to its simplicity, the Morris-Lecar model is widely used in computational neuroscience research. This is the reason we use its analogue, the $I_{Na,p} + I_K$-model, throughout the book.

Hutcheon and Yarom (2000) suggested classifying all currents into amplifying and resonant. There have been no attempts to classify various electrophysiological mechanisms of excitability in neurons, though minimal models, such as the $I_{Na,t}$-model or the $I_{Ca}+I_{K(C)}$-model, would not surprise most researchers. The other models would probably look bizarre to classical electrophysiologists, though they provide a good opportunity to practice geometrical phase plane analysis and support FitzHugh's observation that an N-shaped $V$-nullcline is the key characteristic of neuronal dynamics. Izhikevich (2003) took advantage of this observation and suggested the simple model (5.5, 5.6) that captures the spike generation mechanism of many known neuronal types (see chapter 8).

## Exercises

1. Show that the $I_A$-model cannot have a limit cycle attractor when $I_A$ has instantaneous activation kinetics. (Hint: Use the Bendixson criterion.)

2. When the injected DC current $I$ or the Na$^+$ maximal conductance $g_{Na}$ in the $I_{Na,p}+I_K$-model has a large value, the excited state ($V \approx -20$ mV) becomes stable. Sketch possible intersections of nullclines of the model.

3. Using $I$ as a bifurcation parameter, determine the saddle-node bifurcation diagram of

   - The $I_{Na,t}$-model with parameters as in Fig.5.6a.
   - The $I_A$-model with parameters as in Fig.5.14a.

4. Why is $g$ in Fig.5.22c negative when $V$ is hyperpolarized?

5. In Fig.5.25 we plot the currents that constitute the right-hand side of the voltage equation (5.3),

$$I - I_{fast}(V) \qquad \text{and} \qquad I_{slow}(V) = g(V - E_K) \, ,$$

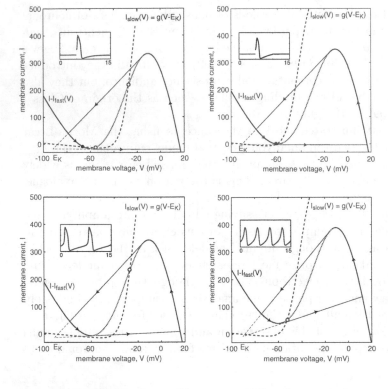

Figure 5.25: Exercise 5: The $(V, I)$-phase plane of the $I_{Na,p} + I_K$-model (compare with Fig.5.4).

on the $(V, I)$ plane. The curves define fast and slow movements of the state of the system. Interpret the figure. (Hint: Treat the curves as "sort-of" nullclines.)

6. Show that the $I_{Cl} + I_K$-model can have oscillations. (Hint: Inject negative DC current so that the voltage-gated $Cl^-$ current becomes inward/amplifying).

7. (NMDA+$I_K$-model) Show that a neuronal model consisting of an NMDA current and a resonant current, (say, $I_K$) can exhibit excitability and periodic spiking.

8. The Nernst potential of an ion is a function of its concentration inside/outside the cell membrane, which may change. Consider the $I_{Na,p} + E_{Na}([Na^+]_{in/out})$-model and show that it can exhibit excitability and oscillations on a slow time scale.

9. Determine when the $I_A$-model has a limit cycle attractor without assuming $\tau_h(V) \ll \tau_m(V)$.

10. **[Ph.D.]** There are $Na^+$-gated and $Cl^-$-gated currents in addition to the $Ca^{2+}$-gated currents considered in this book. In addition, the Nernst potentials may change as concentrations of ions inside/outside the cell membrane change. This may lead to new minimal models. Classify and study all these models.

# Chapter 6

# Bifurcations

Neuronal models can be excitable for some values of parameters, and fire spikes periodically for other values. These two types of dynamics correspond to a stable equilibrium and a limit cycle attractor, respectively. When the parameters change, e.g., the injected DC current in Fig.6.1 ramps up, the models can exhibit a bifurcation – a transition from one qualitative type of dynamics to another. We consider transitions away from equilibrium point in section 6.1 and transitions away from a limit cycle in section 6.2. All these transitions can be reliably observed when only one parameter, in our case $I$, changes. Mathematicians refer to such transitions as bifurcations of *codimension-1*. In this chapter we provide definitions and examples of all codimension-1 bifurcations of an equilibrium and a limit cycle that can occur in two-dimensional systems. In section 6.3 we mention some codimension-1 bifurcations in high-dimensional systems, as well as some codimension-2 bifurcations. In chapter 7 we discuss how the type of bifurcation determines a cell's neurocomputational properties.

## 6.1 Equilibrium (Rest State)

A neuron is excitable because its resting state is near a bifurcation, i.e., near a transition from quiescence to periodic spiking. Typically, such a bifurcation can be revealed by injecting a ramp current, as we do in Fig.6.1. The four bifurcations in the figure have qualitatively different properties, summarized in Fig.6.2. In this section we use analytical and geometrical tools to understand what the differences among the bifurcations are.

Recall (see chapter 4) that an equilibrium of a dynamical system is stable if all the eigenvalues of the Jacobian matrix at the equilibrium have negative real parts. When a parameter, say $I$, changes, one of two events can happen:

1. A negative eigenvalue increases and becomes 0. This happens at the saddle-node bifurcation, and the equilibrium disappears.

2. Two complex-conjugate eigenvalues with negative real parts approach the imaginary axis and become purely imaginary. This happens at the Andronov-Hopf bifurcation, and the equilibrium loses stability but does not disappear.

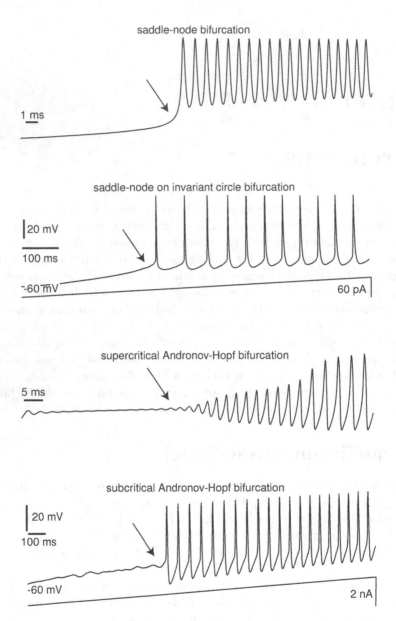

Figure 6.1: Transitions from resting to tonic (periodic) spiking occur via bifurcations of equilibrium (marked by arrows). Saddle-node on invariant circle bifurcation: in vitro recording of pyramidal neuron of rat's primary visual cortex. Subcritical Andronov-Hopf bifurcation: in vitro recording of brainstem mesencephalic V neuron. The other two traces are simulations of the $I_{\mathrm{Na,p}}+I_{\mathrm{K}}$-model.

| Bifurcation of an equilibrium | Fast subthreshold oscillations | Amplitude of spikes | Frequency of spikes |
|---|---|---|---|
| saddle-node | no | nonzero | nonzero |
| saddle-node on invariant circle | no | nonzero | $A\sqrt{I-I_b} \to 0$ |
| supercritical Andronov-Hopf | yes | $A\sqrt{I-I_b} \to 0$ | nonzero |
| subcritical Andronov-Hopf | yes | nonzero | nonzero |

Figure 6.2: Summary of codimension-1 bifurcations of an equilibrium. $I$ denotes the amplitude of the injected current, $I_b$ is the bifurcation value, and $A$ is a parameter that depends on the biophysical details.

Thus, there are only two qualitative events that can happen with a stable equilibrium in a dynamical system of arbitrary dimension: it can either disappear or lose stability. Of course, there could also be a third event: all eigenvalues continue to have negative real parts, in which case the equilibrium remains stable.

Since any equilibrium of a neuronal model is the zero of the steady-state I-V curve $I_\infty(V)$ (the net current at the equilibrium must be zero), analysis of the shape of the I-V curve can provide invaluable information about possible bifurcations of the resting state.

Two typical steady-state I-V curves are depicted in Fig.6.3. The I-V curve in Fig.6.3a has a region with a negative slope and thus may have three equilibria: the left equilibrium is probably stable (though it might be unstable; see exercise 8), the middle is unstable, and the right equilibrium can be stable or unstable, depending on the kinetics of the gating variables (it is stable in the one-dimensional case, i.e., when gating variables have instantaneous kinetics). The I-V curve in Fig.6.3b is monotone. A positive (inward) injected DC current $I$ shifts the I-V curves down. This leads to the disappearance of the equilibrium in Fig.6.3a, but not in Fig.6.3b. Therefore, Fig.6.3a corresponds to the saddle-node bifurcation and Fig.6.3b to the Andronov-Hopf bifurcation. Exactly when the equilibrium loses stability in Fig.6.3b cannot be inferred from the I-V relations (for this, we need to consider the full neuronal model). But what we can infer is that the bifurcation *cannot be* of the saddle-node type. Surprisingly, nonmonotonic I-V curves result in saddle-node bifurcations but do not exclude Andronov-Hopf bifurcations, as the reader is asked to demonstrate in exercise 8. This phenomenon is relevant to the cortical pyramidal neurons considered in chapter 8.

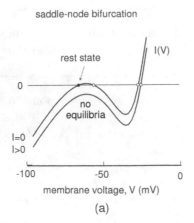

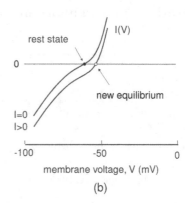

Figure 6.3: Steady-state I-V curves of the $I_{\mathrm{Na,p}}+I_{\mathrm{K}}$-model with high-threshold (left) and low-threshold (right) K$^+$ current (parameters as in Fig.4.1).

### 6.1.1   Saddle-Node (Fold)

We provided the definition of a saddle-node bifurcation in one-dimensional systems in section 3.3.4, and the reader is encouraged to look at that section and at Fig.4.31 before proceeding further.

A $k$-dimensional dynamical system

$$\dot{x} = f(x, b), \qquad x \in \mathbb{R}^k$$

having an equilibrium point $x_{\mathrm{sn}}$ for some value of the bifurcation parameter $b_{\mathrm{sn}}$ (i.e., $f(x_{\mathrm{sn}}, b_{\mathrm{sn}}) = 0$) exhibits *saddle-node* (also known as *fold*) bifurcation if the equilibrium is non-hyperbolic with a simple zero eigenvalue, the function $f$ is non-degenerate, and it is transversal with respect to $b$. The first condition is easy to check:

- *Non-hyperbolicity.* The Jacobian $k \times k$ matrix of partial derivatives at the equilibrium (see section 4.2.2) has exactly one zero eigenvalue, and the other eigenvalues have nonzero real parts.

In general, the remaining two conditions have complicated forms, since they involve projections of the vector field on the *center manifold*, which is tangent to the eigenvector corresponding to the zero eigenvalue of the Jacobian matrix. However, there is a shortcut for conductance-based neuronal models.

Let $\mathbf{I}(V, b)$ denote the steady-state I-V relation, which can be measured experimentally, divided by the membrane capacitance $C$. For example, $\mathbf{I}(V, I) = \{I - I_\infty(V)\}/C$ when the injected DC current $I$ is used as a bifurcation parameter. We replace the multi-dimensional neuronal model with the one-dimensional system $\dot{V} = \mathbf{I}(V, b)$. From $\mathbf{I}(V, b) = 0$ (equilibrium condition) we find $b = I_\infty(V)$. Non-hyperbolicity implies $\mathbf{I}_V(V, b) = 0$, so that the bifurcation occurs at the local maxima and minima of $I_\infty(V)$. We considered all these properties in chapter 3.

- *Non-degeneracy.* The second-order derivative of $\mathbf{I}(V, b_{sn})$ with respect to $V$ is nonzero, that is,

$$a = \frac{1}{2} \frac{\partial^2 \mathbf{I}(V, b_{sn})}{\partial V^2} \neq 0 \qquad (\text{at } V = V_{sn}) . \qquad (6.1)$$

That is, the piece of the I-V curve, $I_\infty(V)$, at the bifurcation point, $V_{sn}$, looks like the square parabola.

- *Transversality.* Function $\mathbf{I}(V, b)$ is non-degenerate with respect to the bifurcation parameter $b$; that is,

$$c = \frac{\partial \mathbf{I}(V_{sn}, b)}{\partial b} \neq 0 \qquad (\text{at } b = b_{sn}) .$$

This condition is always satisfied when the injected DC current $I$ is the bifurcation parameter, because $\partial \mathbf{I}/\partial b = \partial \mathbf{I}/\partial I = 1/C$.

The saddle-node bifurcation has codimension-1 because only one condition (non-hyperbolicity) involves strict equality ("="), and the other two involve inequalities ("$\neq$"). The dynamics of multi-dimensional neuronal systems near a saddle-node bifurcation can be reduced to that of the topological normal form

$$\dot{V} = c(b - b_{sn}) + a(V - V_{sn})^2 , \qquad (6.2)$$

where $V$ is the membrane voltage, and $a$ and $c$ are defined above. In the context of neuronal models, this equation with an after-spike resetting is called the quadratic integrate-and-fire neuron, which we discuss in chapters 3 and 8.

## Example: The $I_{Na,p}+I_K$-model

Let us use the $I_{Na,p}+I_K$-model (4.1, 4.2) with a high-threshold K$^+$ current to illustrate these conditions. The saddle-node bifurcation occurs when the $V$-nullcline touches the $n$-nullcline, as in Fig.6.4. Solving the equations numerically, we find that this occurs when $I_{sn} = 4.51$ and $(V_{sn}, n_{sn}) = (-60.935, 0.0007)$. The Jacobian matrix at the equilibrium,

$$L = \begin{pmatrix} 0.0435 & -290 \\ 0.00015 & -1 \end{pmatrix} ,$$

has two eigenvalues, $\lambda_1 = 0$ and $\lambda_2 = -0.9565$, with corresponding eigenvectors

$$v_1 = \begin{pmatrix} 1 \\ 0.00015 \end{pmatrix} \qquad \text{and} \qquad v_2 = \begin{pmatrix} 1 \\ 0.0034 \end{pmatrix} ,$$

depicted in the inset in Fig.6.4. (It is easy to check that $Lv_1 = 0$ and $Lv_2 = -0.9565v_2$.) The non-degeneracy and transversality conditions yield $a = 0.1887$ and $c = 1$, so that the topological normal form for the $I_{Na,p}+I_K$-model is

$$\dot{V} = (I - 4.51) + 0.1887(V + 61)^2, \qquad (6.3)$$

which can be solved analytically. The corresponding bifurcation diagrams are depicted in Fig.6.5. It is no surprise that there is a fairly good match when $I$ is near the bifurcation value.

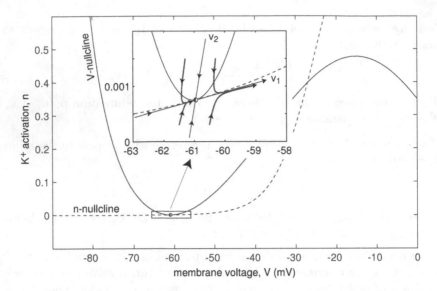

Figure 6.4: Saddle-node bifurcation in the $I_{Na,p}+I_K$-model (4.1, 4.2) with high-threshold K$^+$ current (parameters as in Fig.4.1a) and $I = 4.51$.

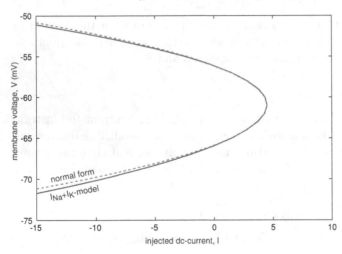

Figure 6.5: Bifurcation diagrams of the topological normal form (6.3) and the $I_{Na,p}+I_K$-model (4.1, 4.2).

## 6.1.2 Saddle-Node on Invariant Circle

As its name indicates, saddle-node on invariant circle bifurcation (also known as SNIC or SNLC bifurcation) is a standard *saddle-node* bifurcation described above with an additional condition: it occurs on an *invariant circle*, compare Fig.6.6a and 6.6b. Here, the invariant circle consists of two trajectories, called heteroclinic trajectories connecting the node and the saddle. It is called invariant because any solution starting on the circle remains on the circle. As the saddle and node coalesce, the small trajectory shrinks and the large heteroclinic trajectory becomes a homoclinic invariant circle, i.e.,

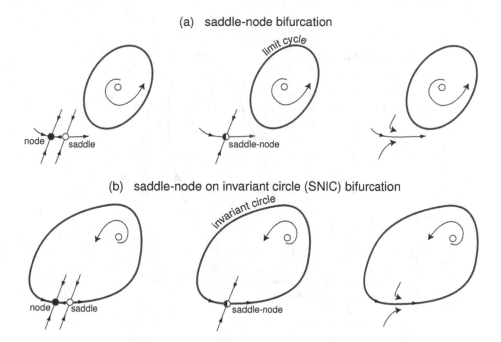

Figure 6.6: Two types of saddle-node bifurcation.

originating and terminating at the same point. When the point disappears, the circle becomes a limit cycle.

Both types of the bifurcation can occur in the $I_{Na,p}+I_K$-model, as we show in Fig.6.7. The difference between the top and the bottom of the figure is the time constant $\tau(V)$ of the K$^+$ current. Since the K$^+$ current has a high threshold, the time constant does not affect dynamics at rest, but it makes a huge difference when an action potential is generated. If the current is fast (top), it activates during the upstroke, thereby decreasing the amplitude of the action potential, and deactivates during the downstroke, thereby resulting in overshoot and another action potential. In contrast, the slower K$^+$ current (bottom) does not have time to deactivate during the downstroke, thereby resulting in undershoot (short afterhyperpolarization), with $V$ going below the resting state.

From the geometrical point of view, the phase portraits in Fig.6.6b and in Fig.6.7 (bottom), have the same topological structure: there is a homoclinic trajectory (an invariant circle) that originates at the saddle-node point, leaves its small neighborhood (to fire an action potential), then reenters the neighborhood, and terminates at the saddle-node point. This homoclinic trajectory is a limit cycle attractor with infinite period, which corresponds to firing with zero frequency. This and other neurocomputational features of saddle-node bifurcations are discussed in the next chapter. Below, we only explore how the frequency of oscillation depends on the bifurcation parameter, e.g., on the injected DC current $I$.

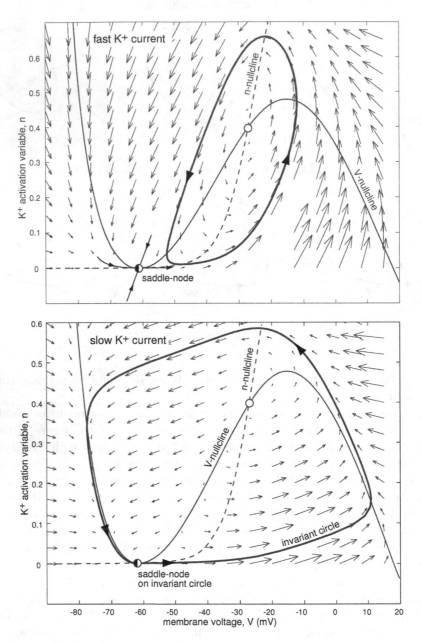

Figure 6.7: Saddle-node bifurcation in the $I_{\mathrm{Na,p}}{+}I_{\mathrm{K}}$-model with a high-threshold K$^+$ current can be off the limit cycle (top) or on the invariant circle (bottom). Parameters are as in Fig.4.1a with $\tau(V) = 0.152$ (top) or $\tau(V) = 1$ (bottom).

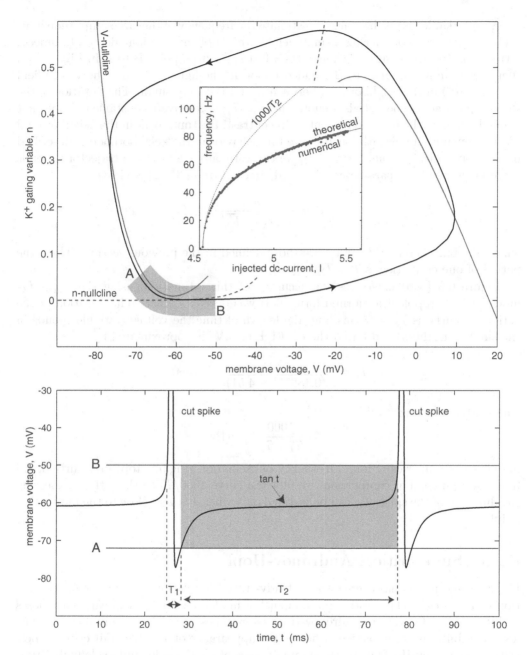

Figure 6.8: The $I_{\mathrm{Na,p}}+I_{\mathrm{K}}$-model can fire a periodic train of action potentials with arbitrary small frequency when it is near a saddle-node on invariant circle bifurcation. The trajectory moves fast from point B to A (a spike) and slowly in the shaded region from point A to B. The segment labeled "tan t" behaves like $\tan t$ in the limit of infinitesimal proximity to the bifurcation.

A remarkable fact is that one can estimate the frequency of the large-amplitude limit cycle attractor by considering a small neighborhood of the saddle-node point. Indeed, a trajectory on the limit cycle generates a fast spike from point B to A in Fig.6.8 and then slowly moves from A to B (shaded region in the figure) because the vector field (the velocity) in the neighborhood between A and B is very small. The duration of the stereotypical action potentials, denoted here as $T_1$, is relatively constant and does not depend much on the injected current $I$. In contrast, the time spent in the neighborhood (A, B) depends significantly on $I$. Since the behavior in the neighborhood is described by the topological normal form (6.2), we can estimate the time the trajectory spends there in terms of the parameters $a$, $b$, and $c$ (see exercise 3). This yields

$$T_2 = \frac{\pi}{\sqrt{ac(b - b_{\mathrm{sn}})}} \ ,$$

where the parameters $a$, $b$, and $c$ are those defined in the previous section. Thus, the period of one oscillation is $T = T_1 + T_2$.

Figure 6.8 (top) illustrates the accuracy of this estimation, using the $I_{\mathrm{Na,p}} + I_{\mathrm{K}}$-model, whose topological normal form (6.3) was derived earlier. The duration of the action potential is $T_1 = 4.7$ ms, and the length of time the voltage variable spends in the shaded neighborhood (A,B) (here $-61 \pm 11$ mV) is approximated by

$$T_2 = \frac{\pi}{\sqrt{0.1887(I - 4.51)}} \qquad \text{(ms)}.$$

The analytical curve

$$\omega = \frac{1000}{T_1 + T_2} \qquad \text{(Hz)}$$

matches the numerically found frequency of oscillation (Fig.6.8, top) in a fairly broad frequency range. For comparison, we plot the curve $1000/T_2$ to show that neglecting the duration of the spike, $T_1$, can be justified only when $I$ is very close to the bifurcation point.

### 6.1.3  Supercritical Andronov-Hopf

If a neuronal model has a monotonic steady-state I-V relation, a saddle-node bifurcation cannot occur. The resting state in such a model does not disappear, but it loses stability, typically via an Andronov-Hopf (sometimes called Hopf) bifurcation. The loss of stability is accompanied either by the appearance of a stable limit cycle (supercritical Andronov-Hopf) or by the disappearance of an unstable limit cycle (subcritical Andronov-Hopf).

Let us consider a two-dimensional system

$$\begin{aligned}
\dot{v} &= F(v, u, b) \\
\dot{u} &= G(v, u, b)
\end{aligned} \tag{6.4}$$

and suppose that $(v, u) = (0, 0)$ is an equilibrium when the bifurcation parameter $b = 0$, that is, $F(0, 0, 0) = G(0, 0, 0) = 0$. This system undergoes an *Andronov-Hopf bifurcation* at the equilibrium if the following three conditions are satisfied:

- *Non-hyperbolicity.* The Jacobian $2 \times 2$ matrix of partial derivatives at the equilibrium (see section 4.2.2),

$$L = \begin{pmatrix} F_v & F_u \\ G_v & G_u \end{pmatrix} ,$$

  has a pair of purely imaginary eigenvalues, $\pm i\omega \in \mathbb{C}$ with $\omega \neq 0$. That is, $\operatorname{tr} L = F_v + G_u = 0$ and $\omega^2 = \det L = F_v G_u - F_u G_v > 0$ at $v = u = b = 0$.

The linear change of variables

$$v = x \qquad \text{and} \qquad F_u u = -F_v x - \omega y \tag{6.5}$$

converts (6.4) into the form

$$\begin{aligned} \dot{x} &= -\omega y + f(x, y) \\ \dot{y} &= \omega x + g(x, y) , \end{aligned} \tag{6.6}$$

where the functions

$$f(x, y) = F(v, u) + \omega y \qquad \text{and} \qquad g(x, y) = -(F_v F(v, u) + F_u G(v, u))/\omega - \omega x$$

have no linear terms in $x$ and $y$. Now we are ready to state the other two conditions:

- *Non-degeneracy.* The parameter

$$a = \frac{1}{16} \left\{ f_{xxx} + f_{xyy} + g_{xxy} + g_{yyy} \right\} + \frac{1}{16\omega} \left\{ f_{xy}(f_{xx} + f_{yy}) - g_{xy}(g_{xx} + g_{yy}) - f_{xx}g_{xx} + f_{yy}g_{yy} \right\} \tag{6.7}$$

  is nonzero.

- *Transversality.* Let $c(b) \pm i\omega(b)$ denote the complex-conjugate eigenvalues of the Jacobian matrix of (6.4) for $b$ near 0, with $c(0) = 0$ and $\omega(0) = \omega$. The real part, $c(b)$, must be non-degenerate with respect to $b$, that is, $c'(0) \neq 0$.

The codimension of Andronov-Hopf bifurcation is *one*, since only one condition involves strict equality ($\operatorname{tr} L = 0$), and the other two involve inequalities ("$\neq$").

The sign of $a$ determines the type of the Andronov-Hopf bifurcation, depicted in Fig.6.9:

- *Supercritical* Andronov-Hopf bifurcation occurs when $a < 0$. It corresponds to a stable limit cycle appearing from a stable equilibrium.

- *Subcritical* Andronov-Hopf bifurcation occurs when $a > 0$. It corresponds to an unstable limit cycle shrinking to a stable equilibrium.

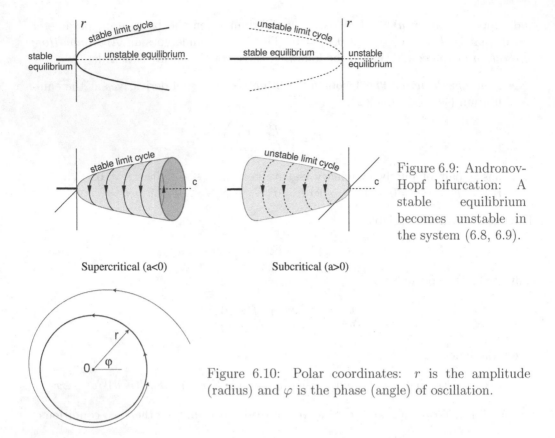

Figure 6.9: Andronov-Hopf bifurcation: A stable equilibrium becomes unstable in the system (6.8, 6.9).

Figure 6.10: Polar coordinates: $r$ is the amplitude (radius) and $\varphi$ is the phase (angle) of oscillation.

Finding $a$ in applications can be challenging. A few useful examples are considered in exercises 14–18.

Any system undergoing an Andronov-Hopf bifurcation can be reduced to the topological normal form by a change of variables (see also exercise 4)

$$\dot{r} = c(b)r + ar^3, \tag{6.8}$$
$$\dot{\varphi} = \omega(b) + dr^2, \tag{6.9}$$

where $r \geq 0$ is the amplitude (radius), and $\varphi$ is the phase (angle) of oscillation, as in Fig.6.10, and $a$, $b$, $c(b)$, and $\omega(b)$ are as above.

The function $c(b)$ in the normal form (6.8, 6.9) determines the stability of the equilibrium $r = 0$ corresponding to a non-oscillatory state (stable for $c < 0$ and unstable for $c > 0$, regardless of the value of $a$). The function $\omega(b)$ determines the frequency of damped or sustained oscillations around this state. The parameter $d$ describes how the frequency of oscillation depends on its amplitude. A state-dependent change of time can remove the term $dr^2$ from (6.9) (Kuznetsov 1995), so many assume $d = 0$ to start with.

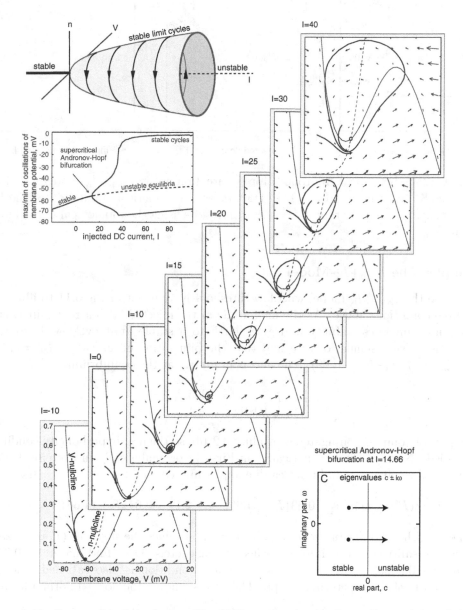

Figure 6.11: Supercritical Andronov-Hopf bifurcation in the $I_{Na,p}+I_K$-model with low-threshold K$^+$ current: As the bifurcation parameter $I$ increases, the equilibrium loses stability and gives birth to a stable limit cycle with growing amplitude. Parameters are as in Fig.4.1b.

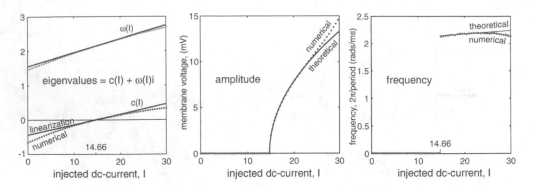

Figure 6.12: Supercritical Andronov-Hopf bifurcation in the $I_{Na,p}+I_K$-model with low-threshold K$^+$ current (see Fig.6.11). Dots represent numerical simulation of the full model, continuous curves represent analytical results using the topological normal form (6.8, 6.9).

## Example: The $I_{Na,p}+I_K$-Model

Let us use the $I_{Na,p}+I_K$-model with low-threshold K$^+$ current in Fig.6.11 to illustrate the three conditions above. As the magnitude of the injected DC current $I$ increases, the equilibrium loses stability and gives birth to a stable limit cycle with growing amplitude. Using simulations we find that the bifurcation occurs when $I_{ah} = 14.66$ and $(V_{ah}, n_{ah}) = (-56.5, 0.09)$. The Jacobian matrix at the equilibrium,

$$L = \begin{pmatrix} 1 & -335 \\ 0.0166 & -1 \end{pmatrix},$$

has a pair of complex conjugate eigenvalues $\pm 2.14$i, so the non-hyperbolicity condition is satisfied. Next, we find numerically (in Fig.6.12 or analytically in exercise 9) that the eigenvalues at the equilibrium can be approximated by

$$c(I) + \omega(I)i \approx 0.03\{I - 14.66\} \pm (2.14 + 0.04\{I - 14.66\})i$$

in a neighborhood of the bifurcation point $I = 14.66$. Since the slope of $c(I)$ is nonzero, the transversality condition is also satisfied. Using exercise 17 we find that $a = -0.0026$ and $d = -0.0029$, so that the non-degeneracy condition is also satisfied, and the bifurcation is of the supercritical type. The corresponding topological normal form is

$$\dot{r} = 0.03\{I - 14.66\}r - 0.0026r^3,$$
$$\dot{\varphi} = (2.14 + 0.04\{I - 14.66\}) - 0.0029r^2.$$

To analyze the normal form, we consider the $r$-equation and neglect the phase variable $\varphi$. From

$$r(c(b) + ar^2) = 0$$

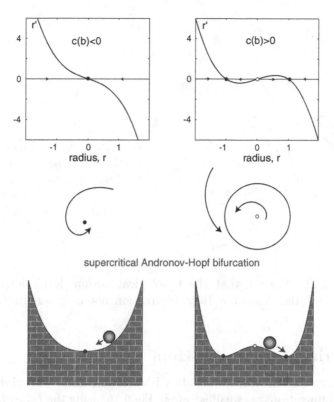

supercritical Andronov-Hopf bifurcation

Figure 6.13: Supercritical Andronov-Hopf bifurcation in (6.8, 6.9) with $c = \pm 1$ and $a = -1$ (negative values of the radial polar coordinate $r$ do not have any physical meaning).

we conclude that $r = 0$ is an equilibrium for any value of $c(b)$. Since

$$(c(b)r + ar^3)_r = c(b) \qquad \text{at } r = 0,$$

the equilibrium is stable for $c(b) < 0$ and unstable for $c(b) > 0$, as we illustrate in Fig.6.13. Indeed, the resting state in the $I_{\text{Na,p}}+I_{\text{K}}$-model is stable when $I < 14.66$ and unstable when $I > 14.66$.

When $c(b) > 0$, the normal form has a family of stable periodic solutions with amplitude

$$r = \sqrt{c(b)/|a|} \qquad \text{and} \qquad \text{(frequency)} = \omega(b) + d\,c(b)/|a| \;.$$

Hence, the $I_{\text{Na,p}}+I_{\text{K}}$-model has a family of periodic attractors with

$$r = \sqrt{0.03\{I - 14.66\}/0.0026}$$

and

$$\text{(frequency)} = (2.14 + 0.04\{I - 14.66\}) - 0.0029 \cdot 0.03\{I - 14.66\}/0.0026 \;,$$

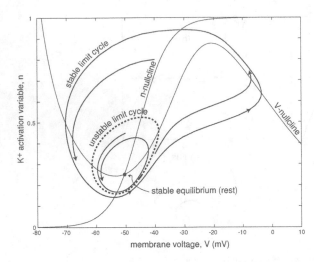

Figure 6.14: Phase portrait of the $I_{Na,p}+I_K$-model: An unstable limit cycle (dashed circle) is often surrounded by a stable one (solid circle) in two-dimensional neuronal models.

depicted in Fig.6.12. We see that the topological normal form describes the full $I_{Na,p}+I_K$-model near the Andronov-Hopf bifurcation not only qualitatively but also quantitatively.

### 6.1.4   Subcritical Andronov-Hopf

Neuronal models with monotonic steady-state I-V relations can often exhibit subcritical Andronov-Hopf bifurcations, as we illustrate in Fig.6.16, using the $I_{Na,p}+I_K$-model having a low-threshold K$^+$ current and a steep activation curve for the Na$^+$ current. The stable equilibrium in such a system is surrounded by an unstable limit cycle (dashed circle), which is often surrounded by another stable cycle, as in Fig.6.14 (not depicted in Fig.6.16 for clarity). As the magnitude of the injected DC current $I$ increases, the unstable cycle shrinks to the stable equilibrium and makes it lose stability. Systems undergoing such a bifurcation satisfy the same three conditions – non-hyperbolicity, non-degeneracy, and transversality – presented in the previous section, and they can be reduced to the topological normal form (6.8, 6.9) with positive $a$.

Analysis of the normal form shows that the stability of the non-oscillatory equilibrium $r = 0$ depends on the sign of $c(b)$:

- When $c(b) < 0$ (see Fig.6.15, left), there is a pair of equilibria, $r = \pm\sqrt{|c(b)|/a}$ corresponding to an unstable periodic solution that shrinks to $r = 0$ as $c(b) \to 0$ and makes the stable equilibrium $r = 0$ lose its stability.

- When $c(b) > 0$ (see Fig.6.15, right), the non-oscillatory state $r = 0$ is unstable, and all trajectories diverge from it.

This behavior can be clearly seen in Fig.6.16.

Finally, note that there is always a bistability (co-existence) of the resting attractor and some other attractor near a subcritical Andronov-Hopf bifurcation in two-

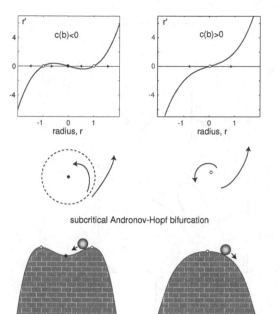

subcritical Andronov-Hopf bifurcation

Figure 6.15: Subcritical Andronov-Hopf bifurcation in (6.8, 6.9) with $c = \pm 1$ and $a = 1$.

dimensional conductance-based models, as in Fig.6.14 (in non-neural models, the trajectories can go to infinity and there need not be bistability). The bistability must also be present at the saddle-node bifurcation of an equilibrium, but may or may not be present at the saddle-node on invariant circle or at a supercritical Andronov-Hopf bifurcation.

## Delayed Loss of Stability

In Fig.6.17a we inject a ramp of current into the $I_{\text{Na,p}}+I_{\text{K}}$-model to drive it slowly through the subcritical Andronov-Hopf bifurcation point $I \approx 48.75$ (see Fig.6.16). We choose the ramp so that the bifurcation occurs exactly at $t = 100$. Even though the focus equilibrium is unstable for $t > 100$, the membrane potential remains near -50 mV, as if the equilibrium were still stable. This phenomenon, discovered by Shishkova (1973), is called *delayed loss of stability*. It is ubiquitous in simulations of smooth dynamical systems near subcritical or supercritical Andronov-Hopf bifurcations.

The mechanism of delayed loss of stability is quite simple. The state of the system is attracted to the stable focus while $t < 100$. Even though the focus loses stability at $t = 100$, the state of the system is infinitesimally close to the equilibrium, so it takes a long time to diverge from it. The longer the convergence to the equilibrium, the longer the divergence from it; hence the noticeable delay. The delay has an upper bound that depends on the smoothness of the dynamical system (Nejshtadt 1985). It can be shortened or even reversed (advanced loss of stability) by weak noise that is always present in neurons. This may explain why the delay has never been seen experimentally despite the fact that it is practically unavoidable in simulations.

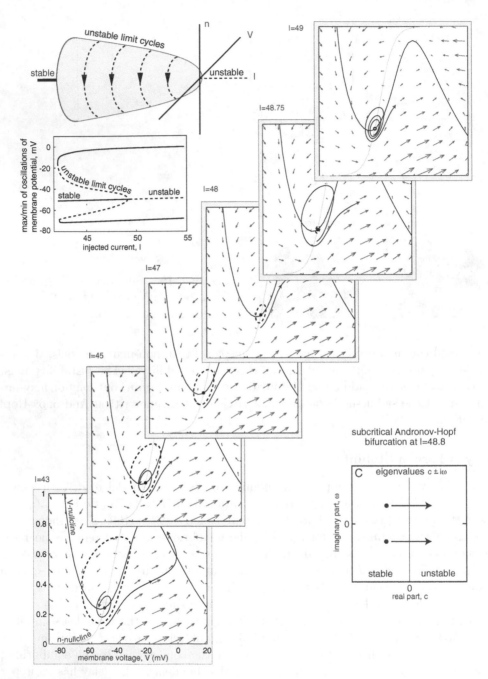

Figure 6.16: Subcritical Andronov-Hopf bifurcation in the $I_{\mathrm{Na,p}}+I_{\mathrm{K}}$-model. As the bifurcation parameter $I$ increases, an unstable limit cycle (dashed circle; see also Fig.6.14) shrinks to an equilibrium and makes it lose stability. Parameters are as in Fig.4.1b, except $g_{\mathrm{L}} = 1$, $g_{\mathrm{Na}} = g_{\mathrm{K}} = 4$, and the Na$^+$ activation function has $V_{1/2} = -30$ mV and $k = 7$.

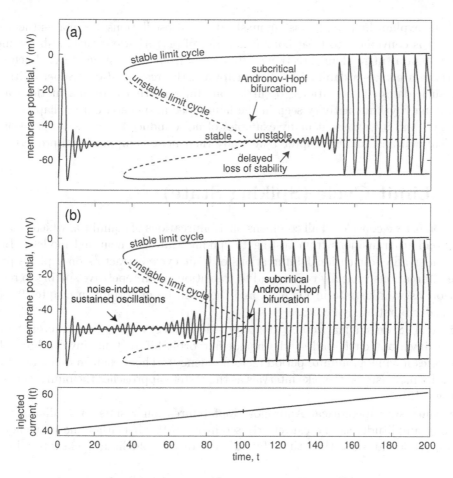

Figure 6.17: Delayed loss of stability (a) and noise-induced sustained oscillations (b) near subcritical Andronov-Hopf bifurcation. Shown are simulations of the $I_{Na,p}+I_K$-model with parameters as in Fig.6.16 and the same initial conditions. Small conductance noise is added in (b) to unmask oscillations.

## Unmasking of Oscillations by Noise

In Fig.6.17b we repeat the same simulation as in Fig.6.17a except that we add a weak conductance noise to the $I_{Na,p}+I_K$-model. Starting with the same initial conditions, the system converges to the stable focus equilibrium, as expected, exhibiting damped oscillations of membrane potential. After a while, however, it diverges from the equilibrium and exhibits sustained waxing and waning oscillations, as if there were a small amplitude limit cycle attractor with a variable amplitude. The oscillations persist until the state of the system escapes from the attraction domain of the stable focus, which is bounded by the unstable limit cycle, to the attraction domain of the large-amplitude stable limit cycle.

Let us explain how weak noise unmasks damped oscillations and makes them sustained. It is convenient to treat noise as a series of perturbations that push the membrane potential in random directions, often away from the resting state. Each such perturbation evokes a damped oscillation toward the resting state. Superposition of many such damped oscillations, occurring at different times, results in the waxing and waning rhythmic activity seen in the figure (see also exercise 3 in chapter 7). In chapters 8 and 9 we present many examples of noise-induced sustained oscillations in biological neurons, and in chapter 7 we study their neurocomputational properties.

## 6.2   Limit Cycle (Spiking State)

In section 6.1 we considered all codimension-1 bifurcations of equilibria, which typically correspond to transitions from resting to spiking states in neuronal models. Below we consider all codimension-1 bifurcations of limit cycle attractors on a phase plane. These bifurcations typically correspond to transitions from repetitive spiking to resting behavior, as we illustrate in Fig.6.19, and they will be important in chapter 9 where we consider bursting dynamics.

In Fig.6.18 we summarize how the bifurcations affect a periodic attractor. Saddle-node on invariant circle and saddle homoclinic orbit bifurcations involve homoclinic trajectories having an infinite period (zero frequency). They result in oscillations with drastically increasing interspike intervals as the system approaches the bifurcation state (see Fig.6.19).

In contrast, supercritical Andronov-Hopf bifurcation results in oscillations with vanishing amplitude, as one can clearly see in Fig.6.19. If neither the frequency nor the amplitude vanishes, then the bifurcation is of the fold limit cycle type. Indeed,

| Bifurcation of a limit cycle attractor | Amplitude | Frequency |
|---|---|---|
| saddle-node on invariant circle | nonzero | $A\sqrt{I-I_{\mathrm{b}}} \to 0$ |
| supercritical Andronov-Hopf | $A\sqrt{I-I_{\mathrm{b}}} \to 0$ | nonzero |
| fold limit cycle | nonzero | nonzero |
| saddle homoclinic orbit | nonzero | $\frac{-A}{\ln|I-I_{\mathrm{b}}|} \to 0$ |

Figure 6.18: Summary of codimension-1 bifurcations of a limit cycle attractor on a plane. $I$ denotes the amplitude of the injected current, $I_{\mathrm{b}}$ is the bifurcation value, and $A$ is a parameter that depends on the biophysical details.

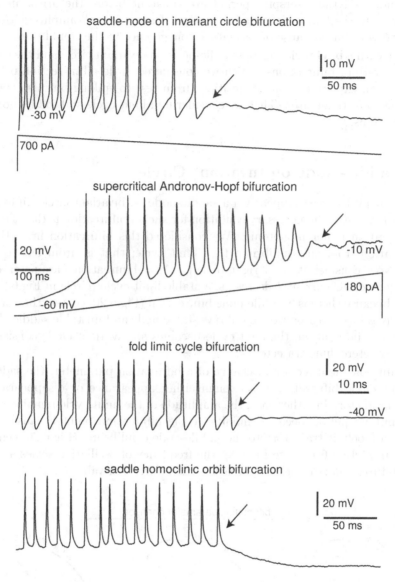

Figure 6.19: Transitions from tonic (periodic) spiking to resting occur via bifurcations of limit cycle attractors (marked by arrows). Saddle-node on invariant circle bifurcation: recording of layer 5 pyramidal neuron in rat's visual cortex. Supercritical Andronov-Hopf bifurcation: excitation block in pyramidal neuron of rat's visual cortex. Fold limit cycle bifurcation: brainstem mesencephalic V neuron of rat. Saddle homoclinic orbit bifurcation: neuron in pre-Boltzinger complex of rat brainstem. (Data provided by C. A. Del Negro and J. L. Feldman.)

the amplitude and the interspike period are constant before the arrow in Fig.6.19 corresponding to the fold limit cycle bifurcation. Damped small-amplitude oscillation after the arrow occurs because of oscillatory convergence to the equilibrium.

We start with a brief review of the saddle-node on invariant circle and the supercritical Andronov-Hopf bifurcations, which we considered in detail in section 6.1. These bifurcations can explain not only transitions from rest to spiking but also transitions from spiking to resting states. Then we consider fold limit cycle and saddle homoclinic orbit bifurcations.

### 6.2.1   Saddle-Node on Invariant Circle

A stable limit cycle can disappear via a saddle-node on invariant circle bifurcation as depicted in Fig.6.20. The necessary condition for such a bifurcation is that the steady-state I-V relation is not monotonic. We considered this bifurcation in section 6.1.2 as a bifurcation from an equilibrium to a limit cycle; that is, from left to right in Fig.6.20. Now consider it from right to left. As a bifurcation parameter changes, e.g., the injected DC current $I$ decreases, a stable limit cycle (circle in Fig.6.20, right) disappears because there is a saddle-node bifurcation (Fig.6.20, center) that breaks the cycle and gives birth to a pair of equilibria– stable node and unstable saddle (Fig.6.20, left). After the bifurcation, the limit cycle becomes an invariant circle consisting of a union of two heteroclinic trajectories.

Depending on the direction of change of a bifurcation parameter, the saddle-node on invariant circle bifurcation can explain either appearance or disappearance of a limit cycle attractor. In either case, the amplitude of the limit cycle remains relatively constant, but its period becomes infinite at the bifurcation point because the cycle becomes a homoclinic trajectory to the saddle-node equilibrium (Fig.6.20, center). As we showed in section 6.1.2 (see Fig.6.8), the frequency of oscillation scales as $\sqrt{I - I_b}$ when the bifurcation parameter approaches the bifurcation value $I_b$.

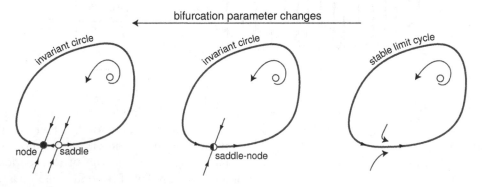

Figure 6.20: Saddle-node on invariant circle (SNIC) bifurcation of a limit cycle attractor.

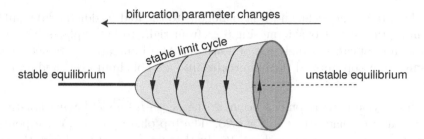

Figure 6.21: Supercritical Andronov-Hopf bifurcation of a limit cycle attractor.

## 6.2.2 Supercritical Andronov-Hopf

A stable limit cycle can shrink to a point via supercritical Andronov-Hopf bifurcation in Fig.6.21, which we considered in section 6.1.3. Indeed, as the bifurcation parameter changes, e.g., the injected DC current $I$ in Fig.6.11 decreases, the amplitude of the limit cycle attractor vanishes, and the cycle becomes a stable equilibrium. As we showed in section 6.1.3 (see Fig.6.12), the amplitude scales as $\sqrt{I - I_b}$ when the bifurcation parameter approaches the bifurcation value $I_b$.

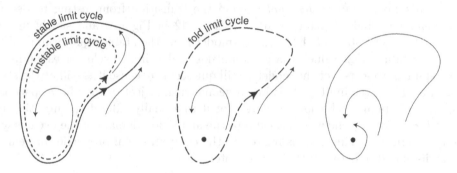

Figure 6.22: Fold limit cycle bifurcation: a stable and an unstable limit cycle approach and annihilate each other.

## 6.2.3 Fold Limit Cycle

A stable limit cycle can appear (or disappear) via the *fold limit cycle* bifurcation depicted in Fig.6.22. Consider the figure from left to right, which corresponds to the disappearance of the limit cycle, and hence to the disappearance of periodic spiking activity. As the bifurcation parameter changes, the stable limit cycle is approached by an unstable one; they coalesce and annihilate each other. At the point of annihilation, there is a periodic orbit, but it is neither stable nor unstable. More precisely, it is stable from the side corresponding to the stable cycle (outside in Fig.6.22), and unstable from the other side (inside in Fig.6.22). This periodic orbit is referred to as a fold (also known as a saddle-node) limit cycle, and it is analogous to the fold (saddle-node) equilibrium studied in section 6.1. Considering Fig.6.22 from right to left explains how a stable limit cycle can appear seemingly out of nowhere: As a bifurcation parameter changes, a fold limit cycle appears and then bifurcates into a stable limit cycle and an unstable one.

Fold limit cycle bifurcation can occur in the $I_{Na,p}+I_K$-model having low-threshold $K^+$ current, as we demonstrate in Fig.6.23. The top phase portrait, corresponding to $I = 43$, is the same as the one in Fig.6.16. In that figure we studied how the equilibrium loses stability via subcritical Andronov-Hopf bifurcation, which occurs when an unstable limit cycle shrinks to a point. We never questioned where the unstable limit cycle came from. Neither were we concerned with the existence of a large-amplitude stable limit cycle corresponding to the periodic spiking state. In Fig.6.23 we study this problem. We decrease the bifurcation parameter $I$ to see what happens with the limit cycles. As $I$ approaches the bifurcation value 42.18, the unstable and stable limit cycles approach and annihilate each other. When $I$ is less than the bifurcation value, there are no periodic orbits, only one stable equilibrium corresponding to the resting state.

Notice that the fold limit cycle bifurcation explains how (un)stable limit cycles appear or disappear, but it *does not* explain the transition from resting to periodic spiking behavior. Indeed, let us start with $I = 42$ in Fig.6.23 and slowly increase the parameter. The state of the $I_{Na,p}+I_K$-model is at the stable equilibrium. When $I$ passes the bifurcation value, a large-amplitude stable limit cycle corresponding to periodic spiking appears, yet the model is still quiescent, because it is still at the stable equilibrium. Thus, the limit cycle is just a geometrical object in the phase space that corresponds to spiking behavior. However, for it to actually exhibit spiking, the state of the system must somehow be pushed into the attraction domain of the cycle, say by external stimulation. This issue is related to the computational properties of neurons, and it is discussed in detail in the next chapter.

In Fig.6.24 we depict the bifurcation diagram of the $I_{Na,p}+I_K$-model. For each value of $I$, we simulate the model forward ($t \to \infty$) to find the stable limit cycle and backward ($t \to -\infty$) to find the unstable limit cycle. Then we plot their amplitudes (maximal voltage minus minimal voltage along the limit cycle) on the $(I, V)$-plane. One can clearly see that there is a fold limit cycle bifurcation (left) and a subcritical Andronov-Hopf bifurcation (right). The left part of the bifurcation diagram looks exactly like the one for saddle-node bifurcation, which explains why the fold limit cycle bifurcation is often referred to as *fold* or *saddle-node of periodics*.

The similarity of the fold limit cycle bifurcation and the saddle-node bifurcation is not a coincidence. Stability of limit cycles can be studied using Floquet theory or Poincare cross-section maps (Kuznetsov 1995), or by brute force (e.g., by reducing the model to an appropriate polar coordinate system). When a limit cycle attractor undergoes fold limit cycle bifurcation, its radius undergoes saddle-node bifurcation. (This is a hint for exercise 10.)

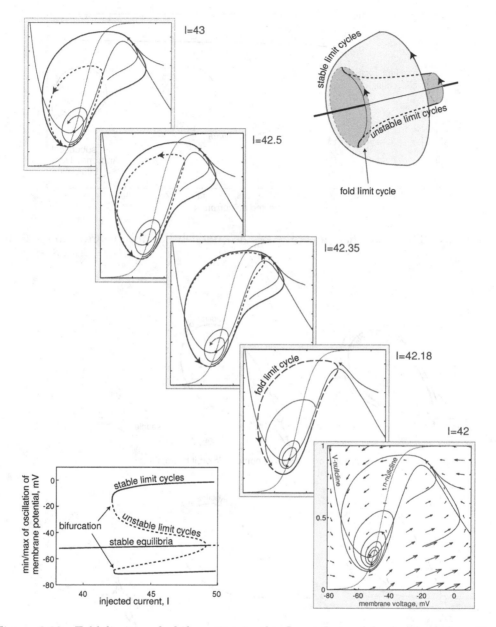

Figure 6.23: Fold limit cycle bifurcation in the $I_{\text{Na,p}}+I_{\text{K}}$-model. As the bifurcation parameter $I$ decreases, the stable and unstable limit cycles approach and annihilate each other. Parameters are as in Fig.6.16.

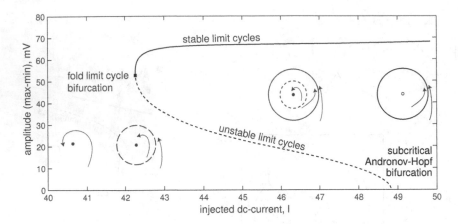

Figure 6.24: Bifurcation diagram of the $I_{\text{Na,p}}+I_{\text{K}}$-model. Parameters are as in Fig.6.16.

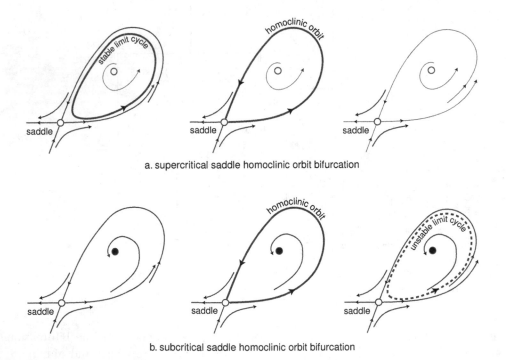

Figure 6.25: Saddle homoclinic orbit bifurcation.

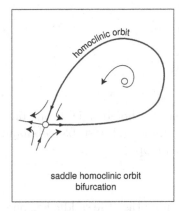 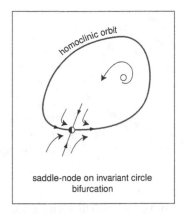

Figure 6.26: Two bifurcations involving homoclinic trajectories to an equilibrium.

## 6.2.4  Homoclinic

A limit cycle can appear or disappear via a saddle homoclinic orbit bifurcation, as depicted in Fig.6.25. As the bifurcation parameter changes, the cycle becomes a homoclinic orbit to the saddle equilibrium, and its period becomes infinite. After the bifurcation, the cycle no longer exists. A necessary condition for such a bifurcation is that the steady-state I-V relation is not monotonic.

One should be careful to distinguish the saddle homoclinic orbit bifurcation from the saddle-node on invariant circle bifurcation depicted in Fig.6.26. Indeed, it might be easy to confuse these bifurcations, since both involve an equilibrium and a large-amplitude homoclinic trajectory that becomes a limit cycle. The key difference is that the equilibrium is a saddle in the former and a saddle-node in the latter. The saddle equilibrium persists as the bifurcation parameter changes, whereas the saddle-node equilibrium disappears or bifurcates into two points, depending on the direction of change of the bifurcation parameter.

Recall that a saddle on a plane has two real eigenvalues of opposite signs. Their sum, $\lambda_1 + \lambda_2$, is called the *saddle quantity*.

- If $\lambda_1 + \lambda_2 < 0$, then the saddle homoclinic orbit bifurcation is *supercritical*, which corresponds to the (dis)appearance of a *stable* limit cycle.

- If $\lambda_1 + \lambda_2 > 0$, then the saddle homoclinic orbit bifurcation is *subcritical*, which corresponds to the (dis)appearance of an *unstable* limit cycle.

Thus, the saddle quantity plays the same role as the parameter $a$ in the Andronov-Hopf bifurcation. The supercritical saddle homoclinic orbit bifurcation is more common in neuronal models than the subcritical one for the reason explained in section 6.3.6. Hence, we consider only the supercritical case below, and we drop the word "supercritical" for the sake of brevity.

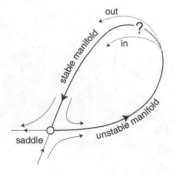

Figure 6.27: Saddle homoclinic orbit bifurcation occurs when the stable and unstable submanifolds of the saddle make a loop.

A useful way to look at the bifurcation is to note that the saddle has one stable and one unstable direction on a phase plane. There are two orbits associated with these directions, called the stable and unstable submanifolds, depicted in Fig.6.27. Typically, the submanifolds miss each other, that is, the unstable submanifold goes either inside or outside the stable one. This could happen for two different values of the bifurcation parameter. One can imagine that as the bifurcation parameter changes continuously from one value to the other, the submanifolds join at some point and form a single homoclinic trajectory that starts and ends at the saddle.

The saddle homoclinic orbit bifurcation is ubiquitous in neuronal models, and it can easily be observed in the $I_{Na,p}+I_K$-model with fast $K^+$ conductance, as we illustrate in Fig.6.28. Let us start with $I = 7$ (top of Fig.6.28) and decrease the bifurcation parameter $I$. First, there is only a stable limit cycle corresponding to periodic spiking activity. When $I$ decreases, a stable equilibrium and an unstable equilibrium appear via saddle-node bifurcation (not shown in the figure), but the state of the model is still on the limit cycle attractor. Further decrease of $I$ moves the saddle equilibrium closer to the limit cycle (case $I = 4$ in the figure), until the cycle becomes an infinite period homoclinic orbit to the saddle (case $I \approx 3.08$), and then disappears (case $I = 1$). At this moment, the state of the system approaches the stable equilibrium, and the tonic spiking stops.

Similar to the fold limit cycle bifurcation, the saddle homoclinic orbit bifurcation explains how the limit cycle attractor corresponding to periodic spiking behavior appears and disappears. However, it does not explain the transition to periodic spiking behavior. Indeed, when $I = 4$ in Fig.6.28, the limit cycle attractor exists, yet the neuron may still be quiescent because its state may be at the stable node. The periodic spiking behavior appears only after external perturbations push the state of the system into the attraction domain of the limit cycle attractor, or $I$ increases further and the stable node disappears via a saddle-node bifurcation.

We can use linear theory to estimate the frequency of the limit cycle attractor near the saddle homoclinic orbit bifurcation. Because the vector field is small near the equilibrium, the periodic trajectory passes slowly through a small neighborhood of the equilibrium, then quickly makes a rotation and returns to the neighborhood, as we illustrate in Fig.6.29. Let $T_1$ denote the time required to make one rotation

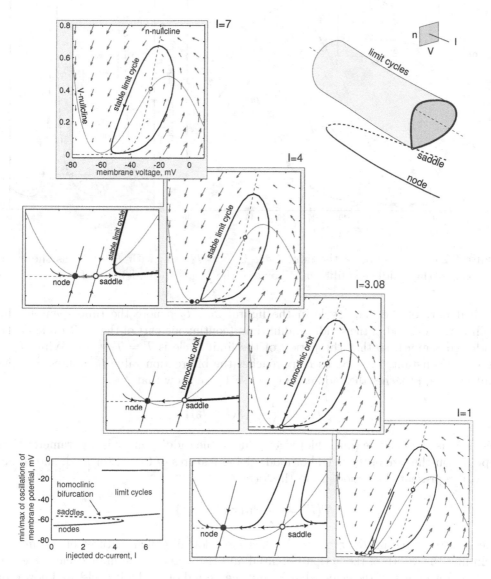

Figure 6.28: Saddle homoclinic orbit bifurcation in the $I_{\mathrm{Na,p}}+I_{\mathrm{K}}$-model with parameters as in Fig.4.1a and fast K$^+$ current ($\tau(V) = 0.16$). As the bifurcation parameter $I$ decreases, the stable limit cycle becomes a homoclinic orbit to a saddle.

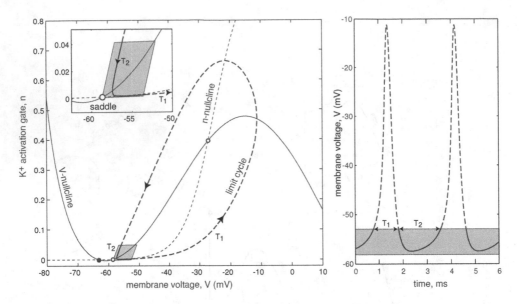

Figure 6.29: The period of the limit cycle is $T = T_1 + T_2$ with $T_2 \to \infty$ as the cycle approaches the saddle equilibrium. Shown is the $I_{\mathrm{Na,p}}+I_{\mathrm{K}}$-model with $I = 3.5$.

(dashed part of the limit cycle in the figure) and $T_2$ denote the time spent in the small neighborhood of the saddle equilibrium (continuous part of the limit cycle in the shadowed region), so that the period of the limit cycle is $T = T_1 + T_2$. While $T_1$ is relatively constant, $T_2 \to \infty$ as $I$ approaches the bifurcation value $I_{\mathrm{b}} = 3.08$, and the limit cycle approaches the saddle. In exercise 11 we show that

$$T_2 = -\frac{1}{\lambda_1} \ln\{\tau(I - I_{\mathrm{b}})\} \, ,$$

where $\lambda_1$ is the positive (unstable) eigenvalue of the saddle, and $\tau$ is a parameter that depends on the size of the neighborhood, global features of the vector field, and so on. We can represent the period, $T$, in the form

$$T(I) = -\frac{1}{\lambda_1} \ln\{\tau_1(I - I_{\mathrm{b}})\} \, ,$$

where a single parameter $\tau_1 = \tau e^{-\lambda_1 T_1}$ accounts for all global features of the model, including the width of the action potential and the shape of the limit cycle. One can easily determine $\tau_1$ if the eigenvalue $\lambda_1$ and the period of the limit cycle are known for at least one value of $I$. The $I_{\mathrm{Na,p}}+I_{\mathrm{K}}$-model has $\tau_1 = 0.2$, as we show in Fig.6.30. Note that the theoretical frequency $1000/T(I)$ matches the numerically found frequency in a broad range. Also note how imprecise the numerical results are (see inset in the figure).

Both the saddle-node on invariant circle bifurcation and the saddle homoclinic orbit bifurcation result in spiking with decreasing frequency, so that their frequency-current

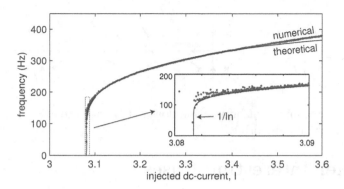

Figure 6.30: Frequency of spiking in the $I_{Na,p}+I_K$-model with parameters as in Fig.6.28 near a saddle homoclinic orbit bifurcation. Dots are numerical results; the continuous curve is $\omega(I) = 1000\lambda(I)/\{-\ln(0.2(I-3.0814))\}$, where the eigenvalue $\lambda(I) = 0.87\sqrt{4.51-I}$ was obtained from the normal form (6.3). The inset shows a magnified region near the bifurcation value $I = 3.0814$.

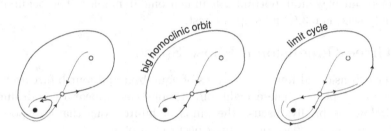

Figure 6.31: Big saddle homoclinic orbit bifurcation.

(F-I) curves go continuously to zero. The key difference is that the former asymptotes as $\sqrt{I-I_b}$, and the latter as $1/\ln(I-I_b)$. The striking feature of the logarithmic decay in Fig.6.30 is that the frequency is greater than 100 Hz and the theoretical curve does not seem to go to zero for all $I$ except those in an infinitesimal neighborhood of the bifurcation value $I_b$. Such a neighborhood is almost impossible to catch numerically, let alone experimentally in real neurons.

Many neuronal models, and even some cortical pyramidal neurons (see Fig.7.42) exhibit a saddle homoclinic orbit bifurcation depicted in Fig.6.31. Here, the unstable manifold of a saddle returns to the saddle along the opposite side, thereby making a big loop; hence the name *big saddle homoclinic orbit* bifurcation. This kind of bifurcation often occurs when an excitable system is near a codimension-2 Bogdanov-Takens bifurcation considered in section 6.3.3, and it has the same properties as the "small" homoclinic orbit bifurcation considered above: it can be subcritical or supercritical, depending on the saddle quantity; it results in a logarithmic F-I curve; and it implies the coexistence of attractors. All methods of analysis of excitable systems near "small" saddle homoclinic orbit bifurcations can also be applied to the case in Fig.6.31.

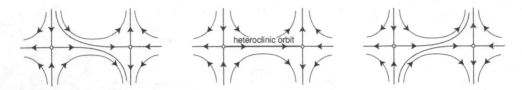

Figure 6.32: Heteroclinic orbit bifurcation does not change the existence or stability of any equilibrium or periodic orbit.

## 6.3    Other Interesting Cases

Saddle-node and Andronov-Hopf bifurcations of equilibria, combined with fold limit cycle, homoclinic orbit bifurcation, and heteroclinic orbit bifurcation (see Fig.6.32), exhaust all possible bifurcations of codimension-1 on a plane. These bifurcations can also occur in higher-dimensional systems. Below we discuss additional codimension-1 bifurcations in three-dimensional phase space, and then we consider some codimension-2 bifurcations that play an important role in neuronal dynamics. The beginning reader may read only section 6.3.6 and skip the rest.

### 6.3.1    Three-Dimensional Phase Space

So far we have considered four bifurcations of equilibria and four bifurcations of limit cycles on a phase plane. These eight bifurcations can appear in multidimensional systems. Below we briefly discuss the kinds of bifurcations that are possible in a three-dimensional phase space but cannot occur on a plane.

First, there are no new bifurcations of *equilibria* in multidimensional phase space. Indeed, what could possibly happen with the Jacobian matrix of an equilibrium of a multidimensional dynamical system? A simple zero eigenvalue would result in a saddle-node bifurcation, and a simple pair of purely imaginary complex-conjugate eigenvalues would result in an Andronov-Hopf bifurcation. Both are exactly the same as in the lower-dimensional systems already considered. Thus, adding dimensions to a dynamical system does not create new possibilities for bifurcations of equilibria.

In contrast, adding the third dimension to a planar dynamical system creates new possibilities for bifurcations of *limit cycles*, some of which are depicted in Fig.6.33. Below we briefly describe these bifurcations.

The *saddle-focus homoclinic orbit* bifurcation in Fig.6.33 is similar to the saddle homoclinic orbit bifurcation considered in section 6.2.4, except that the equilibrium has a pair of complex-conjugate eigenvalues and a nonzero real eigenvalue. The homoclinic orbit originates in the subspace spanned by the eigenvector corresponding to the real eigenvalue (as in Fig.6.33) and terminates along the subspace spanned by the eigenvectors corresponding to the complex-conjugate pair. The reverse direction is also possible. Depending on the direction and the relative magnitude of the eigenvalues, this bifurcation can result in the (dis)appearance or a stable (supercritical) or unstable (subcritical) twisted large-period orbit.

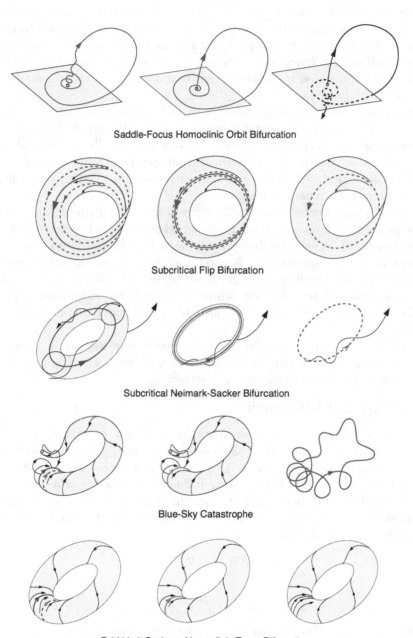

Figure 6.33: Some codimension-1 bifurcations of limit cycles in three-dimensional phase space (modified from Izhikevich 2000a).

The *subcritical flip* bifurcation in Fig.6.33 occurs when a stable periodic orbit is surrounded by an unstable orbit of twice the period. The unstable periodic orbit shrinks to the stable one and makes it lose stability. This bifurcation is similar to the pitchfork bifurcation studied below, except that it has codimension-1 (pitchfork bifurcation has infinite codimension unless one considers dynamical systems with symmetry). A supercritical flip bifurcation is similar, except that an unstable cycle is surrounded by a stable double-period cycle.

The *subcritical Neimark-Sacker* bifurcation in Fig.6.33 occurs when a stable periodic orbit is surrounded by an unstable invariant torus. The latter shrinks and makes the periodic orbit lose its stability. In some sense, which we will not elaborate on here, this bifurcation is similar to the supercritical Andronov-Hopf bifurcation of an equilibrium. The supercritical Neimark-Sacker bifurcation occurs when an unstable orbit is surrounded by a stable invariant torus.

The *blue-sky catastrophe* in Fig.6.33 occurs when a small-amplitude stable limit cycle disappears and a large-amplitude large-period stable orbit appears out of nowhere (from the blue sky). The orbit has an infinite period at the bifurcation, yet it is not homoclinic to any equilibrium. A careful analysis shows that the large orbit is homoclinic to the small limit cycle at the moment the cycle disappears. In some sense, which we elaborate on later, this bifurcation is similar to the saddle-node on invariant circle bifurcation (see exercise 20). In particular, both bifurcations share the same asymptotics.

The *fold limit cycle on homoclinic torus* bifurcation in Fig.6.33 is similar to the blue-sky catastrophe except that the disappearance of the small periodic orbit results in a large-amplitude torus (quasi-periodic) attractor.

### 6.3.2   Cusp and Pitchfork

Recall that an equilibrium $x_b$ of a one-dimensional system $\dot{x} = f(x, b)$ is at a saddle-node bifurcation when $f_x = 0$ (first derivative of $f$) but $f_{xx} \neq 0$ (second derivative of $f$) at the equilibrium. The latter is called the non-degeneracy condition, and it guarantees that the system dynamics is equivalent to that of $\dot{x} = c(b) + x^2$.

If $f_x = 0$ and $f_{xx} = 0$, but $f_{xxx} \neq 0$, then the equilibrium is at the codimension-2 *cusp* bifurcation, and the behavior of the system near the equilibrium can be described by the topological normal form

$$\dot{x} = c_1(b) + c_2(b)x + ax^3,$$

where

$$c_1(b) = f(x_b, b) , \qquad c_2(b) = f_x(x_b, b) , \qquad a = f_{xxx}/6 \neq 0 ,$$

in particular, $c_1 = c_2 = 0$ at the cusp point. The cusp bifurcation is supercritical when $a < 0$ and subcritical otherwise. It is explained by the shape of the surface

$$c_1 + c_2 x + ax^3 = 0 ,$$

depicted in Fig.6.34.

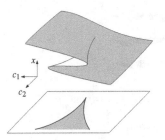

Figure 6.34: Cusp surface.

Let us treat $c_1$ and $c_2$ as independent parameters, and check that there are saddle-node bifurcations in any neighborhood of the cusp point. The bifurcation sets of the topological normal form can easily be found. Differentiating $c_1 + c_2 x + a x^3$ with respect to $x$ gives $c_2 + 3 a x^2$. Equating both of these expressions to zero and eliminating $x$ gives two saddle-node bifurcation curves

$$c_1 = \pm \frac{2}{\sqrt{a}} \left( \frac{c_2}{3} \right)^{3/2},$$

depicted at the bottom of Fig.6.34. Since $c_1 = c_1(b)$ and $c_2 = c_2(b)$, varying the bifurcation parameter $b$ results in a path on the $(c_1, c_2)$-plane. Depending on the shape and location of this path, one can get many one-dimensional bifurcation diagrams. A summary of some special cases is depicted in Fig.6.35, showing that there can be many interesting dynamical regimes in the vicinity of a cusp bifurcation point.

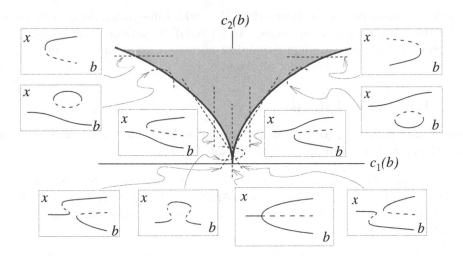

Figure 6.35: Summary of special cases for the supercritical cusp bifurcation. Dotted segments are paths $c_1 = c_1(b)$, $c_2 = c_2(b)$, where $b$ is a one-dimensional bifurcation parameter. The corresponding bifurcation diagrams are depicted in boxes. Continuous curves represent stable solutions, dashed curves represent unstable solutions. (Modified from Hoppensteadt and Izhikevich 1997.)

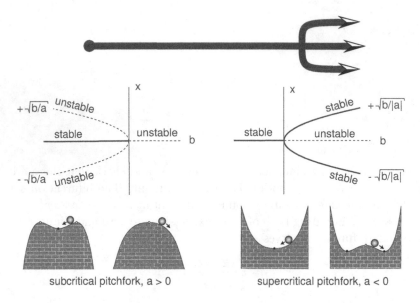

Figure 6.36: Pitchfork bifurcation diagrams.

An important special case is when $c_1 = 0$ and $c_2(b) = b$, so that the topological normal form is

$$\dot{x} = bx + ax^3.$$

This form corresponds to a *pitchfork* bifurcation, whose diagram is depicted in Fig.6.36 (see also the bottom bifurcation diagram in Fig.6.35). This bifurcation has an infinite codimension unless one considers dynamical systems with symmetry, such as, $\dot{x} = f(x, b)$ with $f(-x, b) = -f(x, b)$ for all $x$ and $b$.

### 6.3.3  Bogdanov-Takens

Can an equilibrium undergo Andronov-Hopf and saddle-node bifurcations simultaneously? There are two possibilities, illustrated in Fig.6.37:

- *Fold-Hopf.* The Jacobian matrix at the equilibrium has a pair of pure imaginary complex-conjugate eigenvalues (Andronov-Hopf bifurcation) and one zero eigenvalue (saddle-node bifurcation). In this case the two bifurcations occur in different subspaces.

- *(Bogdanov-Takens)* The Jacobian matrix has two zero eigenvalues. In this case the two bifurcations occur in the same subspace.

The fold-Hopf bifurcations occur in systems having dimension 3 and up, while the Bogdanov-Takens bifurcation can occur in two-dimensional systems. Both bifurcations have codimension-2; that is, they require two bifurcation parameters. Note that the

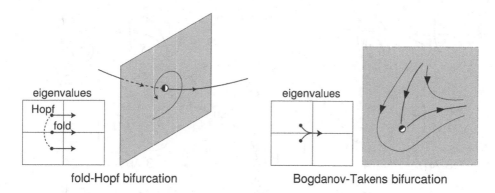

fold-Hopf bifurcation        Bogdanov-Takens bifurcation

Figure 6.37: Two ways an equilibrium can undergo a saddle-node (fold) and an Andronov-Hopf bifurcation simultaneously.

fold-Hopf bifurcation has three eigenvalues with zero real part, whereas the Bogdanov-Takens bifurcation has only two zero eigenvalues. This bifurcation can, on the one hand, be viewed as a saddle-node bifurcation in which another (negative) eigenvalue gets arbitrarily close to zero, and, on the other hand, as an Andronov-Hopf bifurcation in which the imaginary part of the complex-conjugate eigenvalues goes to zero.

The Jacobian matrix of an equilibrium at the Bogdanov-Takens bifurcation satisfies two conditions: $\det L = 0$ (saddle-node bifurcation) and $\operatorname{tr} L = 0$ (Andronov-Hopf bifurcation). For example, it can have the form

$$L = \begin{pmatrix} 0 & 1 \\ 0 & 0 \end{pmatrix} . \tag{6.10}$$

Because of these two conditions, the codimension of this bifurcation is 2. There are also certain non-degeneracy and transversality conditions (see Kuznetsov 1995). The corresponding topological normal form,

$$\begin{aligned} \dot{u} &= v \,, \\ \dot{v} &= a + bu + u^2 + \sigma uv \,, \end{aligned} \tag{6.11}$$

has two bifurcation parameters, $a$ and $b$, and the parameter $\sigma = \pm 1$ determines whether the bifurcation is subcritical or supercritical. This parameter depends on the combination of the second-order partial derivatives with respect to the first variable, and it is nonzero because of the non-degeneracy conditions (Kuznetsov 1995). The bifurcation diagram and representative phase portraits for various $a, b$, and $\sigma$ are depicted in Fig.6.38 (the case $\sigma > 0$ can be reduced to $\sigma < 0$ by the substitutions $t \rightarrow -t$ and $v \rightarrow -v$). A remarkable fact is that the saddle-node and the Andronov-Hopf bifurcations do not occur alone. There is also a saddle homoclinic orbit bifurcation always appearing near the Bogdanov-Takens point.

Bogdanov-Takens bifurcation often occurs in neuronal models with nullclines intersecting as in Fig.6.39a. We show in the next chapter that this bifurcation separates

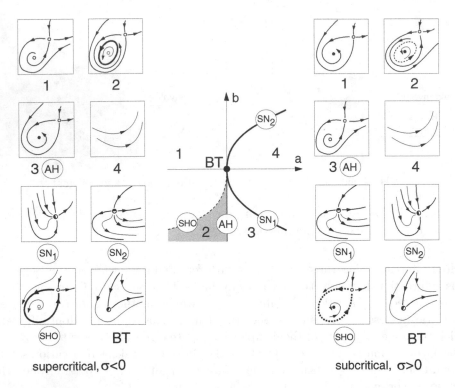

Figure 6.38: Bogdanov-Takens (BT) bifurcation diagram of the topological normal form (6.11). Abbreviations: AH, Andronov-Hopf bifurcation; SN, saddle-node bifurcation; SHO, saddle homoclinic orbit bifurcation.

integrators from resonators, and it can occur in some layer 5 pyramidal neurons of rat visual cortex, as we discuss in section 7.2.11 and 8.2.1. The two equilibria in the lower (left) knee of the fast nullcline in Fig.6.39b are not necessarily a saddle and a stable node, but can be a saddle and an (un)stable focus, as in the phase portraits in Fig.6.38.

Interestingly, the global vector field structure of neuronal models with nullclines as in Fig.6.39a results in the birth of a spiking limit cycle attractor via a big saddle homoclinic orbit bifurcation, so the neuronal model undergoes a cascade of bifurcations, depicted in Fig.6.40, as the amplitude of the injected current $I$ increases. The local phase portraits corresponding to $I_0$, $I_1$, and $I_2$ are topologically equivalent to the phase portrait "1" in Fig.6.38 (right). (The equivalence is local near the left knee; there is no global equivalence because of the extra equilibrium in Fig.6.40 and because of the big homoclinic or periodic orbit.) As $I$ increases, a stable large-amplitude spiking limit cycle appears via a big supercritical homoclinic orbit bifurcation at some $I_1$. It coexists with the stable resting state for all $I_1 < I < I_5$. At some point $I_2$, the saddle quantity, i.e., the sum of its eigenvalues, changes from negative to positive (it is zero at the Bogdanov-Takens bifurcation), so another saddle homoclinic orbit

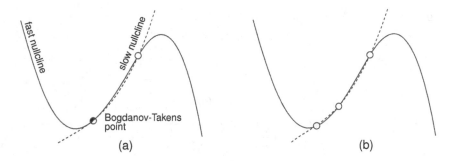

Figure 6.39: Intersection of nullclines of a two-dimensional system, resulting in Bogdanov-Takens bifurcation.

bifurcation (at some $I_3$) occurs, which is subcritical, giving birth to an unstable limit cycle. The phase portrait at $I_3$ is locally topologically equivalent to the one marked SHO in Fig.6.38. Similarly, the phase portrait at $I_4$ is locally equivalent to the one labeled "2" in Fig.6.38. The unstable cycle shrinks to the equilibrium and makes it lose stability via a subcritical Andronov-Hopf bifurcation at some $I_5$, which corresponds to case AH in Fig.6.38. Further increase of $I$ converts the unstable focus into an unstable node, which approaches the saddle and disappears via the saddle-node bifurcation $SN_1$ in Fig.6.38 (not shown in Fig.6.40).

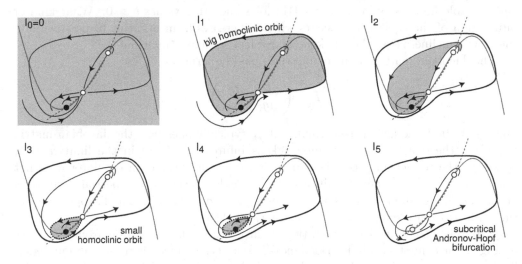

Figure 6.40: Transformations of phase portraits of a neuronal model near the subcritical Bogdanov-Takens bifurcation point as the magnitude of the injected current $I$ increases (here $I_{k+1} > I_k$). Shaded regions are the attraction domains of the equilibrium corresponding to the resting state.

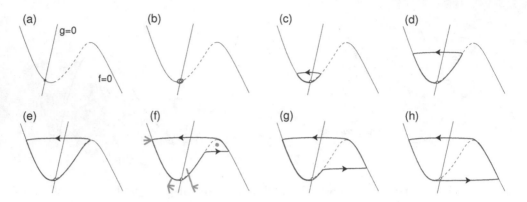

Figure 6.41: Canard (French duck) limit cycles in a relaxation oscillator (hand drawing).

## 6.3.4   Relaxation Oscillators and Canards

Let us consider a relaxation oscillator

$$\begin{aligned}\dot{x} &= f(x, y, b) &&\text{(fast variable)}\\\dot{y} &= \mu g(x, y, b) &&\text{(slow variable)}\end{aligned}$$

with fast and slow nullclines, as in Fig.6.41a, and $\mu \ll 1$. Suppose that there is a stable equilibrium, as in Fig.6.41a, for some values of the bifurcation parameter $b < 0$, and a stable limit cycle, as in Fig.6.41h, for some other values $b > 0$. What kind of bifurcation of the equilibrium occurs when $b$ increases from negative to positive, and the slow nullcline passes the left knee of the fast N-shaped nullcline?

The Jacobian matrix at the equilibrium has the form

$$L = \begin{pmatrix} f_x & f_y \\ \mu g_x & \mu g_y \end{pmatrix}$$

Since $f_x = 0$ at the knee (prove this), but $f_y$ typically does not, the Jacobian matrix resembles the one for the Bogdanov-Takens bifurcation (6.10) in the limit $\mu = 0$. However, the resemblance is only superficial, since the relaxation oscillator does not satisfy the non-degeneracy conditions. In particular, second-order partial derivatives of $\mu g(x, y, b)$ vanish in the limit $\mu \to 0$, resulting in $\sigma = 0$ and in the disappearance of the term $u^2$ from the topological normal form (6.11).

A purely geometrical consideration confirms that the transition from Fig.6.41a to Fig.6.41h cannot be of the Bogdanov-Takens type, since there is a unique equilibrium and no possibility for a saddle-node bifurcation, which always accompanies the Bogdanov-Takens bifurcation. Actually, the equilibrium loses stability via an Andronov-Hopf bifurcation that occurs when

$$\text{tr } L = f_x + \mu g_y = 0 \qquad \text{and} \qquad \det L = \mu(f_x g_y - f_y g_x) > 0 \, .$$

The loss of stability typically happens not at the left knee, where $f_x = 0$, but a little to the right of the knee, where $f_x = -\mu g_y > 0$ (because $g_y < 0$ in neuronal models). We saw this phenomenon in section 4.2.6 when we considered FitzHugh-Nagumo model.

An interesting observation is that the period of damped or sustained oscillations near the Andronov-Hopf bifurcation point in Fig.6.41b is of the order $1/\sqrt{\mu}$, because the frequency $\omega = \sqrt{\det L} \approx \sqrt{\mu}$, whereas the period of large-amplitude relaxation oscillation is of the order $1/\mu$, because it takes $1/\mu$ units of time to slide up and down along the branches of the fast nullcline in Fig.6.41h. Thus, the period of small subthreshold oscillations of a neural model may have no relation to the period of spiking, if the model has many time scales.

The Andronov-Hopf bifurcation can be supercritical or subcritical, depending on the functions $f$ and $g$; see exercise 14 and exercise 18. Figure 6.41 depicts the supercritical case. In the subcritical case, stable and unstable limit cycles are typically born via fold limit cycle bifurcation; then the unstable limit cycle goes through the shapes as in Fig.6.41g, f, e, d, c, and b, and finally shrinks to a point.

## Canards

The distinctive feature of limit cycles in Fig.6.41c–6.41g is that they follow the unstable branch (dashed curve) of the fast nullcline before jumping to the left or to the right (stable) branch. Due to the relaxation nature of the system, the vector field is horizontal outside the N-shape fast nullcline, so any transition from Fig.6.41b to Fig.6.41h must gradually go through the stages in Fig.6.41c–6.41g. Because the cycle in Fig.6.41f resembles a *duck*, at least in the eyes of the French mathematicians E. Benoit, J.-L. Callot, F. Diener, and M. Diener, who discovered this phenomenon in 1977, it is often called a *canard (French duck) cycle*.

In general, any trajectory that follows the unstable branch is called a *canard trajectory*. Canard trajectories play an important role in defining thresholds for resonator neurons, as we discuss in section 7.2.5. It takes on the order of $1/\mu$ units of time to slide along the unstable branch of the fast nullcline. A small perturbation to the left or to the right can result in an immediate jump to the corresponding stable branch of the nullcline. Hence, the initial conditions should be specified with an unrealistic precision of the order of $e^{-1/\mu}$ to follow the unstable branch, which explains why the canard trajectories are difficult to catch numerically, let alone experimentally. Consequently, the canard cycles, though stable, exists in an exponentially small region of values of the parameter $b$. A typical simulation shows a sudden explosion of a stable limit cycle from small (Fig.6.41b) to large (Fig.6.41h) as the parameter $b$ is slowly varied. In summary, canard cycles in two-dimensional relaxation oscillators play an important role of thresholds, but they are fragile and rather exceptional.

In contrast, canard trajectories in three-dimensional relaxation oscillators (one fast and two slow variables) are generic in the sense that they exist in a wide range of parameter values. A simple way to see this is to treat $b$ as the second slow variable. Then there is a set of initial conditions corresponding to the canard trajectories. Studying canards in $\mathbb{R}^3$ goes beyond the scope of this book (see bibliographical notes).

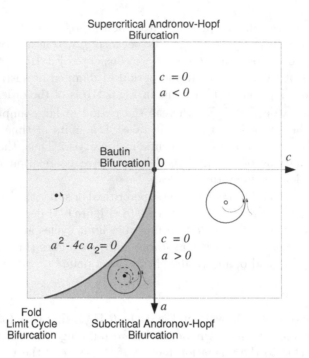

Figure 6.42: Supercritical Bautin bifurcation in (6.12); see also Fig.9.42 (left).

## 6.3.5 Bautin

What happens when a subcritical Andronov-Hopf bifurcation becomes supercritical, that is, when the parameter $a$ in the topological normal form for Andronov-Hopf bifurcation (6.8, 6.9) changes sign? The bifurcation becomes degenerate when $a = 0$, and the behavior of the system is described by the topological normal form for *Bautin bifurcation*, which we write here in the complex form

$$\dot{z} = (c + i\omega)z + az|z|^2 + a_2 z|z|^4, \tag{6.12}$$

where $z \in \mathbb{C}$ is a complex variable, and $c, a$, and $a_2$ are real parameters. The parameters $a$ and $a_2$ are called the first and second *Liapunov* (often spelled *Lyapunov*) *coefficients*. The Bautin bifurcation occurs when $a = c = 0$ and $a_2 \neq 0$, and hence it has codimension-2. It is subcritical when $a_2 > 0$ and supercritical otherwise. If $a_2 = 0$, then one needs to consider the next term $a_3 z|z|^6$, not shown in the normal form (6.12), to get a bifurcation of codimension-3, and so on.

We can easily determine bifurcations of the topological normal form. First of all, (6.12) undergoes Andronov-Hopf bifurcation when $c = 0$, which is supercritical for $a < 0$ and subcritical otherwise. Moreover, if $a$ and $a_2$ have different signs, then (6.12) undergoes fold limit cycle bifurcation when

$$a^2 - 4ca_2 = 0 \,,$$

as we illustrate in Fig.6.42. Thus, both Andronov-Hopf and fold limit cycle bifurcations occur simultaneously at the Bautin point $a = c = 0$. Many two-dimensional neuronal models, such as the $I_{\mathrm{Na,p}}+I_{\mathrm{K}}$-model with low-threshold K$^+$ current, are relatively near this bifurcation, which explains why the unstable limit cycle involved in the subcritical Andronov-Hopf bifurcation is usually born via fold limit cycle bifurcation. There is some evidence that rodent trigeminal interneurons, dorsal root ganglion neurons, and mes V neuron in the brainstem are also near this bifurcation; see section 9.3.3.

## 6.3.6  Saddle-Node Homoclinic Orbit

Let us compare the saddle-node on invariant circle bifurcation and the saddle homoclinic orbit bifurcation depicted in Fig.6.43 (top). In both cases there is a homoclinic orbit (i.e., a trajectory that originates and terminates at the same equilibrium). However, the equilibria are of different types, and the orbit returns to them along different directions. Now suppose a system undergoes both bifurcations simultaneously, as we illustrate in Fig.6.43 (bottom). Such a bifurcation, called *saddle-node homoclinic orbit* bifurcation, has codimension-2, since two strict conditions must be satisfied. First, the equilibrium must be at the saddle-node bifurcation point, i.e., must have the eigenvalue $\lambda_1 = 0$. Second, the homoclinic trajectory must return to the equilibrium along the noncentral direction, i.e., along the stable direction corresponding to the negative eigenvalue $\lambda_2$. Since the saddle-node quantity, $\lambda_1 + \lambda_2$, is always negative, this bifurcation always results in the (dis)appearance of a *stable* limit cycle.

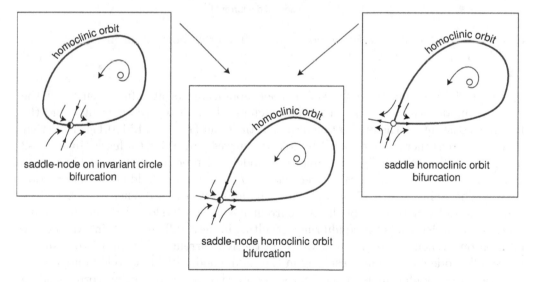

Figure 6.43: Saddle-node homoclinic orbit bifurcation occurs when a system undergoes a saddle-node on invariant circle and saddle homoclinic orbit bifurcations simultaneously.

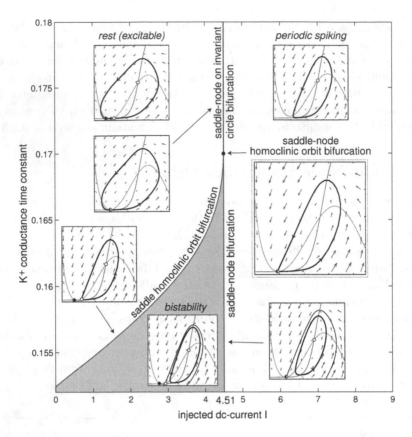

Figure 6.44: Unfolding of saddle-node homoclinic orbit bifurcation in the $I_{\text{Na,p}}+I_{\text{K}}$-model with parameters as in Fig.6.28.

In Fig.6.44 we illustrate the saddle-node homoclinic orbit bifurcation using the $I_{\text{Na,p}}+I_{\text{K}}$-model with two bifurcation parameters: the injected DC current $I$ and the K$^+$ time constant $\tau$. The bifurcation occurs at the point $(I, \tau) = (4.51, 0.17)$. Note that there are three other codimension-1 bifurcation curves converging to this codimension-2 point, as we illustrate in Fig.6.45. Since the model undergoes a saddle-node bifurcation at $I = 4.51$ and any $\tau$, the straight vertical line $I = 4.51$ is the saddle-node bifurcation curve. The point $\tau = 0.17$ on this line separates two cases. When $\tau > 0.17$, the activation and deactivation of the K$^+$ current is sufficiently slow that the membrane potential $V$ undershoots the equilibrium, resulting in the saddle-node *on* invariant circle bifurcation. When $\tau < 0.17$, deactivation of the K$^+$ current is fast, and $V$ overshoots the saddle-node equilibrium, resulting in the saddle-node *off* limit cycle bifurcation.

Shaded triangular areas in the figures denote the parameter region corresponding to the bistability of stable equilibrium and a limit cycle attractor (resting and spiking states). Let us decrease the parameter $I$ and cross such a region from right to left. When $I = 4.51$, a saddle equilibrium and a node equilibrium appear. Further

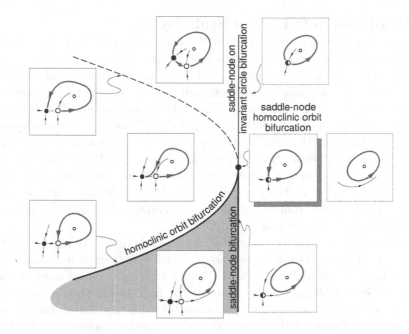

Figure 6.45: Unfolding of saddle-node homoclinic orbit bifurcation.

decreasing $I$ moves the saddle equilibrium rightward and the limit cycle leftward, until they merge. This occurs on the saddle homoclinic orbit bifurcation curve, which is determined numerically in Fig.6.44.

Neuronal models exhibiting saddle-node homoclinic bifurcations can be reduced to a topological normal form

$$\dot{V} = c(b - b_{\text{sn}}) + a(V - V_{\text{sn}})^2, \qquad \text{if } V(t) = V_{\text{max}}, \text{ then } V(t) \leftarrow V_{\text{reset}}, \qquad (6.13)$$

which is similar to that for saddle-node bifurcation (6.2), except that there is a reset $V \leftarrow V_{\text{reset}}$ when the membrane voltage reaches a certain large value $V_{\text{max}}$. Any sufficiently large $V_{\text{max}}$ will work equally well, even $V_{\text{max}} = +\infty$, because $V$ reaches $+\infty$ in a finite time (see exercise 3). Using $V_{\text{max}} = 30$ and results of section 6.1.1, the topological normal form for the $I_{\text{Na,p}} + I_{\text{K}}$-model is

$$\dot{V} = (I - 4.51) + 0.1887(V + 61)^2, \qquad \text{if } V(t) = 30, \text{ then } V(t) \leftarrow V_{\text{reset}}.$$

The saddle-node homoclinic bifurcation occurs when $I = 4.51$ and $V_{\text{reset}} = -61$. This normal form is called the quadratic integrate-and-fire neuron; see chapters 3 and 8.

The topological normal form (6.13) is a useful equation, as will be seen in the rest of the book. It describes quantitative and qualitative features of neuronal dynamics remarkably well, yet it has only one non-linear term. This makes it suitable for real-time simulations of huge numbers of neurons. Its bifurcation structure is studied in exercise 12 (see also Fig.8.3), and the reader should at least look at the solution at the end of the book.

### 6.3.7   Hard and Soft Loss of Stability

Bifurcation is a qualitative change of the phase portrait of a system. Not all changes are equally dramatic, however. Some are hardly noticeable. For example, consider an equilibrium undergoing a supercritical Andronov-Hopf bifurcation: as a bifurcation parameter changes, the equilibrium loses stability and a small-amplitude stable limit cycle appears, as in Fig.6.11. The state of the system remains near the equilibrium; it just exhibits small-amplitude oscillations around it. We can change the parameter in the opposite direction, and then the limit cycle shrinks to a point and the system returns to the equilibrium. In neurons, such a bifurcation does not lead to an immediate spike. The neuron remains quiescent; it just exhibits subthreshold small-amplitude sustained oscillations. Such a loss of stability is called *soft*: the equilibrium is no longer stable, but its small neighborhood remains attractive. Supercritical pitchfork, cusp, and flip bifurcations correspond to soft loss of stability.

In contrast, if the equilibrium loses stability via subcritical Andronov-Hopf bifurcation, the state of the system diverges from it, which results in an immediate spike or some kind of large-amplitude jump. Such a loss of stability is called *hard*: neither the equilibrium nor its neighborhood is attractive. The hard loss of stability usually leads to noticeable or catastrophic changes in systems behavior, and the stability boundary is called *dangerous* (Bautin 1949). Changing the bifurcation parameter in the opposite direction will make the equilibrium stable again, but may not bring the state of the system back to equilibrium. Saddle-node bifurcation is hard unless it is on an invariant circle. In this case, the loss of stability is catastrophic, i.e., leading to noticeable spikes, but reversible. Saddle homoclinic orbit bifurcation is hard. In general, most bifurcations in neurons, or at least in neuronal models, are hard.

## Review of Important Concepts

- Stable equilibrium (resting state) in a typical neuronal model can
  – disappear via saddle-node bifurcation, which can be *off* or *on* invariant circle or
  – lose stability via Andronov-Hopf bifurcation, which can be supercritical or subcritical.
  These four cases are summarized in Fig.6.46.

- Stable limit cycle (periodic spiking state) in a typical two-dimensional neuronal model can
  – be cut by saddle-node on invariant circle bifurcation
  – shrink to a point via supercritical Andronov-Hopf bifurcation
  – disappear via fold limit cycle bifurcation or
  – disappear via saddle homoclinic orbit bifurcation.
  These four cases are summarized in Fig.6.47.

- Some atypical (codimension-2) bifurcations may play important roles in neuronal dynamics.

- Bogdanov-Takens bifurcation separates integrators from resonators.

# Bibliographical Notes

Though bifurcation theory can be traced back to Poincare and Andronov, it is a relatively new branch of mathematics. The first attempt to apply it to neuroscience was in 1955, when Richard FitzHugh concluded his paper on mathematical modeling of threshold phenomena by saying that many neuronal properties

> . . . are invariant under continuous, one-to-one transformations of the coordinates of phase space and fall within the domain of topology, a branch of mathematics which may be intrinsically better fitted for the preliminary description and classification of biological systems than analysis, which includes differential equations. This suggestion is of little practical value at present, since too little is known of the topology of vector fields in many-dimensional spaces, at least to those interested in theoretical biology. Nevertheless, the most logical procedure in the description of a complex biological system might be to characterize the topology of its phase space, then to establish a set of physically identifiable coordinates in the space, and finally to fit differential equations to the trajectories, instead of trying to reach this final goal at one leap.

It is remarkable that FitzHugh was explicitly talking about topological equivalence and bifurcations, though he never called them such, years before these mathematical notions were firmly established. This book continues the line of research initiated by FitzHugh and further developed by Rinzel and Ermentrout (1989).

In this chapter we provided a fairly detailed exposition of bifurcation theory. What we covered should be sufficient not only for understanding the rest of the book, but also for navigating through bifurcation papers concerned with computational neuroscience. More bifurcation theory, including bifurcations in mappings $x_{n+1} = f(x_n, b)$, can be found in the excellent book *Elements of Applied Bifurcation Theory* by Yuri Kuznetsov (1995; new ed., 2004), which, however, might be a bit technical for a nonmathematician. Some of the bifurcations considered in this chapter, such as the blue-sky catastrophe, are classified as "exotic" by Kuznetsov (1995), though the catastrophe was recently found in a model of a leech heart interneuron (Shilnikov and Cymbalyuk 2005).

There is no unified naming scheme for the bifurcations, mostly because they were discovered and rediscovered independently in many fields and in many countries. For example, the Andronov-Hopf bifurcation was known to A. Poincare, so some scientists refer to it as the Poincare-Andronov-Hopf bifurcation. Many refer to it as just the Hopf bifurcation due to the fault of the famous Russian mathematician Vladimir Igorevich Arnold and the famous French mathematician Rene Thom. According to Arnold's account, he was visited by Thom in the 1960s. While there were discussing various bifurcations, Arnold put too much emphasis on Hopf's "recent" (1942) paper. As a result of Arnold's misattribution, Thom popularized the bifurcation as the Hopf bifurcation. In Fig.6.49 we provide some common alternative names for the bifurcations considered in this chapter. The complete list of names of known bifurcations is very long, and it resembles the list of faculty members of the Department of Radiophysics at Gorky State University, in what is now Nizhnii Novgorod, Russia. The department was founded by A. A. Andronov in 1945 (see Fig. 6.50).

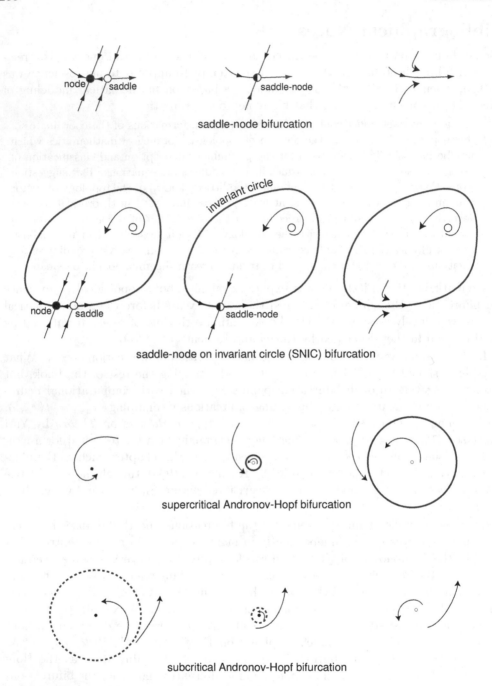

Figure 6.46: Summary of all codimension-1 bifurcations of a stable equilibrium (resting state).

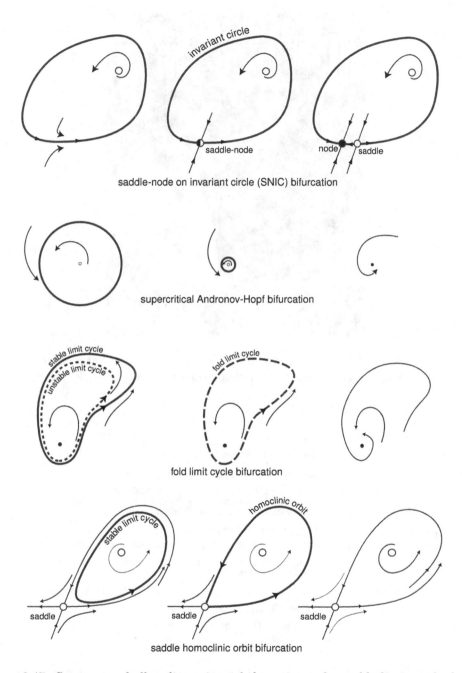

Figure 6.47: Summary of all codimension-1 bifurcations of a stable limit cycle (tonic spiking state) on a plane.

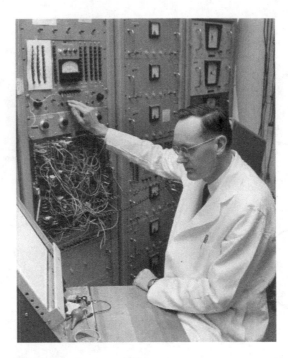

Figure 6.48: Richard FitzHugh with analog computer at the National Institute of Health, Bethesda, Maryland, ca. 1960. (Photograph provided by R. FitzHugh).

| bifurcation | alternative names |
|---|---|
| saddle-node | fold, limit point, saddle-node off limit cycle |
| saddle-node on invariant circle | SNIC, saddle-node on limit cycle (SNLC), circle, saddle-node homoclinic, saddle-node central homoclinic, saddle-node infinite period (SNIPer), homoclinic |
| Andronov-Hopf | Hopf, Poincare-Andronov-Hopf |
| saddle homoclinic orbit | homoclinic, saddle-loop, saddle separatrix loop, Andronov-Leontovich |
| fold limit cycle | saddle-node of limit cycles, double limit cycle, fold cycle, saddle-node (fold) of periodics |
| saddle-node homoclinic orbit | saddle-node noncentral homoclinic, saddle-node separatrix-loop |
| Bogdanov-Takens | Takens-Bogdanov, double-zero |
| Bautin | degenerate Hopf, generalized Hopf |
| flip | period doubling |

Figure 6.49: Popular alternative names for some of the bifurcations considered in this chapter.

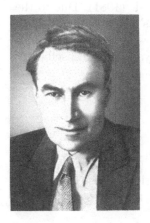

Figure 6.50: The founder of the Russian school of nonlinear dynamics, Aleksander Aleksandrovich Andronov (1901–1952) in 1950. (Picture provided by M. I. Rabinovich.)

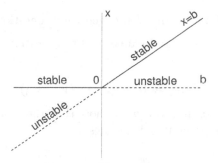

Figure 6.51: Transcritical bifurcation in $\dot{x} = x(b - x)$.

The division of bifurcations into subcritical and supercritical may be confusing to a novice. For example, some scientists erroneously think that supercritical bifurcations result in the appearance of attractors (stable equilibria, limit cycles, etc.), and subcritical bifurcations result in their disappearance. Let us emphasize here that the appearance or disappearance of an equilibrium or a limit cycle depends on the direction of change of the bifurcation parameter. For example, the subcritical pitchfork bifurcation in Fig.6.36 can result in the appearance of a stable equilibrium $x = 0$ if $b$ decreases past 0. Our classification of bifurcations into subcritical and supercritical is consistent with the following widely accepted rule: let the bifurcation parameter change in the direction leading to the increase in the number of objects (equilibria, limit cycles). The bifurcation is *supercritical* if stable objects appear, *subcritical* if unstable objects appear, and *transcritical* (as in Fig.6.51) if equal numbers of stable and unstable objects appear or disappear. The condition for supercritical (subcritical) Andronov-Hopf bifurcation, (6.7), is taken from Guckenheimer and Holmes (1983).

Delayed loss of stability was first described by Shishkova (1973), and studied in detail by Nejshtadt (1985) (many find his paper difficult to read). An alternative description is given by Arnold et al. (1994) and Baer et al. (1989).

Canard (French duck) solutions were reported by Benoit et al. (1981). Due to the recent political climate in the USA, some refer to "French ducks" as "freedom ducks", probably to emphasize that "French = freedom". Canards in $\mathbb{R}^3$ were studied by Benoit (1984), Samborskij (1985; in $\mathbb{R}^n$), and more recently by Szmolyan and Wechselberger (2001, 2004) and Wechselberger (2005).

## Exercises

1. (Transcritical bifurcation) Justify the bifurcation diagram in Fig.6.51.

2. Show that the non-degeneracy and transversality conditions are necessary for the saddle-node bifurcation. That is, present a system that does not exhibit saddle-node bifurcation, but satisfies

   (a) the non-hyperbolicity and non-degeneracy conditions or

   (b) the non-hyperbolicity and transversality conditions.

3. Consider the model
   $$\dot{V} = c(b - b_{sn}) + a(V - V_{sn})^2,$$

   with positive $a$ and $c$, and $b > b_{sn}$. Show that the sojourn time in a bounded neighborhood of the point $V = V_{sn}$ scales as

   $$T = \frac{\pi}{\sqrt{ac(b - b_{sn})}}$$

   when $b$ is near $b_{sn}$. (Hint: Find the solution that starts at $-\infty$ and terminates at $+\infty$.)

4. Show that the two-dimensional system

   $$\begin{aligned}
   \dot{u} &= c(b)u - \omega(b)v &+ (au - dv)(u^2 + v^2)\,, & \qquad (6.14)\\
   \dot{v} &= \omega(b)u + c(b)v &+ (du + av)(u^2 + v^2)\,, & \qquad (6.15)
   \end{aligned}$$

   the complex-valued system

   $$\dot{z} = (c(b) + i\omega(b))z + (a + id)z|z|^2\,,$$

   and the polar-coordinate system

   $$\begin{aligned}
   \dot{r} &= c(b)r + ar^3,\\
   \dot{\varphi} &= \omega(b) + dr^2
   \end{aligned}$$

   are equivalent.

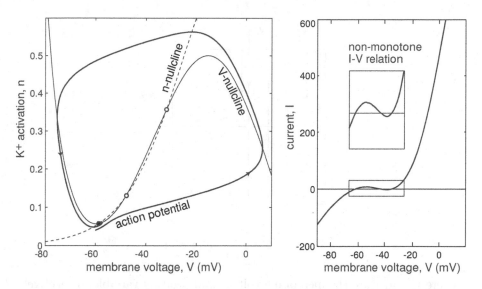

Figure 6.52: exercise 8: This $I_{\mathrm{Na,p}}+I_{\mathrm{K}}$-model has a non-monotonic I-V relation, yet the resting state becomes unstable via Andronov-Hopf bifurcation before disappearing via saddle-node bifurcation. Parameters are as in Fig.4.1a, except that $E_{\mathrm{leak}} = -78$ mV and $n_\infty(V)$ has $k = 12$ mV.

5. Show that the non-degeneracy and transversality conditions are necessary for the Andronov-Hopf bifurcation. That is, present a system that does not exhibit the Andronov-Hopf bifurcation, but satisfies

    (a) the non-hyperbolicity and non-degeneracy conditions or

    (b) the non-hyperbolicity and transversality conditions.

6. Show that the system (6.14, 6.15) with $c(b) = b$, $\omega(b) = 1$, $a \neq 0$ and $d = 0$ exhibits Andronov-Hopf bifurcation. Check all three conditions.

7. Determine the stability of the limit cycle near an Andronov-Hopf bifurcation. (Hint: Consider the equilibrium $r = \sqrt{|c/a|}$ in the topological normal form (6.8)).

8. The model in Fig.6.52 has a non-monotonic I-V relation. Nevertheless, the resting state *loses stability* via Andronov-Hopf bifurcation before disappearing via saddle-node bifurcation. Draw representative phase portraits of the model. Is the system near Bogdanov-Takens bifurcation?

9. Consider a generic two-dimensional conductance-based model

$$\dot{V} = I - I(V, x) , \qquad (6.16)$$
$$\dot{x} = (x_\infty(V) - x)/\tau(V) , \qquad (6.17)$$

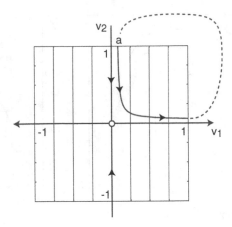

Figure 6.53: See exercise 11.

where $V$ and $x$ are the membrane voltage and a gating variable, respectively, $I$ is the injected DC current, and $I(V, x)$ is the instantaneous I-V relation, which of course depends on the gating variable $x$. Here the membrane capacitance $C = 1$ for the sake of simplicity. Show that the eigenvalues at an equilibrium $c \pm \omega$ are given by

$$c = (I_V(V, x) + 1/\tau(V))/2$$

and

$$\omega = \sqrt{c^2 - I'_\infty(V)/\tau(V)}$$

where $I_\infty(V) = I(V, x_\infty(V))$ is the steady-state I-V relation of the model. In particular, the frequency at the Andronov-Hopf bifurcation is

$$\text{(frequency)} = \sqrt{I'_\infty(V)/(C\tau(V))} \, ,$$

where $C$ is the membrane capacitance.

10. Determine when the system

$$z' = (a + \omega i)z + z|z|^2 - z|z|^4 \, , \qquad z \in \mathbb{C}$$

undergoes fold limit cycle bifurcation.

11. Consider a square neighborhood of a saddle equilibrium in Fig.6.53 (compare with the inset in Fig.6.29). Here $v_1$ and $v_2$ are eigenvectors with eigenvalues $\lambda_2 < 0 < \lambda_1$. Suppose the limit cycle enters the square at the point $a = \tau(I - I_b)$, where $\tau > 0$ is some parameter. Determine the amount of time the trajectory spends in the square as a function of $I$.

12. Determine the bifurcation diagram of the topological normal form (6.13) for saddle-node homoclinic bifurcation.

13. Prove that the system

$$\begin{aligned}\dot{v} &= I + v^2 - u\,,\\ \dot{u} &= a(bv - u)\end{aligned}$$

with $a > 0$ undergoes

- saddle-node bifurcation when $b^2 = 4I$,
- Andronov-Hopf bifurcation when $a < b$ and $a^2 - 2ab + 4I = 0$,
- Bogdanov-Takens bifurcation when $a = b = 2\sqrt{I}$.

Use the results of exercise 15 to prove that the Andronov-Hopf bifurcation in the model above is always subcritical.

14. Use (6.7) to prove that the relaxation oscillator

$$\begin{aligned}\dot{v} &= f(v) - u\\ \dot{u} &= \mu(v - b)\end{aligned}$$

with an N-shaped fast nullcline $u = f(v)$ undergoes Andronov-Hopf bifurcation when $f'(b) = 0$ (i.e., exactly at the knee; what is so special about this model?). Show that the bifurcation is supercritical when $f'''(b) < 0$ and subcritical when $f'''(b) > 0$.

15. Prove that the Andronov-Hopf bifurcation point in

$$\begin{aligned}\dot{v} &= F(v) - u\\ \dot{u} &= \mu(bv - u)\end{aligned}$$

satisfies $F' = \mu$ and $b > \mu$. Use (6.7) to show that

$$a = \{F''' + (F'')^2/(b - \mu)\}/16\,.$$

16. Prove that the Andronov-Hopf bifurcation point in

$$\begin{aligned}\dot{v} &= F(v) - u\\ \dot{u} &= \mu(G(v) - u)\end{aligned}$$

satisfies $F' = \mu$ and $G' > \mu$. Use (6.7) to show that

$$a = \{F''' + F''(F'' - G'')/(G' - \mu)\}/16\,.$$

17. Prove that the Andronov-Hopf bifurcation point in

$$\begin{aligned}\dot{v} &= F(v) - (v + 1)u\\ \dot{u} &= \mu(G(v) - u)\end{aligned}$$

satisfies $F' = \mu$ and $G' > \mu$. Use (6.7) to show that

$$a = \{F''' + \mu - (F'' - \mu)(1 + \mu[G'' - F'' + 2\mu]/\omega^2)\}/16\,.$$

18. Use (6.7) to show that a two-dimensional relaxation oscillator

$$\dot{v} = F(v, u)$$
$$\dot{u} = \mu G(v, u)$$

at an Andronov-Hopf bifurcation point has

$$a = \frac{1}{16} \left\{ F_{vvv} + F_{vv} \left[ \frac{F_{vv}G_u - F_u G_{vv}}{F_u G_v} - \frac{F_{vu}}{F_u} \right] \right\} + \mathcal{O}(\sqrt{\mu}) \ .$$

19. **[M.S.]** A leaky integrate-and-fire model has the same asymptotic firing rate $(1/ln)$ as a system near saddle homoclinic orbit bifurcation. Explore the possibility that integrate-and-fire models describe neurons near such a bifurcation.

20. **[M.S.]** (blue-sky catastrophe) Prove that

$$\dot{\varphi} = \omega, \quad \dot{x} = a + x^2, \qquad \text{if } x = +\infty, \quad \text{then } x \leftarrow -\infty, \quad \text{and} \quad \varphi \leftarrow 0 \ ,$$

is the canonical model (see section 8.1.5) for blue-sky catastrophe. This model without the reset of $\varphi$ is canonical for the fold limit cycle on homoclinic torus bifurcation. The model with the reset $x \leftarrow b + \sin \varphi$ is canonical for the Lukyanov-Shilnikov bifurcation of a fold limit cycle with non-central homoclinics (Shilnikov and Cymbalyuk 2004, Shilnikov et al. 2005). Here, $\varphi$ is the phase variable on the unit circle and $a$ and $b$ are bifurcation parameters.

21. **[M.S.]** Define topological equivalence and the notion of a bifurcation for piecewise continuous flows.

22. **[Ph.D.]** Use the definition in the exercise above to classify codimension-1 bifurcations in piecewise continuous flows.

23. **[M.S.]** The bifurcation sequence in Fig.6.40 seems to be typical in two-dimensional neuronal models. Develop the theory of Bogdanov-Takens bifurcation with a global reentrant orbit.

24. **[Ph.D.]** Develop an automated dynamic clamp protocol (Sharp et al. 1993) that analyzes bifurcations in neurons in vitro, similar to what AUTO, XPPAUT, and MATCONT do in models.

# Chapter 7

# Neuronal Excitability

Neurons are excitable in the sense that they are typically at rest but can fire spikes in response to certain forms of stimulation. What kind of stimulation is needed to fire a given neuron? What is the evoked firing pattern? These are the questions concerning the neuron's computational properties, e.g., whether they are integrators or resonators, their firing frequency range, the spike latencies (delays), the coexistence of resting and spiking states, etc. From the dynamical systems point of view, neurons are excitable because they are near a bifurcation from resting to spiking activity. The type of bifurcation, and not the ionic currents per se, determines the computational properties of neurons. In this chapter we continue our effort to understand the relationship between bifurcations of the resting state and the neurocomputational properties of excitable systems.

## 7.1  Excitability

A textbook definition of neuronal excitability is that a "subthreshold" synaptic input evokes a small graded postsynaptic potential (PSP), while a "superthreshold" input evokes a large all-or-none action potential, which is an order of magnitude larger than the amplitude of the subthreshold response. Unfortunately, we cannot adopt this definition to define excitability of dynamical systems because many systems, including some neuronal models discussed in chapter 4, have neither all-or-none action potentials nor firing thresholds. Instead, we employ a purely geometrical definition.

From the geometrical point of view, a dynamical system with a stable equilibrium is *excitable* if there is a large-amplitude piece of trajectory that starts in a small neighborhood of the equilibrium, leaves the neighborhood, and then returns to the equilibrium, as we illustrate in Fig.7.1 (left).

In the context of neurons, the equilibrium corresponds to the resting state. Because it is stable, all trajectories starting in a sufficiently small region of the equilibrium, much smaller than the shaded neighborhood in the figure, converge back to the equilibrium. Such trajectories correspond to subthreshold PSPs. In contrast, the large trajectory in the figure corresponds to firing a spike. Therefore, superthreshold PSPs are those that

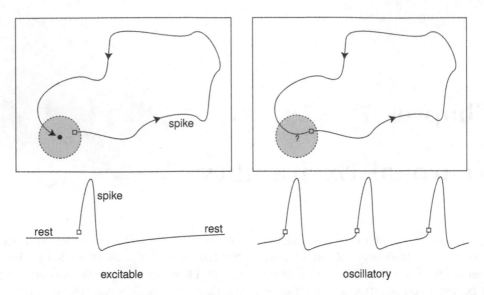

Figure 7.1: Left: An abstract definition of excitability. There is a spike trajectory that starts near a stable equilibrium and returns to it. Right: Excitable systems are near bifurcations. A modification of the vector field in the small shaded region can result in a periodic trajectory.

push the state of the neuron to or near the beginning of the large trajectory (small square in Fig.7.1), thereby initiating the spike. These inputs can be injected by an experimenter via an attached electrode, or they can represent the total synaptic input from the other neurons in the network, or both.

## 7.1.1   Bifurcations

The definition in Fig.7.1 is quite general, and it does not make any assumptions regarding the details of the vector field inside or outside of the small shaded neighborhood. Let us use the theory presented in chapter 6 to show that such an excitable system is near a bifurcation from resting to oscillatory dynamics.

- *Bifurcation of a limit cycle.* The vector field in the small shaded neighborhood of the equilibrium can be modified slightly so that the spike trajectory enters the square and becomes periodic, as in Fig.7.1 (right). That is, the dynamical system goes through a bifurcation resulting in the appearance of a limit cycle.

What happens to the stable equilibrium, denoted as "?" in the figure? Depending on the type of the bifurcation of the limit cycle, the equilibrium may disappear or may lose stability. This happens when the limit cycle appears via saddle-node on an invariant circle or a supercritical Andronov-Hopf bifurcation, respectively. Both cases are depicted in Fig.7.2.

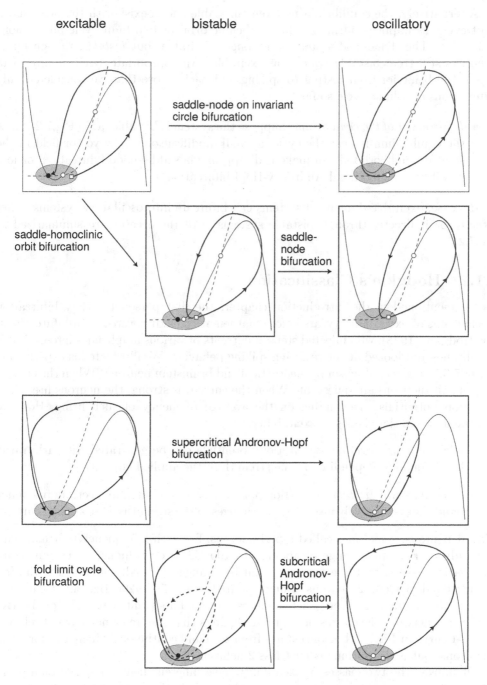

Figure 7.2: Excitable dynamical systems bifurcate into oscillatory ones either directly or indirectly, via bistable systems.

Alternatively, the equilibrium may remain stable and coexist with the newly born limit cycle, as happens during saddle homoclinic orbit or fold limit cycle bifurcations in Fig.7.2. The dynamical system is no longer excitable, but *bistable*, though many scientists still treat bistable systems as excitable. An appropriate synaptic input can switch the behavior from resting to spiking and back. Note that we considered only bifurcations of a limit cycle so far.

- *Bifurcation of the equilibrium.* Suppose the system is bistable, as in Fig.7.2. Since the equilibrium is near the cycle, a small modification of the vector field in the shaded neighborhood can make it disappear via saddle-node bifurcation, or lose stability via subcritical Andronov-Hopf bifurcation.

In any case, excitable dynamical systems can bifurcate into oscillatory systems either directly or indirectly through bistable systems. All these cases are summarized in Fig.7.2.

## 7.1.2  Hodgkin's Classification

As we mentioned in the introduction chapter, the first person to study bifurcation mechanisms of excitability (years before mathematicians discovered such bifurcations) was Hodgkin (1948), who injected steps of currents of various amplitudes into excitable membranes and looked at the resulting spiking behavior. We illustrate his experiments in Fig.7.3, using recordings of rat neocortical and brainstem neurons. When the current is weak, the neurons are quiescent. When the current is strong, the neurons fire trains of action potentials. Depending on the average frequency of such firing, Hodgkin identified two major classes of excitability:

- *Class 1 neural excitability.* Action potentials can be generated with arbitrarily low frequency, depending on the strength of the applied current.

- *Class 2 neural excitability.* Action potentials are generated in a certain frequency band that is relatively insensitive to changes in the strength of the applied current.

Class 1 neurons, sometimes called type I neurons, fire with a frequency that may vary smoothly over a broad range of about 2 to 100 Hz or even higher. The important observation here is that the frequency can be changed tenfold. In contrast, the frequency band of Class 2 neurons is quite limited, e.g., $150 - 200$ Hz, but it can vary from neuron to neuron. The exact numbers are not important here. The qualitative distinction between the classes noted by Hodgkin is that the frequency-current relation (the F-I curve in Fig.7.3, bottom) starts from zero and continuously increases for Class 1 neurons, but is discontinuous for Class 2 neurons.

Obviously, the two classes of excitability have different neurocomputational properties. Class 1 excitable neurons can smoothly encode the strength of an input, e.g., the strength of the applied DC current or the strength of the incoming synaptic bombardment, into the frequency of their spiking output. Class 2 neurons cannot do that.

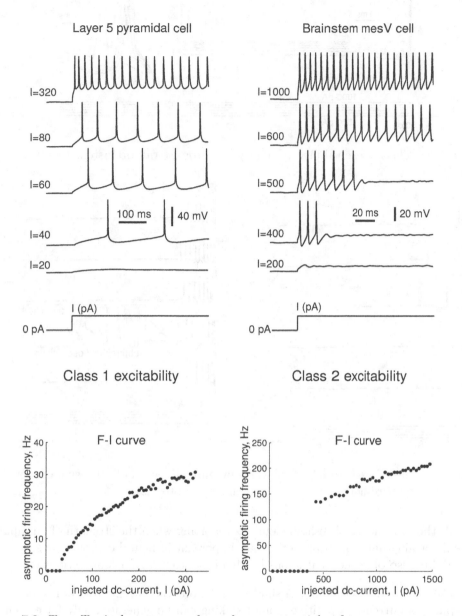

Figure 7.3: Top: Typical responses of membrane potentials of two neurons to steps of DC current of various magnitudes $I$. Bottom: Corresponding frequency-current (F-I) relations are qualitatively different. Shown are recordings of layer 5 pyramidal neurons from rat primary visual cortex (left) and mesV neuron from rat brainstem (right). The asymptotic frequency is $1000/T_\infty$, where $T_\infty$ is taken to be the interval between the last two spikes in a long spike train.

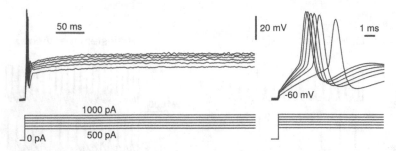

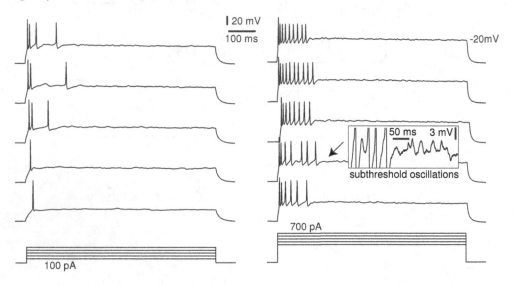

Figure 7.4: Class 3 excitability of a mesV neuron of rat brainstem (contrast with Fig.7.3).

Figure 7.5: Class 3 excitability of a layer 5 pyramidal neuron of rat visual cortex. The inset shows subthreshold oscillations of membrane potential.

Instead, they can act as threshold elements reporting when the strength of an input is above a certain value. Both properties are important in neural computations.

Hodgkin also observed that axons left in oil or seawater for long periods exhibited

- *Class 3 neural excitability.* A single action potential is generated in response to a pulse of current. Repetitive (tonic) spiking can be generated only for extremely strong injected currents or not at all.

Two examples of Class 3 excitable systems are depicted in Fig.7.4 and Fig.7.5. The mesV neuron in the figure fires a phasic spike at the onset of the pulse of current, and then remains quiescent. Even injecting pulses as high as 1000 pA, which result in spike trains in another mesV neuron in Fig.7.3, cannot evoke multiple spikes in this neuron. Similarly, the pyramidal neuron in Fig.7.5 cannot sustain tonic spiking even when the injected current is ten times stronger than the neuron's rheobase. Ironically, neurons exhibiting such a behavior would most likely be discarded as "sick" or "unhealthy", though the neurons analyzed in the figures looked normal from any other point of view. We will study the dynamic mechanism of this class of excitability and show that it may have nothing to do with sickness.

It will shortly be clear that this classification is of limited value except that it points to the fact that neurons should be distinguished according not only to ionic mechanisms of excitability but also to dynamic mechanisms, in particular to the type of bifurcation of the resting state.

### 7.1.3 Classes 1 and 2

Let us consider the strength of the applied current in Hodgkin's experiments as being a bifurcation parameter. Instead of changing the parameter abruptly, as in Fig.7.3, we change it slowly in Fig.7.6 (both figures show recordings of the same neurons). In section 7.1.5 we explain the fundamental difference between these two protocols.

When the current ramps up, the resting potential increases until a bifurcation occurs, resulting in loss of stability or disappearance of the equilibrium corresponding to the resting state, and the neuron activity becomes oscillatory. Note that the pyramidal neuron in Fig.7.6 starts to fire with a small frequency, which then increases according to the F-I curve in Fig.7.3 (a slower current ramp is needed to span the entire frequency range of the F-I curve). In contrast, the brainstem neuron starts to fire with a high frequency that remains relatively constant even though the magnitude of the injected current increases.

Among all four codimension-1 bifurcations of equilibrium, discussed in chapter 6 and mentioned in Fig.7.2, only saddle-node on invariant circle bifurcation results in a

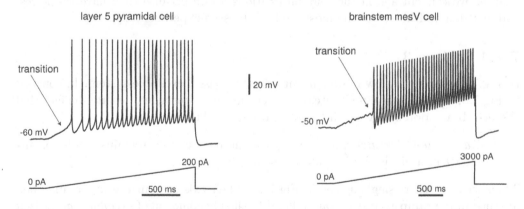

Figure 7.6: As the magnitude of injected DC current increases, the neurons bifurcate from resting to repetitive spiking behavior. Shown are recordings of the neurons in Fig.7.3. Note that the ratio of the first and last interspike intervals of the pyramidal cell is much greater than that of the mesV neuron.

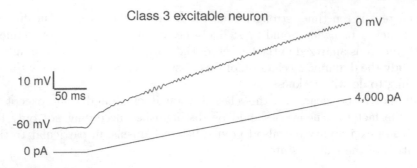

Figure 7.7: A Class 3 excitable brainstem mesV neuron does not fire in response to a ramp current, even though the injected current is stronger than the one in Fig.7.4.

limit cycle attractor with arbitrarily small frequency and continuous F-I curve. The other three bifurcations result in limit cycle attractors with relatively large frequencies and discontinuous F-I curves. Therefore,

- *Class 1 neural excitability* corresponds to the resting state disappearing via saddle-node on invariant circle bifurcation.

- *Class 2 neural excitability* corresponds to the resting state disappearing via saddle-node (*off* invariant circle) bifurcation or losing stability via subcritical or supercritical Andronov-Hopf bifurcations.

Of course, the resting state can lose stability or disappear via other bifurcations having higher codimension, sometimes leading to counterintuitive results (e.g., Class 1 excitability near Andronov-Hopf bifurcation; see exercise 6 and section 7.2.11). In this chapter we concentrate on the four bifurcations above because they have the lowest codimension and hence are the most likely to be seen experimentally.

### 7.1.4  Class 3

In Fig.7.7 we inject a slow ramp current into the Class 3 excitable system. In contrast to Fig.7.6, no spiking and no bifurcation occur in this experiment, despite the fact that the membrane potential goes all the way to 0 mV. Therefore,

- *Class 3 neural excitability* occurs when the resting state remains stable for any fixed $I$ in a biophysically relevant range.

Then why are there single spikes in Fig.7.4? Their existence in the figure and their absence in the ramp experiment are related to the phenomenon of *accommodation* that we now describe.

Let us consider a neuron having a transient Na$^+$ current with relatively fast inactivation. If a sufficiently slow ramp of current is injected, the current has enough time to inactivate, and no action potentials can be generated. Such a neuron accommodates

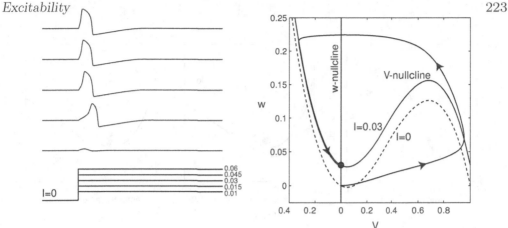

Figure 7.8: Class 3 excitability in FitzHugh-Nagumo model (4.11, 4.12) with $a = 0.1, b = 0.01, c = 0$. The model fires a single spike for any pulse of current.

to the slow ramp. In contrast, a quick membrane depolarization due to a strong step of current does not give enough time for Na$^+$ inactivation, thereby resulting in a spike. During the spike, the current inactivates quickly and precludes any further action potentials. Instead of inactivating the Na$^+$ current, we could have used a low-threshold persistent K$^+$ current, or any other resonant current, to illustrate the phenomenon of accommodation.

From the dynamical systems point of view, slow ramp results in quasi-static dynamics so that all gating variables follow their steady-state values, $x = x_\infty(V)$, and the membrane potential follows its I-V curve. As long as the equilibrium corresponding to the resting state is stable, the neuron is at rest. Even global bifurcations resulting in the appearance of stable limit cycles do not change that. Only when the equilibrium bifurcates (loses stability or disappears), does the neuron change its behavior, e.g., jumps to a limit cycle attractor and starts to fire spikes. Class 3 excitable systems do not fire in response to slow ramps because the resting state does not bifurcate.

In contrast, a pulse of current changes the phase portrait in a rather abrupt manner, as we illustrate in Fig.7.8, using the FitzHugh-Nagumo model with vertical slow nullcline. Injecting $I$ shifts the fast nullcline upward. Though no bifurcation can occur in the model, and the resting state is stable for any value of $I$, its location suddenly shifts when $I$ jumps. The trajectory from the old equilibrium, $(0,0)$, to the new one goes through the right branch of the cubic $V$-nullcline, thereby resulting in a single spike. Since the new equilibrium $(0, 0.03)$ is a global attractor and no limit cycles exist, periodic spiking cannot be generated. In exercise 7 we explore the relationship between Class 3 excitability and Andronov-Hopf bifurcation (note the subthreshold oscillations of membrane potential of the pyramidal neuron in Fig.7.5). We see that injecting ramps of current is not equivalent to injecting pulses of current. The system goes through a bifurcation of the equilibrium in the former, but may bypass it and jump somewhere else in the latter.

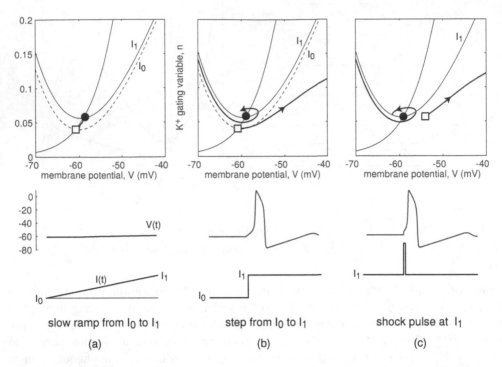

Figure 7.9: The difference between ramp, step, and shock stimulations is in the resetting of initial condition.

## 7.1.5   Ramps, Steps, and Shocks

In Fig.7.9 we elaborate the differences among injecting slow ramps, steps, and shocks (i.e., brief pulses) of current. In the first two cases the magnitude of the injected current changes from $I_0$ to $I_1$, while in the third case the current is $I_1$ except for the infinitesimally brief moment when it has an infinitely large strength. In all three cases the dynamics of the model can be understood via analysis of its phase portrait at $I = I_1$. The key difference among the stimulation protocols is how they reset the initial condition.

At the beginning of the slow ramp in Fig.7.9a, the state of the neuron is at the stable equilibrium. As the current slowly increases, the equilibrium slowly moves, and the trajectory follows it. When the current reaches $I = I_1$, the trajectory is at the new equilibrium, so no response is evoked because the equilibrium is stable. In contrast, when the current is stepped from $I_0$ to $I_1$ in Fig.7.9b, the location of the equilibrium changes instantaneously, but the membrane potential and the gating variables do not have time to catch up. To understand the response of the model to the step, we need to consider its dynamics at $I = I_1$ with the initial condition set to the location of the old equilibrium (marked by the white square in the figure). Such a step evokes a spike response even though the new equilibrium is stable. Finally, shocking the neuron

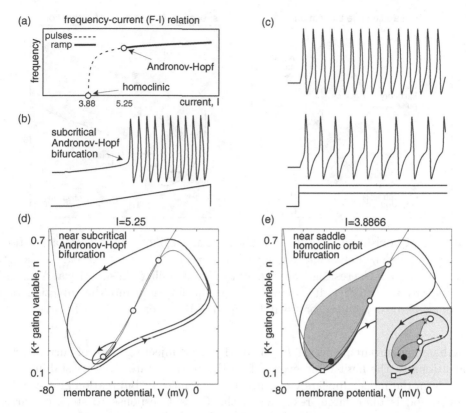

Figure 7.10: The $I_{\text{Na,p}}+I_{\text{K}}$-model undergoes subcritical Andronov-Hopf bifurcation, yet can exhibit low-frequency firing when steps (but not ramps) of current are injected. Parameters: $C = 1$, $I = 0$, $E_{\text{L}} = -66.2$, $g_{\text{L}} = 2$, $g_{\text{Na}} = 5$, $g_{\text{K}} = 4.5$, $m_{\infty}(V)$ has $V_{1/2} = -30$ and $k = 10$, $n_{\infty}(V)$ has $V_{1/2} = -34$ and $k = 13$, and $\tau(V) = 1$, $E_{\text{Na}} = 60$ mV and $E_{\text{K}} = -90$ mV. The shaded region is the attraction domain of the resting state. The inset shows a distorted drawing of the phase portrait.

results in an instantaneous increase of its membrane potential to a new value. (As an exercise, prove that the magnitude of the increase equals the product of pulse width and pulse height divided by the membrane capacitance.) This shifts the initial condition horizontally to a new point, marked by the white square in Fig.7.9c, and results in a spike response.

Now, let us revisit the Hodgkin experiments and demonstrate the fundamental difference between the stimulation protocols. In Fig.7.10a, b, and c we simulate the $I_{\text{Na,p}}+I_{\text{K}}$-model and show that it is Class 2 excitable in response to ramps of current but Class 1 excitable in response to steps of current. The apparent contradiction is resolved in Fig.7.10d and e, where we consider the model's phase portraits. Notice the coexistence of the resting state and a limit cycle attractor. The resting state loses stability via subcritical Andronov-Hopf bifurcation at $I = 5.25$, so the emerging

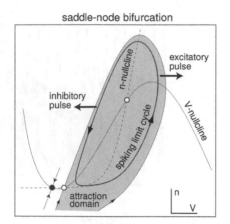
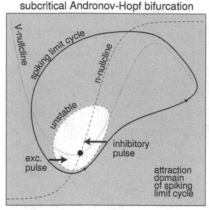

Figure 7.11: Coexistence of stable equilibrium and spiking limit cycle attractor in the $I_{\mathrm{Na,p}}+I_{\mathrm{K}}$-model. Left: The resting state is about to disappear via saddle-node bifurcation. Right: The resting state is about to lose stability via subcritical Andronov-Hopf bifurcation. Right (left) arrows denote the location and the direction of an excitatory (inhibitory) pulse that switches spiking behavior to resting behavior.

spiking has non-zero frequency at $I \approx 5.25$. However, injecting steps of current results in transitions to the limit cycle even before the resting state loses its stability. The limit cycle in the model appears via saddle homoclinic orbit bifurcation at $I \approx 3.8866$, and its period is quite large, resulting in the Class 1 response to steps of current. The F-I curves for homoclinic bifurcations have logarithmic scaling, so small-frequency oscillations are difficult to catch numerically, let alone experimentally.

The surprising discrepancy in Fig.7.10a occurs because the resting state of the $I_{\mathrm{Na,p}}+I_{\mathrm{K}}$-model is near the Bogdanov-Takens bifurcation (i.e., the model is near a transition from resonator to integrator). Such a bifurcation was recorded, though indirectly, in some neocortical pyramidal neurons, as we will show later in this chapter and in chapter 8. Another surprising example of Andronov-Hopf bifurcation with Class 1 excitability is presented in exercise 6. To avoid such surprises, we adopt the ramp definition of excitability throughout the book.

## 7.1.6  Bistability

When transition from the resting to the spiking state occurs via saddle-node (off invariant circle) or subcritical Andronov-Hopf bifurcation, there is a coexistence of a stable equilibrium and a stable limit cycle attractor just before the bifurcation, as we illustrate in Fig.7.11. We refer to such systems as bistable. They have a remarkable neurocomputational property: bistable systems can be switched from one state to the other by an appropriately timed brief stimulus. Rinzel (1978) predicted such a behavior in the Hodgkin-Huxley model, and then bistability and hysteresis were found

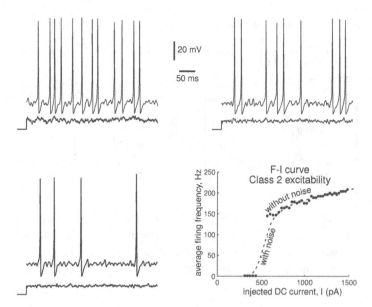

Figure 7.12: Examples of noise-induced low-frequency firings of a Class 2 excitable system. The F-I curve may look like the one for Class 1 excitability. Shown are recordings of brainstem mesV neuron.

experimentally in the squid axon (Guttman et al. 1980). What was really surprising for many neuroscientists is that neurons can be switched from repetitive spiking to resting by brief *depolarizing* shock stimuli.

This phenomenon is illustrated in Fig.7.11. Each shaded area in the figure denotes the attraction domain of a spiking limit cycle attractor. Obviously, the state of the resting neuron must be pushed into the shaded area to initiate periodic spiking. Similarly, the state of the periodically spiking neuron must be pushed out of the shaded area to stop the spiking. As the arrows in the figure indicate, both excitatory and inhibitory stimuli can do that, depending on their timing relative to the phase of spiking oscillation. This protocol can be used to test bistability experimentally. (As an exercise, use geometrical and electrophysiological arguments to explain why a system with high-threshold slow persistent inward current can be bistable but cannot be switched from one mode to another by brief pulses of current.) Bistable behavior reveals itself indirectly when a neuron is kept close to the bifurcation, e.g., when the injected DC current is just below the rheobase. Noisy perturbations can switch the neuron from resting to spiking state, thereby creating an irregular spike train consisting of short bursts of spikes. Such *stuttering* spiking have been observed in many neurons, including some regular spiking (RS) and fast spiking (FS) neocortical neurons, as we discuss in chapter 8. The mean firing frequency during stuttering is proportional to the amplitude of the injected current and it can be quite low even for a Class 2 excitable system, as we illustrate in Fig.7.12. Thus, caution should be used when experimentally determining the class of excitability; only spike trains with regular interspike periods should be accepted to measure the F-I relations.

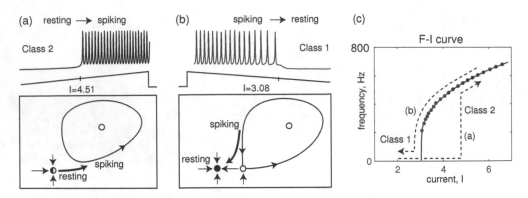

Figure 7.13: (a) The frequency of emerging oscillations at the transition "resting $\rightarrow$ spiking" defines the class of excitability. (b) The frequency of disappearing oscillations at the transition "spiking $\rightarrow$ resting" defines the class of spiking. (c) The $I_{\mathrm{Na,p}}+I_{\mathrm{K}}$-model with high-threshold $K^+$ current exhibits class 2 excitability but class 1 spiking. Its F-I curve has a hysteresis.

## 7.1.7    Class 1 and 2 Spiking

The class of excitability is determined by the frequency of emerging oscillations at the transition "resting $\rightarrow$ spiking", as in Fig.7.13a. Let us look at the frequency of disappearing oscillations at the transition "spiking $\rightarrow$ resting". To induce such a transition, we inject a strong pulse of DC current of slowly decreasing amplitude, as in Fig.7.13b. Similarly to the Hodgkin classification of excitability, we say that a neuron has *Class 1 spiking* if the frequency-current (F-I) curve at the transition "spiking $\rightarrow$ resting" decreases to zero, as in Fig.7.13c, and *Class 2 spiking* if it stops at a certain non-zero value.

The class of excitability coincides with the class of spiking when the transitions "resting $\leftrightarrow$ spiking" occur via saddle-node on invariant circle bifurcation or supercritical Andronov-Hopf bifurcation. Indeed, if the current ramps are sufficiently slow, the neuron as a dynamical system goes through the same bifurcation, but in the opposite direction. The classes may differ when the bifurcation is of the saddle-node (off invariant circle) type or the subcritical Andronov-Hopf type because of the bistability of the resting and spiking states. Such a bistability results in the hysteresis behavior of the system when the injected current $I$ increases and decreases slowly, which may result in the hysteresis of the F-I curve. For example, the transition "resting $\rightarrow$ spiking" in Fig.7.13a occurs via saddle-node bifurcation at $I = 4.51$, and the frequency of spiking equals the frequency of the limit cycle attractor, which is non-zero at this value of $I$. Decreasing $I$ results in the transition "spiking $\rightarrow$ resting" via the saddle homoclinic orbit bifurcation in Fig.7.13b, and in the oscillations with zero frequency at $I = 3.08$. Thus, the F-I behavior of the model in this figure (and in Fig.7.10) exhibits Class 2 excitability but Class 1 spiking. Because of the logarithmic scaling of the F-I curve at the saddle homoclinic bifurcation (see section 6.2.4), experimentally estimating the zero value of the F-I curves is challenging.

Interestingly, steps of injected DC current, as in Fig.7.10c, induce the transition "resting → spiking". But because the model in the figure is near a codimension-2 Bogdanov-Takens bifurcation, the steps test the frequency of the limit cycle attractor at the bifurcation "spiking → resting", as in Fig.7.10e; that is, they test the class of spiking! The F-I curve in response to steps in the figure is the same as the F-I curve in response to a slowly decreasing current ramp. (As an exercise, explain why this is true for Fig.7.10 but not for Fig.7.13.)

To summarize, we define the class of excitability according to the frequency of emerging spiking of a neuron in response to a slowly increasing current ramp. The class of excitability corresponds to a bifurcation of the resting state (equilibrium) resulting in the transition "resting → spiking". We define the class of spiking according to the frequency of disappearing spiking of a neuron in response to a slowly decreasing current ramp. The class of spiking corresponds to the bifurcation of the limit cycle, resulting in the transition "spiking → resting". Stimulating a neuron with ramps (and pulses) is the first step in exploring the bifurcations in the neuron dynamics. Combined with the test for the existence of subthreshold oscillations of the membrane potential, it tells whether the neuron is an integrator or a resonator, and whether it is monostable or bistable, as we discuss next.

## 7.2 Integrators vs. Resonators

In this book we classify excitable systems based on two features: the coexistence of resting and spiking states and the existence of subthreshold oscillations. The former feature divides all systems into *monostable* and *bistable*. The latter feature divides all systems into *integrators* (no oscillations) and *resonators*. These features uniquely determine the type of bifurcation of the resting state, as we summarize in Fig.7.14. For example, a bistable integrator corresponds to a saddle-node bifurcation, whereas monostable resonator corresponds to a supercritical Andronov-Hopf bifurcation. Integrators and resonators have drastically different neurocomputational properties, summarized in Fig.7.15 and discussed next (the I-V curves are discussed in chapter 6).

coexistence of resting and spiking states

| | YES (bistable) | NO (monostable) |
|---|---|---|
| subthreshold oscillations — NO (integrator) | saddle-node | saddle-node on invariant circle |
| subthreshold oscillations — YES (resonator) | subcritical Andronov-Hopf | supercritical Andronov-Hopf |

Figure 7.14: Classification of neurons into monostable/bistable integrators/resonators according to the bifurcation of the resting state.

| properties | integrators | | resonators | |
|---|---|---|---|---|
| bifurcation | saddle-node on invariant circle | saddle-node | subcritical Andronov-Hopf | supercritical Andronov-Hopf |
| excitability | class 1 | class 2 | class 2 | class 2 |
| oscillatory potentials | no | | yes | |
| frequency preference | no | | yes | |
| I-V relation at rest | non-monotone | | monotone | |
| spike latency | large | | small | |
| threshold and rheobase | well-defined | | may not be defined | |
| all-or-none action potentials | yes | | no | |
| co-existence of resting and spiking | no | yes | yes | no |
| post-inhibitory spike or facilitation (brief stimuli) | no | | yes | |
| inhibition-induced spiking | no | | possible | |

Figure 7.15: Summary of neurocomputational properties.

## 7.2.1   Fast Subthreshold Oscillations

According to the definition, resonators have oscillatory potentials, whereas integrators do not. This feature is so important that many of the other neuronal properties discussed later are mere consequences of the existence or absence of such oscillations.

Fast subthreshold oscillations, as in Fig.7.16, are typically due to a fast low-threshold persistent $K^+$ current. At rest, there is a balance of all inward currents and this partially activated $K^+$ current. A brief depolarization further activates the $K^+$ current and results in fast afterhyperpolarization. While the cell is hyperpolarized, the current deactivates below its steady-state level, the balance is shifted toward the inward currents, and the membrane potential depolarizes again. And so on.

The existence of fast subthreshold oscillatory potentials is a distinguishable feature of neurons near an Andronov-Hopf bifurcation. Indeed, the resting state of such a neuron is a stable focus. When it is stimulated by a brief synaptic input or an injected pulse of current, the state of the system deviates from the focus equilibrium, then returns to the equilibrium along a spiral trajectory, as depicted in Fig.7.16 (top), thereby producing a damped oscillation. The frequency of such an oscillation is the imaginary part of the complex-conjugate eigenvalues at the equilibrium (see section 6.1.3), and it can be as large as 200 Hz in mammalian neurons.

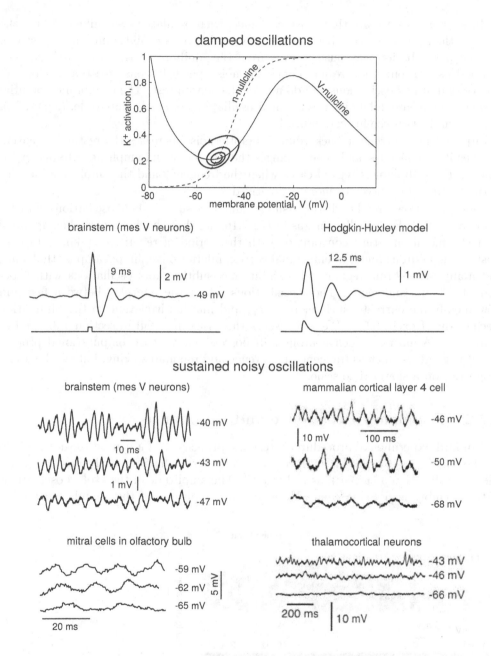

Figure 7.16: Examples of fast damped (top) and sustained (bottom) subthreshold oscillations of membrane potential in neurons and their voltage dependence. (Modified from Izhikevich et al. 2003).

In exercise 3 we prove that noise can make such oscillations sustained. While the state of the system is perturbed and returns to the focus equilibrium, another strong random perturbation may push it away from the equilibrium, thereby starting a new damped oscillation. As a result, persistent noisy perturbations create a random sequence of damped oscillations and do not let the neuron rest. The membrane potential of such a neuron exhibits noisy sustained oscillations of small amplitude, depicted in Fig.7.16 and discussed in section 6.1.4.

Injected DC current or background synaptic noise increases the resting potential, changes its eigenvalues, and hence changes the frequency and amplitude of noisy oscillations. Fig.7.16 depicts typical cases when the frequency and the amplitude increase as the resting state becomes more depolarized.

One should be careful to distinguish *fast* and *slow* subthreshold oscillations of membrane potential. Fast oscillations, as in Fig.7.16, are those having a period comparable with the membrane time constant or with the period of repetitive spiking. In contrast, some neurons found in entorhinal cortex, inferior olive, hippocampus, thalamus, and many other brain regions can exhibit slow subthreshold oscillations with a period of 100 ms and more. These oscillations reflect the interplay between fast and slow membrane currents, such as $I_h$ or $I_T$, and may be irrelevant to the bifurcation mechanism of excitability. We will discuss this issue in detail in section 7.3.3 and in chapter 9. Amazingly, such neurons still possess many neurocomputational properties of resonators, such as frequency preference and rebound spiking, but exhibit these properties on a slower time scale.

## 7.2.2   Frequency Preference and Resonance

A standard experimental procedure to test the propensity of a neuron to subthreshold oscillations is to stimulate it with a sinusoidal current having slowly increasing frequency (called a *zap current*), as in Fig.7.17. The amplitude of the evoked oscillations of the membrane potential, normalized by the amplitude of the stimulating oscilla-

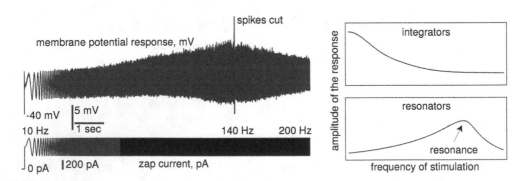

Figure 7.17: Response of the mesV neuron to injected zap current sweeping through a range of frequencies. Integrators and resonators have different responses.

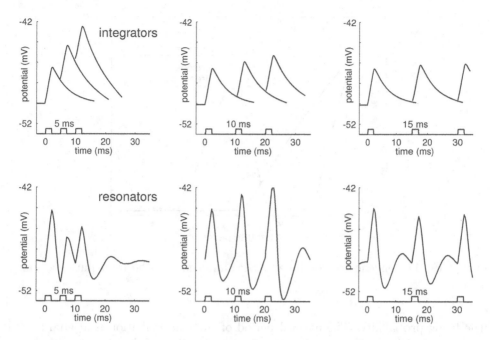

Figure 7.18: Responses of integrators (top) and resonators (bottom) to input pulses having various inter-pulse periods.

tory current, is called the neuronal *impedance* – a frequency domain extension of the concept of resistance. The impedance profile of integrators is decreasing while that of resonators has a peak corresponding to the frequency of subthreshold oscillations, around 140 Hz in the mesV neuron in the figure. Thus, integrators act as low-pass filters while resonators act as band-pass filters to periodic signals.

Instead of sinusoidal stimulation, consider more biological stimulation with pulses of current simulating synaptic bombardment. The response of any neuron to input pulses depends on the frequency content of these pulses. In Fig.7.18 we use triplets with various inter-pulse periods to illustrate the issue. The pulses may arrive from three different presynaptic neurons or from a single presynaptic neuron firing short bursts.

In Fig.7.18 (top) we show that integrators prefer high-frequency inputs. The first pulse in each triplet evokes a postsynaptic potential (PSP) that decays exponentially. The PSP evoked by the second pulse adds to the first one, and so on. The dependence of the combined PSP amplitude on the inter-pulse period is shown in Fig.7.19. Apparently, the integrator acts as a coincidence detector because it is most sensitive to the pulses arriving simultaneously.

Resonators also can detect coincidences, as one can see in Fig.7.19. In addition, they can detect resonant inputs. Indeed, the first pulse in each triplet in Fig.7.18 (bottom), evokes a damped oscillation of the membrane potential, which results in an oscillation

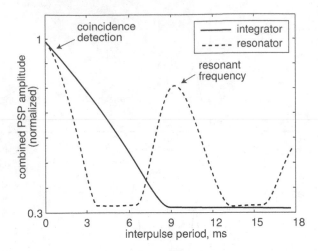

Figure 7.19: Dependence of combined PSP amplitude on the inter-pulse period; see Fig.7.18.

of the firing probability. The natural period of such an oscillation is around 9 ms for the mesencephalic V neuron used in the figure. The effect of the second pulse depends on its timing relative to the first pulse: if the interval between the pulses is near the natural period, which is 10 ms in Fig.7.18 and Fig.7.20, the second pulse arrives during the rising phase of oscillation, and it increases the amplitude of oscillation even further. In this case the effects of the pulses add up. The third pulse increases the amplitude of oscillation even further, thereby increasing the probability of an action potential, as in Fig.7.20.

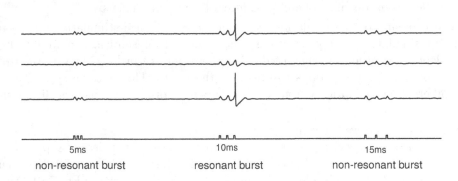

Figure 7.20: Experimental observations of selective response to a resonant (10 ms interspike period) burst in mesencephalic V neurons in brainstem having subthreshold membrane oscillations with a natural period around 9 ms; see also Fig.7.18. Three consecutive voltage traces are shown to demonstrate some variability of the result. (Modified from Izhikevich et al. 2003).

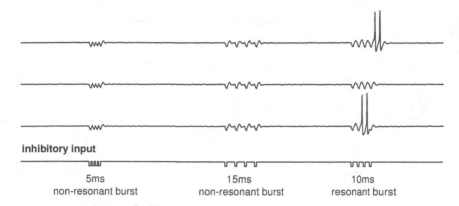

Figure 7.21: Experimental observations of selective response to inhibitory resonant burst in mesencephalic V neurons in brainstem having oscillatory potentials with the natural period around 9 ms. (Modified from Izhikevich et al. 2003).

If the interval between pulses is near half the natural period, e.g., 5 ms in Fig.7.18 and Fig.7.20, the second pulse arrives during the falling phase of oscillation, and it leads to a decrease in oscillation amplitude. The spikes effectively cancel each other in this case. Similarly, the spikes cancel each other when the interpulse period is 15 ms, which is 60 percent greater than the natural period. The same phenomenon occurs for inhibitory synapses, as we illustrate in Fig.7.21. Here the second pulse increases (decreases) the amplitude of oscillation if it arrives during the falling (rising) phase.

We study the mechanism of such frequency preference in exercise 4, and present its geometrical illustration in Fig.7.22. There, we depict a projection of the phase portrait

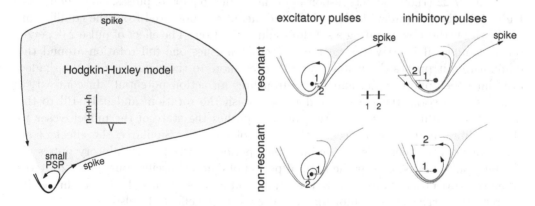

Figure 7.22: (Left) Projection of trajectories of the Hodgkin-Huxley model on a plane. (Right) Phase portrait and typical trajectories during resonant and non-resonant response of the model to excitatory and inhibitory doublets of spikes. (Modified from Izhikevich 2000a).

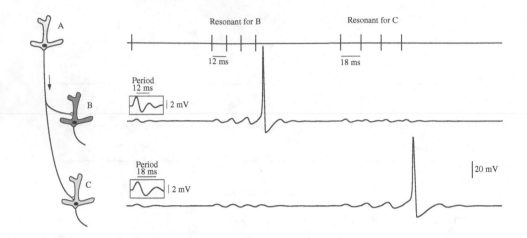

Figure 7.23: Selective communication via bursts. Neuron A sends bursts of spikes to neurons B and C, which have different natural periods (12 ms and 18 ms, respectively; both are simulations of the Hodgkin-Huxley model). As a result of changing the interspike frequency, neuron A can selectively affect either B or C without changing the efficacy of synapses. (Modified from Izhikevich 2002).

of the Hodgkin-Huxley model having a stable focus equilibrium. The model does not have a true threshold, as we discuss in section 7.2.4. To fire a spike, a perturbation must push the state of the model beyond the shaded figure that is bounded by two trajectories, one of which corresponds to a small postsynaptic potential (PSP), while the other corresponds to a spike.

Figure 7.22 (right) depicts responses of the model to pairs of pulses, called doublets. Pulse 1 in the excitatory doublet shifts the membrane potential from the equilibrium to the right, thereby initiating a subthreshold oscillation. The effect of pulse 2 depends on its timing: if it arrives when the trajectory finishes one full rotation around the equilibrium, it pushes the voltage variable even more to the right, beyond the shaded area into the spiking zone, and the neuron fires an action potential. In contrast, if it arrives too soon, the trajectory does not finish the rotation, and it is still to the left of the equilibrium. In this case, pulse 2 pushes the state of the model closer to the equilibrium, thereby canceling the effect of pulse 1. Similarly, the effect of an inhibitory doublet depends on the interspike period between the inhibitory pulses. If the interpulse period is near the natural period of damped oscillations, pulse 2 arrives when the trajectory finishes one full rotation, and it adds to pulse 1, thereby firing the neuron. If it arrives too soon or too late, it cancels the effect of pulse 1.

Quite often, the frequency of subthreshold oscillations depends on their amplitudes, for instance, oscillations in the Hodgkin-Huxley model slow down as they become larger. In this case, the optimal input is a resonant burst with a slowly decreasing (adapting) interspike frequency. We will see many examples of such bursts in chapter 9.

The fact that resonator neurons prefer inputs with "resonant" frequencies is not interesting by itself. What makes it interesting is the observation that the same input can be resonant for one neuron and non-resonant for another, depending on their natural periods. For example, in Fig.7.23 neurons B and C have different periods of subthreshold oscillations: 12 and 18 ms, respectively. By sending a burst of spikes with an interspike interval of 12 ms, neuron A can elicit a response in neuron B, but not in neuron C. Similarly, the burst with an interspike interval of 18 ms elicits a response in neuron C, but not in neuron B. Thus, neuron A can selectively affect either neuron B or neuron C merely by changing the intra-burst (interspike within a burst) frequency without changing the efficacy of synaptic connections. In contrast, integrators do not have this property.

## 7.2.3  Frequency Preference in Vivo

Figures 7.20 and 7.21 convincingly demonstrate the essence of frequency preference and resonance phenomenon *in vitro*, when the neuron is quiescent and "waiting" for the resonant burst to come. What if the neuron is under a constant bombardment of synaptic input, as happens in vivo, firing ten or so spikes per second? Would it be able to tell the difference between the resonant and non-resonant inputs?

To address this question, we performed a frozen-noise experiment pioneered by Bryant and Segundo (1976) and depicted in Fig.7.24. We generated a noisy signal (frozen noise in Fig.7.24a) and saved it into the memory of the program that injects current into a neuron. Then we injected the stored signal into the neuron 50 times to see how reliable its spike response was. Despite the in vivo-like activity in Fig.7.24b, the spike raster in Fig.7.24c shows vertical clusters indicating that the neuron prefers to fire at certain "scheduled" moments of time corresponding to certain features of the frozen noise input.

In Fig.7.24d–g, we added bursts of three spikes to the frozen noise. The amplitudes of the bursts were constant (less than 10 percent of the frozen noise amplitude), but the interspike periods were different. The idea was to see whether the response of the neuron would be any different when the burst period was near the neuronal intrinsic period of 6.7 ms (see the inset in Fig.7.24b). As one would expect, the non-resonant bursts with 4 ms and 9 ms periods remained undetected by the neuron, since the spike rasters in Fig.7.24d and g are essentially the same as in Fig.7.24c. The resonant burst with 7 ms period in Fig.7.24f produced the most significant deviation from Fig.7.24c (marked by the black arrow), indicating that the neuron is most sensitive to the resonant input. Typically, the resonant burst does not make the neuron fire extra spikes, but only changes the timing of "scheduled" spikes. Injecting resonant bursts at different moments results in other interesting phenomena, such as extra spikes and the omission of "scheduled" spikes (not shown here), or no effect at all. Finally, there is a subtle but noticeable effect of the resonant (7 ms) and nearly resonant (6 ms) bursts even 100 ms after the stimulation (white arrows in the figure), for which we have no explanation.

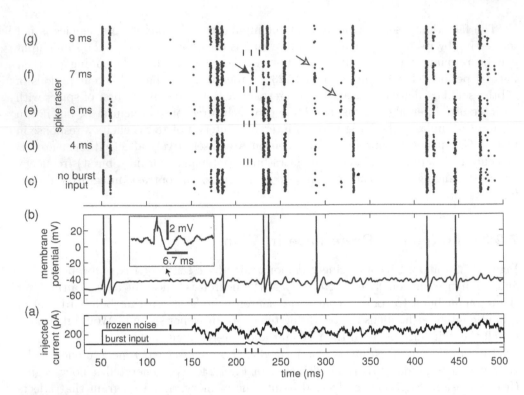

Figure 7.24: Frozen noise experiments demonstrate frequency preference and resonance to embedded bursts. (a) A random signal (frozen noise) is injected into a neuron (b) in vitro to simulate in vivo conditions. The neuron responds with some spike-timing variability, depicted in (c). (d–g) Burst input is added to the frozen noise. Note that the neuron is most sensitive to the input having the resonant period 7 ms, which is near the period of subthreshold oscillation (6.7 ms). Shown are in vitro responses of mesencephalic V neuron of rat brainstem recorded by the author, Niraj S. Desai, and Betsy C. Walcott. The order of stimulation was the first line of c, d, e, f, g, then the second line of c, d, e, f, g, then the third line, and so on, to avoid slow artifacts.

## 7.2.4   Thresholds and Action Potentials

A common misconception is that all neurons have firing thresholds. Moreover, great effort has been made to determine such thresholds experimentally. Typically, a neuron is stimulated with brief current pulses of various amplitudes to elicit various degrees of depolarization of the membrane potential, as we illustrate in Fig.7.25 using the Hodgkin-Huxley model. Small "subthreshold" depolarizations decay while large "superthreshold" or "suprathreshold" depolarizations result in action potentials. The maximal value of the subthreshold depolarization is taken to be the firing threshold value for that neuron. Indeed, the neuron will fire a spike if depolarized just above that value.

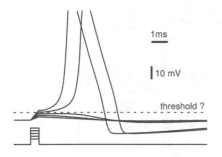

Figure 7.25: Finding the threshold in the Hodgkin-Huxley model.

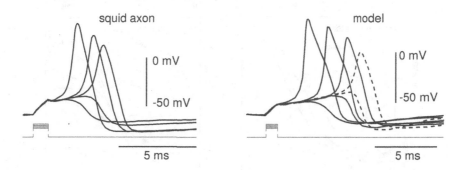

Figure 7.26: Variable-size action potentials in squid giant axon and revised Hodgkin-Huxley model (Clay 1998) in response to brief steps of currents of variable magnitudes. (Data provided by John Clay.)

The notion of a firing threshold is simple and attractive, especially when teaching neuroscience to undergraduates. Everybody, including the author of this book, uses it to describe neuronal properties. Unfortunately, it is wrong. First, the problem is in the definition of an action potential. Are the two dashed curves in Fig.7.26 action potentials? What about a curve in between (not shown in the figure)? Suppose we define an action potential to be any deviation from the resting potential, say by 20 mV. Is the concept of a firing threshold well defined in this case? Unfortunately, the answer is still NO.

The membrane potential value that separates subthreshold depolarizations from action potentials (whatever the definition of an action potential is) depends on the prior activity of the neuron. For example, if a neuron having transient $Na^+$ current has just fired an action potential, the current is partially inactivated, and a subsequent depolarization above the firing threshold may not evoke another action potential. Conversely, if the neuron was briefly hyperpolarized and then released from hyperpolarization, it could fire a rebound postinhibitory spike, as we discuss later in this chapter (see Fig.7.29). Apparently, releasing from hyperpolarization does not qualify as a superthreshold stimulation. Why, then, did the neuron fire?

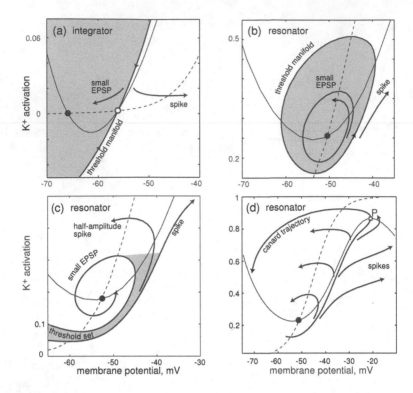

Figure 7.27: Threshold manifolds and sets in the $I_{\text{Na,p}}+I_\text{K}$-model. Parameters in (a) are as in Fig.4.1a, and in (b), (c), and (d) as in Fig.6.16 with $I = 45$ (b) and $I = 42$ (c and d).

## 7.2.5 Threshold manifolds

The problem of formulating a mathematical definition of firing thresholds was first tackled by FitzHugh (1955). Using geometrical analysis of neural models, he noticed that thresholds, if they exist, are never numbers but manifolds, e.g., curves in two-dimensional systems. We illustrate his concept in Fig.7.27, using phase plane analysis of the $I_{\text{Na,p}}+I_\text{K}$-model.

Integrators do have well-defined threshold manifolds. Since an integrator neuron is near a saddle-node bifurcation, whether on or off an invariant circle, there is a saddle point with its stable manifold (see Fig.7.27a). This manifold separates two regions of the phase space, and for this reason is often called a *separatrix*. Depending on the prior activity of the neuron and the size of the input, its state can end up in the shaded area and generate a subthreshold potential, or in the white area and generate an action potential. An intermediate-size input cannot reduce the size of the action potential; it can only delay its occurrence. In the extreme case, a perturbation can put the state vector precisely on the threshold manifold, and the system converges to the saddle, at least in theory. Since the saddle is unstable, small noise present in neurons pushes the state either to the left or to the right, resulting in either a long subthreshold potential or a large-amplitude spike with a long latency, as we discuss in section 7.2.9 and show in Fig.7.34. Finally, note that a neuron has a single threshold value of membrane potential only when its threshold manifold is a straight line orthogonal to the $V$ axis.

Resonators may or may not have well-defined threshold manifolds, depending on the type of bifurcation. Consider a resonator neuron in the bistable regime; that is, sufficiently near a subcritical Andronov-Hopf bifurcation with an unstable limit cycle separating the resting and the spiking states, as in Fig.7.27b. Such an unstable cycle acts as a threshold manifold. Any perturbation that leaves the state of the neuron inside the attraction domain of the resting state, which is the shaded region bounded by the unstable cycle, results in subthreshold potentials. Any perturbation that pushes the state of the neuron outside the shaded region results in an action potential. In the extreme case, a perturbation may put the state right on the unstable limit cycle. Then, the neuron exhibits unstable "threshold" oscillations, at least in theory. In practice, such oscillations cannot be sustained because of noise, and they will either subside or result in spikes.

The bistable regime near subcritical Andronov-Hopf bifurcation is the only case in which a resonator can have a well-defined threshold manifold. In all other cases, including the supercritical Andronov-Hopf bifurcation, resonators do not have well-defined thresholds. We illustrate this in Fig.7.27c. A small deviation from the resting state produces a trajectory corresponding to a "subthreshold" potential. A large deviation produces a trajectory corresponding to an action potential. We refer to the shaded region between the two trajectories as a threshold set. It consists of trajectories corresponding to partial-amplitude action potentials, such as those in Fig.7.26. No single curve separates small potentials from action potentials, so there is no well-defined threshold manifold.

FitzHugh (1955) noticed that the threshold set can be quite thin in some models, including the Hodgkin-Huxley model. In particular, the difference between the trajectories corresponding to small potentials and action potentials can be as small as 0.0001 mV, which is smaller than the noisy fluctuations of the membrane potential. Thus, to observe an intermediate-amplitude spike in such models, one needs to simulate the models with accuracy beyond the limits of uncertainty that appear when the physical interpretation of the model is considered. As a result, for any practical purpose such models exhibit all-or-none behavior, with the threshold set looking like a threshold manifold. FitzHugh referred to this as being a *quasi-threshold* phenomenon.

Quasi-thresholds are related to the special canard trajectory depicted in Fig.7.27d. The trajectory follows the unstable branch of the cubic nullcline all the way to the right knee point P. The flow near the trajectory is highly unstable; any small perturbation pushes the state of the system to the left or to the right, resulting in a "subthreshold" or "superthreshold" response. The solutions depicted in Fig.7.26 (right) try to follow such a trajectory. An easy way to compute the trajectory in two-dimensional relaxation oscillators is to start with the point P and integrate the system backward ($t \to -\infty$). We discuss canard solutions in detail in section 6.3.4.

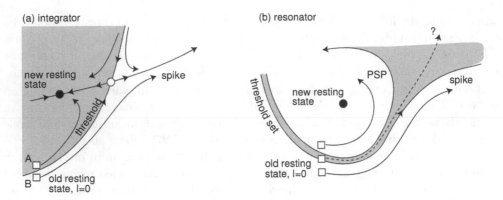

Figure 7.28: Integrators have a well-defined rheobase current, while resonators may not.

### 7.2.6   Rheobase

The neuronal rheobase, that is, the minimal amplitude of a current of infinite duration that makes the neuron fire, measures the "current threshold" of the neuron. Integrators have a well-defined rheobase, while resonators may not. To see this, consider an integrator neuron in Fig.7.28a receiving a current step that instantly changes its phase portrait. In particular, the current moves the equilibrium from the old location corresponding to $I = 0$ (white square in the figure) to a new location (black circle). Whether the neuron fires or not depends on the location of the old equilibrium relative to the stable manifold to the saddle, which plays the role of the new threshold. In case A the neuron does not fire; in case B it fires even though the resting state is still stable. The neuronal rheobase is the amplitude of the current $I$ that puts the threshold exactly on the location of the old equilibrium. Such a value of $I$ always exists, and it often corresponds to the saddle-node bifurcation value. Note that the rheobase current results in a spike with infinite latency, at least theoretically.

A resonator neuron may not have a well-defined rheobase simply because it may not have well-defined threshold. Indeed, the dotted line in Fig.7.28b may correspond to a subthreshold or superthreshold response, depending on where it is in the threshold set. Stimulating such a neuron with "rheobase" current produces spikes with finite latencies but partial amplitudes. A bistable resonator (near subcritical Andronov-Hopf bifurcation) may have a well-defined rheobase because it has a well-defined threshold – the small-amplitude unstable limit cycle.

### 7.2.7   Postinhibitory Spike

Prolonged injection of a hyperpolarizing current and then sudden release from hyperpolarization can produce a rebound postinhibitory response in many neurons. The hyperpolarizing current is often called an anodal current, release from the hyperpolarization is called anodal break, and rebound spiking is called anodal break excitation

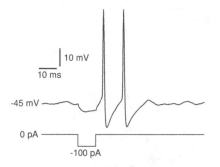

Figure 7.29: Rebound spikes in response to a brief hyperpolarizing pulse in a brainstem mesV neuron having fast subthreshold oscillations of membrane potential.

(FitzHugh 1976). Note that firing of a neuron follows a sudden increase of injected current, whether it is a positive step or a release from a negative step.

Often, postinhibitory responses are caused by the "hyperpolarization-activated" h-current, which slowly builds up and, upon termination of the hyperpolarization, drives the membrane potential over the threshold manifold (or threshold set). Alternatively, the rebound response can be caused by slow deinactivation of $Na^+$ or $Ca^{2+}$ currents, or slow deactivation of a $K^+$ current that is partially activated at rest and prevents firing. In any case, such a rebound response relies on slow currents and long or strong hyperpolarizing steps; it does not depend on the bifurcation mechanism of excitability, and it can occur in integrators or resonators.

Some neurons can exhibit rebound spikes after short and relatively weak hyperpolarizing currents, as we illustrate in Fig.7.29. The negative pulse deactivates a fast low-threshold resonant current (e.g., $K^+$ current) that is partially activated at rest. Upon release from the hyperpolarization, there is a deficit of the outward current and the net membrane current results in rebound depolarization and possibly a spike. Such a response occurs on the fast time scale, and it does depend on the bifurcation mechanism of excitability.

In Fig.7.30 we show why integrators cannot fire rebound spikes in response to short stimulation, while resonators typically can. A brief excitatory pulse of current depolarizes the membrane and brings it closer to the threshold manifold, as in Fig.7.30a. Consequently, an inhibitory pulse hyperpolarizes the membrane and increases the distance to the threshold manifold. The dynamics of such a neuron is consistent with the intuition that excitation facilitates spiking and inhibition prevents it.

Contrary to our intuition, however, inhibition can also facilitate spiking in resonator neurons because the threshold set may wrap around the resting state, as in Fig.7.30b. A sufficiently strong inhibitory pulse can push the state of the neuron beyond the threshold set, thereby evoking a rebound action potential. If the inhibitory pulse is not strong, it still can have an excitatory effect, since it brings the state of the system closer to the threshold set. For example, it can enhance the effect of subsequent excitatory pulses, as we illustrate in Fig.7.31. The excitatory pulse here is subthreshold if applied alone. However, it becomes superthreshold if preceded by an inhibitory pulse. The timing of pulses is important here, as we discussed in section 7.2.2. John Rinzel suggested calling this phenomenon a *postinhibitory facilitation*.

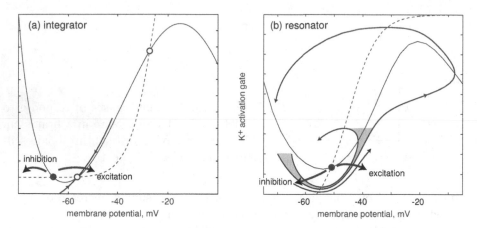

Figure 7.30: Direction of excitatory and inhibitory input in integrators (a) and resonators (b).

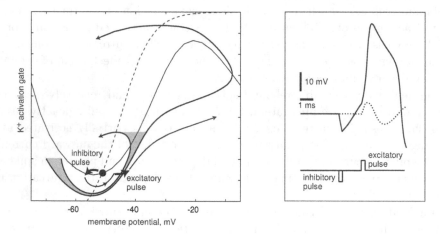

Figure 7.31: Postinhibitory facilitation: A subthreshold excitatory pulse can become superthreshold if it is preceded by an inhibitory pulse.

## 7.2.8 Inhibition-Induced Spiking

In Fig.7.32 (left) we use the $I_{Na,t}$-model introduced in chapter 5 to illustrate an interesting property of some resonators: inhibition-induced spiking. Recall that the model consists of an Ohmic leak current and a transient $Na^+$ current with instantaneous activation and relatively slow inactivation kinetics. It can generate action potentials due to the interplay between the amplifying gate $m$ and the resonant gate $h$.

We widened the activation function $h_\infty(V)$ so that the $Na^+$ current is largely inactivated at the resting state; see the inset in Fig.7.32 (right). Indeed, $h = 0.27$ when $I = 0$. Even though such a system is excitable, it cannot fire repetitive action potentials when a positive step of current (e.g., $I = 10$) is injected. Depolarization produced

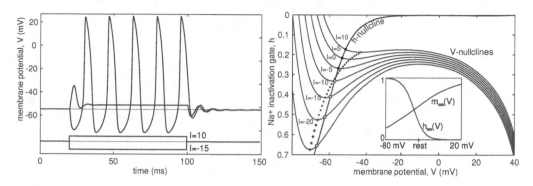

Figure 7.32: Inhibition-induced spiking in the $I_{\mathrm{Na,t}}$-model. Parameters are the same as in Fig.5.6b, except $g_{\mathrm{leak}} = 1.5$ and $m_\infty(V)$ has $k = 27$.

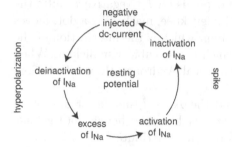

Figure 7.33: Mechanism of inhibition-induced spiking in the $I_{\mathrm{Na,t}}$-model.

by the injected current inactivates the Na$^+$ current so much that no repetitive spikes are possible. Such a system is Class 3 excitable.

Remarkably, injection of a negative step of current (e.g., $I = -15$ in the figure) results in a periodic train of action potentials! How is it possible? Inhibition-induced spiking or bursting is possible in neurons having slow h-current or T-current, such as the thalamocortical relay neurons. (We discuss these and other examples in the next chapter.) The $I_{\mathrm{Na,t}}$-model does not have such currents, yet it can fire in response to inhibition.

Figure 7.33 summarizes the ionic mechanism of inhibition-induced spiking. The resting state in the model corresponds to the balance of the outward leak current and a partially activated, partially inactivated inward Na$^+$ current. When the membrane potential is hyperpolarized by the negative injected current, two processes take place: the Na$^+$ current both deinactivates (variable $h$ increases) and deactivates (variable $m = m_\infty(V)$ decreases). Since $m_\infty(V)$ is flatter than $h_\infty(V)$, deinactivation is stronger than deactivation and the Na$^+$ conductance, $g_{\mathrm{Na}}mh$, increases. This leads to an imbalance of the inward current and to the generation of the first spike. During the spike, the current inactivates completely, and the leak and negative injected currents repolarize and then hyperpolarize the membrane. During the hyperpolarization, clearly seen in the figure, the Na$^+$ current deinactivates and is ready for the generation of the next spike.

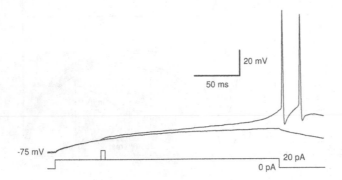

Figure 7.34: Long latencies
and threshold crossing of
layer 5 neuron recorded in
vitro of rat motor cortex.

To understand the dynamic mechanism of such an inhibition-induced spiking, we
need to consider the geometry of the nullclines of the model, depicted in Fig.7.32
(right). Note how the position of the $V$-nullcline depends on $I$. Negative $I$ shifts the
nullcline down and leftward so that the vertex of its left knee, marked by a dot, moves
to the left. As a result, the equilibrium of the system, which is the intersection of the
$V$- and $h$-nullclines, moves toward the middle branch of the cubic $V$-nullcline. When
$I = -2$, the equilibrium loses stability via supercritical Andronov-Hopf bifurcation,
and the model exhibits periodic activity.

Instead of the $I_{\mathrm{Na,t}}$-model, we could have used the $I_{\mathrm{Na}} + I_{\mathrm{K}}$-model or any other
model with a low-threshold resonant gating variable. The key point here is not the ionic
basis of the spike generation mechanism, but its dynamic attribute – the Andronov-
Hopf bifurcation. Even the FitzHugh-Nagumo model (4.11, 4.12) can exhibit this
phenomenon (see exercise 1).

### 7.2.9   Spike Latency

In Fig.7.34 we illustrate an interesting neuronal property - *latency to first spike*. A
barely superthreshold stimulation evokes action potentials with a significant delay,
which could be as large as a second in some cortical neurons. Usually, such a delay is
attributed to slow charging of the dendritic tree or to the action of the A-current, which
is a voltage-gated transient $K^+$ current with fast activation and slow inactivation. The
current activates quickly in response to a depolarization and prevents the neuron from
immediate firing. With time, however, the A-current inactivates and eventually allows
firing. (A slowly activating $Na^+$ or $Ca^{2+}$ current would achieve a similar effect.)

In Fig.7.35 we explain the latency mechanism from the dynamical systems point
of view. Long latencies arise when neurons undergo saddle-node bifurcation, depicted
in Fig.7.35 (left). When a step of current is delivered, the $V$-nullcline moves up so
that the saddle and node equilibria that existed when $I = 0$ coalesce and annihilate
each other. Although there are no equilibria, the vector field remains small in the
shaded neighborhood, as if there were still a ghost of the resting equilibrium there (see
section 3.3.5). The voltage variable increases and passes that neighborhood. As we
discussed in exercise 3 of chapter 6, the passage time scales as $1/\sqrt{I - I_\mathrm{b}}$, where $I_\mathrm{b}$
is the bifurcation point (see Fig.6.8). Hence, the spike is generated with a significant

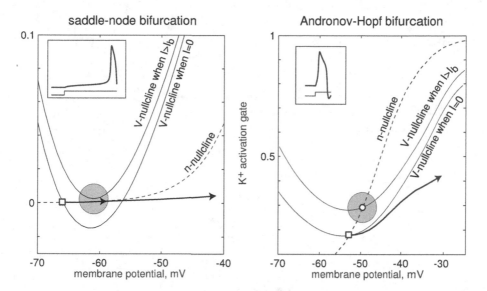

Figure 7.35: Bifurcation mechanism of latency to first spike when the injected DC current steps from $I = 0$ to $I > I_b$, where $I_b$ is a bifurcation value. The shaded circle denotes the region where vector field is small. Phase portraits of the $I_{Na,p}+I_K$-model are shown.

latency. If the bifurcation is on an invariant circle, then the state of the neuron returns to the shaded neighborhood after each spike, resulting in firing with small frequency, a characteristic of Class 1 excitability (see Fig.7.3). In contrast, if the saddle-node bifurcation is *off* an invariant circle, then the state does not return to the neighborhood, and the firing frequency can be large, as in Fig.7.34 or in the neostriatal and basal ganglia neurons reviewed in section 8.4.2.

We see that the existence of long spike latencies is an innate neurocomputational property of integrators. It is still not clear how or when the brain uses it. Two of the most plausible hypotheses are 1) that neurons encode the strength of input into spiking latency, and 2) that neuronal responses become less sensitive to noise, since only prolonged inputs can cause spikes.

Interestingly, resonators do not exhibit long latencies even though there is a neighborhood where the vector field is small and even zero, as we show in Fig.7.35 (right). When the current pulse is applied, the $V$-nullcline moves up and the voltage variable accelerates. However, it misses the shaded neighborhood, and the neuron fires an action potential practically without any latency. In exercise 5 we discuss why some models near Andronov-Hopf bifurcation, including the Hodgkin-Huxley model in Fig.7.26, seem to exhibit small but noticeable latencies. In section 8.2.7 we show that latencies could result from slow charging of the dendritic compartment. In this case, integrator neurons exhibit latency to the first spike, while resonator neurons may exhibit latency to the second spike (after they fire the first, transient spike).

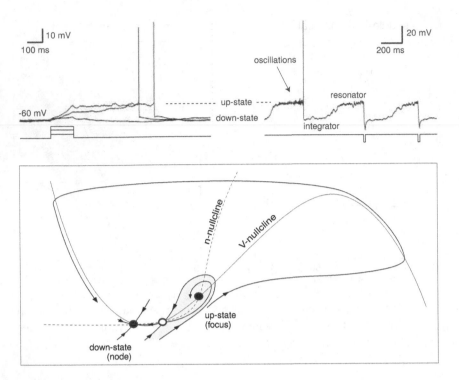

Figure 7.36: Bistability of the up-state and down-state of mitral cells in rat main olfactory bulb. The cells are integrators in the down-state and resonators in the up-state. Membrane potential recordings are modified from Heyward et al. (2001). The shaded area denotes the attraction domain of the up-state.

## 7.2.10   Flipping from an Integrator to a Resonator

One of the reasons we provided so many examples of neuronal systems in chapter 5 was to convince the reader that all neuronal models can exhibit both saddle-node and Andronov-Hopf bifurcations, depending on the parameters describing the ionic currents. Since the kinetics of ionic currents in neurons can change during development or due to the action of neuromodulators, neurons can switch from being integrators to being resonators.

In Fig.7.36 we illustrate an interesting case: mitral cells in rat main olfactory bulb can exhibit bistability of membrane potential. That is, the potential can be in two states: down-state around −60 mV, and up-state around −50 mV (Heyward et al. 2001). A sufficiently strong synaptic input can shift the cell between these states in a matter of milliseconds. An amazing observation is that the down-state is a stable node and the up-state is a stable focus, as we illustrate at the bottom of the figure and study in detail in section 8.4.5. As a result, mitral cells can be quickly switched from being integrators to being resonators by synaptic input.

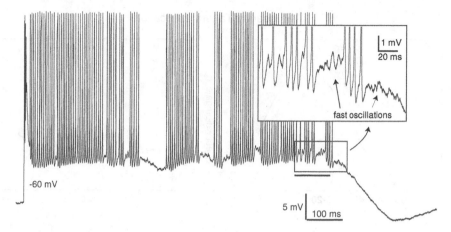

Figure 7.37: Fast subthreshold oscillations during complex spikes of cerebellar Purkinje neuron of a guinea-pig. (Data was by Yonatan Loewenstein.)

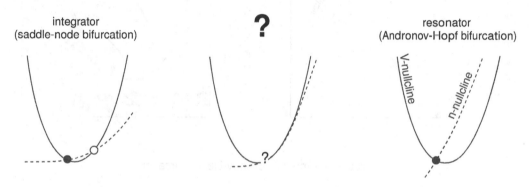

Figure 7.38: Is there an intermediate mode between integrators and resonators?

A similar phenomenon was observed in a cerebellar Purkinje neuron (see Fig.7.37). It acts as an integrator in the down-state, but has fast ($> 100$ Hz) subthreshold oscillations in the up-state, and hence can act as a resonator.

Cortical pyramidal neurons can also exhibit up- and down-states, though the states are not intrinsic, but induced by the synaptic activity. Since the neurons are depolarized in the up-state, there is an interesting possibility that fast $K^+$ conductances are partially activated and the fast $Na^+$ inactivation gate is partially inactivated so that the neuron exhibits fast subthreshold oscillations and acts as a resonator. That is, integrator neurons can switch to the resonator mode when in the up-state. This possibility needs to be tested experimentally.

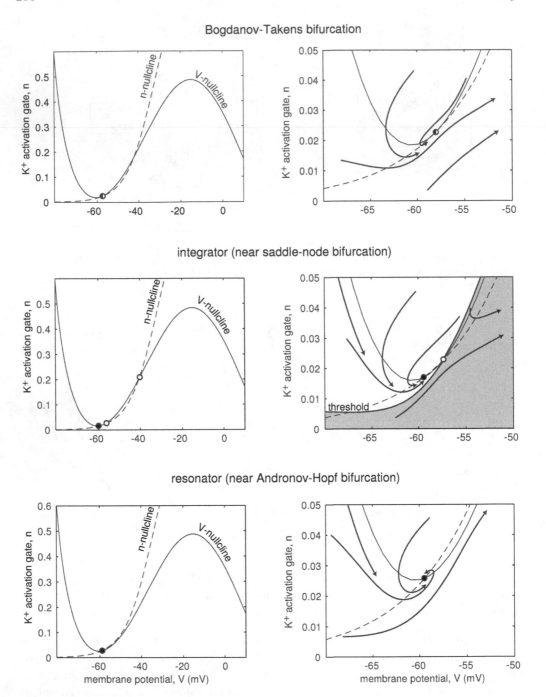

Figure 7.39: Bogdanov-Takens bifurcation in the $I_{Na}+I_K$-model (4.1, 4.2). Parameters are as in Fig.4.1a, except $n_\infty(V)$ has $k = 7$ mV and $V_{1/2} = -31.64$ mV, $E_{leak} = -79.42$ and $I = 5$. Integrator: $V_{1/2} = -31$ mV and $I = 4.3$. Resonator: $V_{1/2} = -34$ mV and $I = 7$.

## 7.2.11   Transition Between Integrators and Resonators

Consider the $I_{Na}+I_K$-model or any other minimal model from chapter 5 that can exhibit saddle-node or Andronov-Hopf bifurcation, depending on the parameter values. Let us start with the $I_{Na}+I_K$-model near saddle-node bifurcation, and hence in the integrator mode. The intersection of its nullclines at the left knee is similar to the one in Fig.7.38 (left). Now, slowly change the parameters toward the values corresponding to the Andronov-Hopf bifurcation with the nullclines intersecting as in Fig.7.38 (right). At some point, the behavior of the model must change from integrator to resonator mode. Is the change sudden, or is it gradual?

Any qualitative change of the behavior of the system is a bifurcation. Such a bifurcation should somehow combine the saddle-node and the Andronov-Hopf cases. That is, it should have a zero eigenvalue, and a pair of complex-conjugate eigenvalues with zero real part. Since the $I_{Na}+I_K$-model is two-dimensional, these two conditions are satisfied only when the model undergoes the Bogdanov-Takens bifurcation considered in section 6.3.3. This bifurcation has codimension-2, that is, it can be reliably observed when two parameters are changed – in this case, $E_{leak}$ and the half-voltage, $V_{1/2}$, of $n_\infty(V)$.

The top of Fig.7.39 depicts the phase portrait of the $I_{Na}+I_K$-model at the Bogdanov-Takens bifurcation. Note that the nullclines are tangent near the left knee, but the tangency is degenerate. A small change of the parameter $V_{1/2}$ can result in either a saddle and a node (middle of the figure) or a focus equilibrium (bottom of the figure). The neuron acts as an integrator in the former case and as a resonator in the latter case.

Due to the proximity to a codimension-2 bifurcation, the behavior of the $I_{Na}+I_K$-model is quite degenerate. That is, it can exhibit features that are normally not observed. For example, the integrator can exhibit postinhibitory spiking, as in Fig.7.40. This occurs because the shaded region in the figure, bounded by the stable manifold

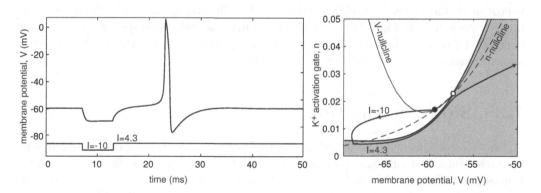

Figure 7.40: Postinhibitory spike of an integrator neuron near Bogdanov-Takens bifurcation; see Fig.7.39.

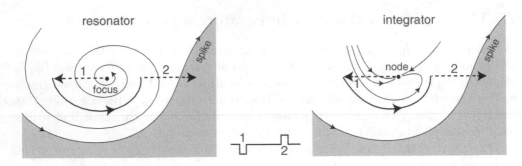

Figure 7.41: Postinhibitory facilitation – enhancement of subthreshold depolarizing pulse (2) by preceding inhibitory pulse (1) – can occur in integrator neurons near Bogdanov-Takens bifurcation.

of the saddle, goes to the left of the resting state. An inhibitory pulse of current that hyperpolarizes the membrane potential to $V < -65$ mV and deactivates the $K^+$ current to $n < 0.005$ pushes the point $(V, n)$ to the shaded region (i.e., beyond the threshold). Upon release from inhibition, the integrator neuron produces a rebound spike and then returns to the resting state.

Integrator neurons can also exhibit frequency preference and resonance, as illustrated in Fig.7.41. The postinhibitory facilitation in resonator neurons in Fig.7.41a was described in section 7.2.7. It may occur in integrator neurons when the node equilibrium has nearly equal eigenvalues and nearly parallel eigenvectors, as in Fig.7.41b. The former are about to become complex-conjugate resulting in rotation of the vector field around the equilibrium, and hence in the postinhibitory rebound response to the first (inhibitory) pulse.

Resonator neurons near a Bogdanov-Takens bifurcation can fire spikes with noticeable latencies. This occurs because the $V$-nullcline follows the $n$-nullcline at the focus equilibrium in Fig.7.39 (bottom). Such a proximity creates a "tunnel" with a small vector field that slows the spiking trajectory. Finally, the neuron can exhibit an oscillation (marked P in Fig.7.42, bottom) before firing a spike in response to a pulse of current. Of course, these behaviors are difficult to catch experimentally, because the system must be near a codimension-2 bifurcation.

# 7.3  Slow Modulation

So far we have considered neuronal models having voltage- or $Ca^{2+}$-gated conductances operating on a fast time scale comparable with the duration of a spike. Such conductances participate directly or indirectly in the generation of each spike and subsequent repolarization of the membrane potential. In addition, neurons have dendritic trees and some slow conductances and currents that may not be involved in the spike generation mechanism directly, but rather may modulate it. For example, some cortical

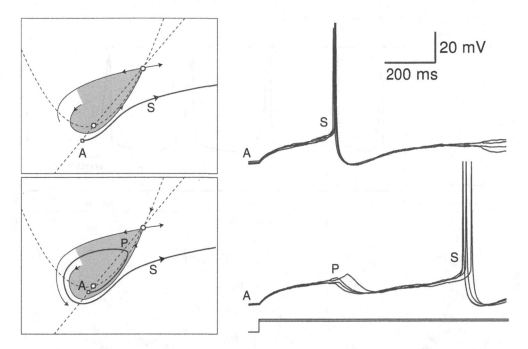

Figure 7.42: Proximity to Bogdanov-Takens bifurcation in layer 5 pyramidal neuron of rat primary visual cortex results in slow subthreshold oscillation before a spike. Shown are a hand-drawn phase portrait and in vitro recordings obtained while an automated procedure was testing the neuronal rheobase.

pyramidal neurons have $I_h$, and all thalamocortical neurons have $I_h$ and $I_{Ca(T)}$. Activation and inactivation kinetics of these currents are too slow to participate in the generation of the upstroke or downstroke of a spike, but the currents can modulate the spiking pattern (e.g., they can transform it into bursting).

To illustrate the phenomenon of slow modulation, we use the $I_{Na,p}+I_K+I_{K(M)}$-model

$$
C\dot{V} = \overbrace{I - g_L(V-E_L) - g_{Na}m_\infty(V)(V-E_{Na}) - g_K n(V-E_K)}^{I_{Na,p}+I_K\text{-model}} - \overbrace{g_M n_M(V-E_K)}^{I_{K(M)}}
$$
$$
\dot{n} = (n_\infty(V) - n)/\tau(V)
$$
$$
\dot{n}_M = (n_{\infty,M}(V) - n_M)/\tau_M(V) \quad \text{(slow K}^+ \text{ M-current),}
$$

(7.1)

whose excitable and spiking properties are similar to those of the $I_{Na,p}+I_K$-submodel on a short time scale. However, the long-term behavior of the two models may be quite different. For example, the K$^+$ M-current may result in frequency adaptation during a long train of action potentials. It can change the shape of the I-V relation of the model and result in slow oscillations, postinhibitory spikes, and other resonator properties even when the $I_{Na,p}+I_K$-submodel is an integrator. All these interesting phenomena are discussed in this section.

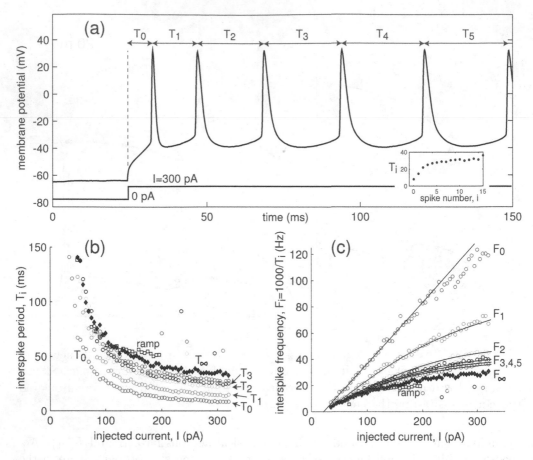

Figure 7.43: Spike frequency adaptation in layer 5 pyramidal cell (see Fig.7.3). Ramp data are from Fig.7.6.

In general, models having fast and slow currents, such as (7.1), can be written in the fast-slow form

$$
\begin{aligned}
\dot{x} &= f(x, u) & \text{(fast spiking)}, \\
\dot{u} &= \mu g(x, u) & \text{(slow modulation)},
\end{aligned}
\tag{7.2}
$$

where the vector $x \in \mathbb{R}^m$ describes fast variables responsible for spiking. It includes the membrane potential $V$ and activation and inactivation gating variables for fast currents, among others. The vector $u \in \mathbb{R}^k$ describes relatively slow variables that modulate fast spiking, e.g., the gating variable of a slow $K^+$ current, the intracellular concentration of $Ca^{2+}$ ions, etc. The small parameter $\mu$ represents the ratio of time scales between spiking and its modulation. Such systems often result in bursting activity, and we study them in detail in chapter 9.

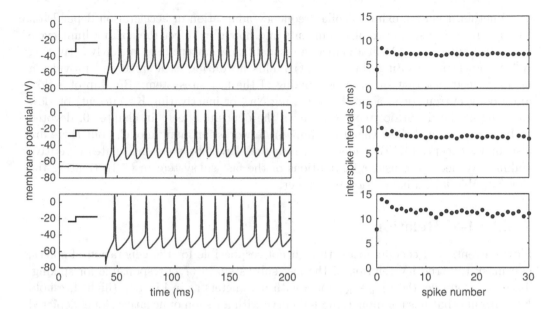

Figure 7.44: Spike-frequency acceleration of a cortical fast spiking (FS) interneuron. Data kindly provided by Barry Connors.

## 7.3.1  Spike Frequency Modulation

Slow currents can modulate the instantaneous spiking frequency of a long train of action potentials, as we illustrate in Fig.7.43a, using recordings of a layer 5 pyramidal neuron. The neuron generates a train of spikes with increasing interspike interval (see inset in the figure) in response to a long pulse of injected DC current. In Fig.7.43b we plot the instantaneous interspike intervals $T_i$, that is, the time intervals between spikes $i$ and $i + 1$, as a function of the magnitude of injected current $I$. Notice that $T_i(I) < T_{i+1}(I)$, meaning that the intervals increase with each spike. The function $T_0(I)$ describes the latency of the first spike, and $T_\infty(I)$ describes the steady-state (asymptotic) interspike period. The instantaneous frequencies, defined as $F_i(I) = 1000/T_i(I)$ (Hz), are depicted in Fig.7.43c. Since the neuron is Class 1 excitable, the F-I curves are square-root parabolas (see section 6.1.2). Note that $F_0(I)$ is nearly a straight line, probably reflecting the passive charging of the dendritic tree.

Decrease of the instantaneous spiking frequency, as in Fig.7.43, is referred to as *spike-frequency adaptation*. This is a prominent feature of cortical pyramidal neurons of the regular spiking (RS) type (Connors and Gutnick 1990), as well as of many other types of neurons discussed in chapter 8. In contrast, cortical fast spiking (FS) interneurons (Gibson et al. 1999) exhibit *spike frequency acceleration*, depicted in Fig.7.44, that is, the instantaneous interspike intervals decrease, and the frequency increases with each spike.

Whether a neuron exhibits spike frequency adaptation or acceleration depends on the nature of the slow current or currents and how they affect the spiking limit cycle of the fast subsystem. At first glance, a resonant slow current (e.g., a slowly activating $K^+$ or slowly inactivating $Na^+$ current) builds up during each spike and provides a negative feedback that should slow spiking of the fast subsystem. Buildup of a slow amplifying current (e.g., a slowly activating $Na^+$ or inactivating $K^+$ current) or slow charging of the dendritic tree should have the opposite effect. In chapter 9, devoted to bursting, we will show that this simple rule works for many models, but there are also many exceptions. To understand how the slow subsystem modulates repetitive spiking, we need to consider bifurcations of the fast subsystem in (7.2), treating the slow variable $u$ as a bifurcation parameter.

## 7.3.2    I-V Relation

Slow currents and conductances, though not responsible for the generation of spikes, can mask the true I-V relation of the fast subsystem in (7.2) responsible for spiking. Take, for example, the $I_{Na,p}+I_K$-model with parameters as in Fig.4.1a (high-threshold $K^+$ current) that has nonmonotonic I-V curve with a region of negative slope, depicted in Fig.7.45a. Such a system is near saddle-node on invariant circle bifurcation and it acts as an integrator. Now add a slow $K^+$ M-current with an I-V relation depicted as a dashed curve in the figure and a time constant $\tau_M = 100$ ms. The spike generating mechanism of the combined $I_{Na,p}+I_K+I_{K(M)}$-model is described by the fast $I_{Na,p}+I_K$-submodel, so that the neuron continues to have integrator properties, at least on the

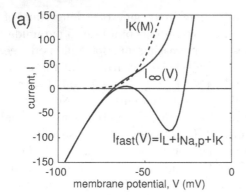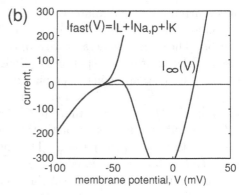

Figure 7.45: Slow conductances can mask the true I-V relation of the spike generating mechanism. (a) The $I_{Na,p}+I_K$-model with parameters as in Fig.4.1a has a nonmonotonic I-V curve $I_{fast}(V)$. Addition of the slow $K^+$ M-current with parameters as in section 2.3.5 and $g_M = 5$ (dashed curve) makes the asymptotic I-V relation, $I_\infty(V)$, of the full $I_{Na,p}+I_K+I_{K(M)}$-model monotonic. (b) Addition of a slow inactivation gate to the $K^+$ current of the $I_{Na,p}+I_K$-model with parameters as in Fig.4.1b results in a nonmonotonic asymptotic I-V relation of the full $I_{Na,p}+I_A$-model.

millisecond time scale. However, the asymptotic I-V relation $I_\infty(V)$ is dominated by the strong $I_{K(M)}(V)$ and is monotonic, as if the $I_{Na,p}+I_K+I_{K(M)}$-model were a resonator. The model can indeed exhibit some resonance properties, such as postinhibitory (rebound) responses, but only on the long time scale of hundreds of milliseconds, which is the time scale of the slow $K^+$ M-current.

Similarly, we can take a resonator model with a monotonic I-V relation and add a slow amplifying current or a gating variable to get a non-monotonic $I_\infty(V)$, as if the model becomes an integrator. For example, in Fig.7.45b we use the $I_{Na,p}+I_K$-model with parameters as in Fig.4.1b (low-threshold $K^+$ current) and adds an inactivation gate to the persistent $K^+$ current, effectively transforming it into transient A-current. If the inactivation kinetics is sufficiently slow, the $I_{Na,p}+I_A$-model retains resonator properties on the millisecond time scale, which is the time scale of individual spikes. However, its asymptotic I-V relation, depicted in Fig.7.45b, becomes non-monotonic. Besides spike-frequency acceleration, the model acquires another interesting property: bistability. A single spike does not inactivate $I_A$ significantly. A burst of spikes can inactivate the $K^+$ A-current to such a degree that repetitive spiking becomes sustained. Slow inactivation of the A-current is believed to facilitate the transition from down-states to up-states in neocortical and neostriatal neurons.

When a neuronal model consists of conductances operating on drastically different time scales, it has multiple I-V relations, one for each time scale. We illustrate this phenomenon in Fig.7.46, using the $I_{Na,p}+I_K+I_{K(M)}$-model with an activation time constant of 0.01 ms for $I_{Na,p}$, 1 ms for $I_K$, and 100 ms for $I_{K(M)}$. The upstroke of an action potential is described only by leak and persistent $Na^+$ currents, since the $K^+$ currents do not have enough time to activate during such a short event. During the upstroke, the model can be reduced to a one-dimensional system (see chapter 3) with instantaneous I-V relation $I_0(V) = I_{leak} + I_{Na,p}(V)$ depicted in Fig.7.46a. The dynamics during and immediately after the action potential is described by the fast $I_{Na,p}+I_K$-subsystem with its I-V relation $I_{fast}(V) = I_0(V) + I_K(V)$. Finally, the asymptotic I-V relation, $I_\infty(V) = I_{fast}(V) + I_{K(M)}(V)$, takes into account all currents in the model.

The three I-V relations determine the fast, medium, and asymptotic behavior of a neuron in a voltage-clamp experiment. If the time scales are well separated (they are in Fig.7.46), all three I-V relations can be measured from a simple voltage-clamp experiment, depicted in Fig.7.46b. We hold the model at $V = -70$ mV and step the command voltage to various values. The values of the current, taken at $t = 0.05$ ms, $t = 5$ ms, and $t = 500$ ms in Fig.7.46b, result in the instantaneous, fast, and steady-state I-V curves, respectively. Notice that the data in Fig.7.46b are plotted on the logarithmic time scale. Various magnifications using the linear time scale are depicted in Fig.7.46c,d, and e. Numerically obtained values of the three I-V relations are depicted as dots in Fig.7.46a. They approximate the theoretical values quite well because there is a 100-fold separation of time scales in the model.

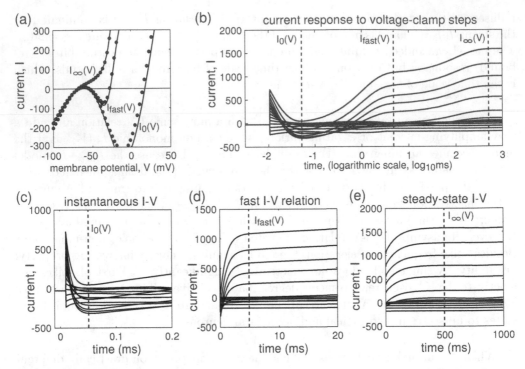

Figure 7.46: (a) The $I_{Na,p}+I_K+I_{K(M)}$-model in Fig.7.45a has three I-V relations: Instantaneous $I_0(V) = I_{leak}(V) + I_{Na,p}(V)$ describes spike upstroke dynamics. The curve $I_{fast}(V) = I_0(V) + I_K(V)$ is the I-V relation of the fast $I_{Na,p}+I_K$-subsystem responsible for the spike generation mechanism. The curve $I_\infty(V) = I_{fast}(V) + I_{K(M)}(V)$ is the steady-state (asymptotic) I-V relation of the full model. Dots denote values obtained from a simulated voltage-clamp experiment in (b); note the logarithmic time scale. Magnifications of current responses are shown in (c – e). Simulated time constants: $\tau_{Na,p}(V) = 0.01$ ms, $\tau_K(V) = 1$ ms, $\tau_M(V) = 100$ ms.

### 7.3.3  Slow Subthreshold Oscillation

Interactions between fast and slow conductances can result in low-frequency subthreshold oscillation of membrane potential, such as the one in Fig.7.47, even when the fast subsystem is near a saddle-node bifurcation, acts as an integrator, and cannot have subthreshold oscillations. The oscillation in Fig.7.47 is caused by the interplay between activation and inactivation of the slow $Ca^{2+}$ T-current and the inward h-current, and it is a precursor of bursting activity (which we consider in detail in chapter 9).

There are at least three different mechanisms of *slow* subthreshold oscillations of membrane potential of a neuron.

- The fast subsystem responsible for spiking has a small-amplitude subthreshold limit cycle attractor. The period of the limit cycle may be much larger than the

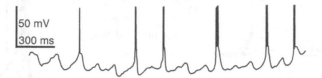

Figure 7.47: Slow subthreshold oscillation of membrane potential of cat thalamocortical neuron evoked by slow hyperpolarization. (Modified from Roy et al. 1984.)

time scale of the slowest variable of the fast subsystem when the cycle is near a saddle-node on invariant circle, saddle homoclinic orbit bifurcation, or Bogdanov-Takens bifurcation (considered in chapter 6). In this case, no slow currents or conductances modulating the fast subsystem are involved. However, such a cycle must be near the bifurcation; hence the low-frequency subthreshold oscillation exists in a narrow parameter range and it is difficult to be seen experimentally.

- The I-V relation of the fast subsystem has an N-shape in the subthreshold voltage range, so that there are two stable equilibria corresponding to two resting states (as, e.g., in Fig.7.36). A slow resonant variable switches the fast subsystem between those two states via a hysteresis loop, resulting in a subthreshold slow relaxation oscillation.

- If the fast subsystem has a monotonic I-V relation, then a stable subthreshold oscillation can result from the interplay between slow variables.

The first case does not need any slow variables; the second case needs only one slow variable; and the third case may need at least two.

## 7.3.4   Rebound Response and Voltage Sag

A slow resonant current can cause a neuron to fire a rebound spike or a burst in response to a sufficiently long hyperpolarizing current, even when the spike generating mechanism of the neuron is near a saddle-node bifurcation and hence has the neurocomputational properties of an integrator. For example, the cortical pyramidal neuron in Fig.7.48a has a slow resonant current $I_h$, which is opened by hyperpolarization. A short pulse of current does not open enough of $I_h$ and results only in a small subthreshold rebound potential. In contrast, a long pulse of current opens enough $I_h$, resulting in a strong inward current that produces the voltage sag and, upon termination of stimulation, drives the membrane potential over the threshold.

Similarly, the thalamocortical neuron in Fig.7.48b has a low-threshold $Ca^{2+}$ T-current $I_{Ca(T)}$ that is partially activated but completely inactivated at rest. A negative pulse of current hyperpolarizes the neuron and deinactivates the T-current, thereby making it available to generate a spike. Note that there is no voltage sag in Fig.7.48b because the T-current is deactivated at low membrane potentials. Upon termination of the long pulse of current, the membrane potential returns to the resting state around

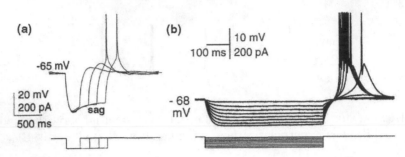

Figure 7.48: Rebound responses to long inhibitory pulses in (a) pyramidal neuron of sensorimotor cortex of juvenile rat (modified from Hutcheon et al. 1996) and (b) rat auditory thalamic neurons. (Modified from Tennigkeit et al. 1997.)

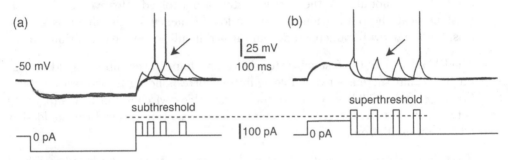

Figure 7.49: Postinhibitory facilitation (a) and post-excitatory depression (b) in a layer 5 pyramidal neuron (IB type) of rat visual cortex recorded in vitro in response to a long hyperpolarizing pulse.

−68 mV, and the $Ca^{2+}$ T-current activates (but does not have time to inactive) and drives the neuron over the threshold. A distinctive feature of thalamocortical neurons is that they fire a rebound burst of spikes in response to strong negative currents.

Even when the rebound depolarization is not strong enough to elicit a spike, it may increase the excitability of the neuron, so that it fires a spike to an otherwise subthreshold stimulus, as in Fig.7.49a. This type of postinhibitory facilitation relies on the slow currents, and not on the resonant properties of the spike generation mechanism (as in Fig.7.31). Figure 7.49b demonstrates the inverse property, post-excitatory depression, that is, a decreased excitability after a transient depolarization. In this seemingly counterintuitive case, a superthreshold stimulation becomes subthreshold when it is preceded by a depolarized pulse, because the pulse partially inactivates the $Na^+$ current and/or activates the $K^+$ current.

## 7.3.5   AHP and ADP

The membrane potential may undergo negative and positive deflections right after the spike, as illustrated in Fig.7.50 and Fig.7.51. These are known as *afterhyperpolarizations* (AHP) and *afterdepolarizations* (ADP). The latter are sometimes called

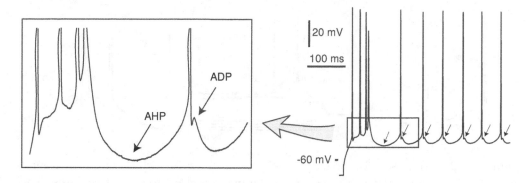

Figure 7.50: Afterhyperpolarizations (AHP) and afterdepolarizations (ADP) in intrinsically bursting (IB) pyramidal neurons of the rat motor cortex, recorded in vitro.

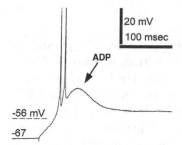

Figure 7.51: Rebound spikes and afterdepolarization (marked ADP) at the break of hyperpolarizing current in thalamocortical neurons of the cat dorsal lateral geniculate nucleus. (Data modified from Pirchio et al. 1997; resting potential is $-56$ mV, holding potential is $-67$ mV.)

*depolarizing afterpotentials* (DAP). A great effort is usually made to determine the ionic basis of AHPs and ADPs, since it is often implicitly assumed that they are generated by slow currents that turn on right after the spike, such as the slow $Ca^{2+}$-gated $K^+$current $I_{AHP}$ or the slow persistent $Na^+$ current, respectively. Below we discuss these and other mechanisms.

Let us consider the AHP first. Each spike in the initial burst in Fig.7.50 presumably activates a slow voltage- or $Ca^{2+}$-dependent outward $K^+$ current, which eventually stops the burst and hyperpolarizes the membrane potential. During the AHP period, the slow outward current deactivates, and the neuron can fire again. The neuron can switch from bursting to tonic spiking mode due to the incomplete deactivation of the slow current. The same explanation holds if we replace "activation of outward" with "inactivation of inward" current.

Similarly, slow inactivation of the transient $Ca^{2+}$ T-current explains the rebound response and the long afterdepolarization (marked ADP) in Fig.7.51: The current was deinactivated by the preceding hyperpolarization, so upon release from the hyperpolarization, it quickly activates and slowly inactivates, thereby producing a slow depolarizing wave on which fast spikes can ride. The ADP seen in the figure is the tail of the wave.

Probably the most common mechanism of ADPs is due to the dendritic spikes, at least in pyramidal neurons of neocortex considered in chapter 8. In Fig.7.52a we

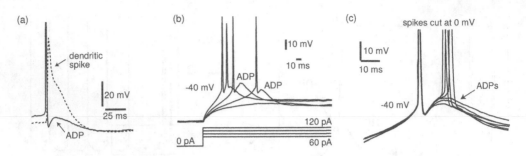

Figure 7.52: (a) A somatic spike evokes a dendritic spike, which in turn produces afterdepolarization (ADP) in the soma of the pyramidal neuron of rat somatosensory cortex (in vitro recording was provided Greg Stuart and Maarten Kole). (b) and (c) Increased level of depolarization in another neuron (the same as in Fig.7.49) converts ADP to a second spike.

depict a dual somatic/dendritic recording of the membrane potential of a pyramidal neuron. The somatic spike backpropagates into the dendritic tree, activates voltage-gated conductances there, and results in a slower dendritic spike. The latter depolarizes the soma and produces a noticeable ADP. Recordings of another neuron in Fig.7.52b and c show that if there is an additional source of depolarization, such as the injected DC current, the ADPs can grow and result in a second spike. This may evoke another dendritic spike, another ADP or spike, and so on. Such a somatic-dendritic ping-pong (Wang 1999; Doiron et al. 2002) results in a bursting activity discussed in section 8.2.2.

In contrast, adult CA1 pyramidal neurons in hippocampus generate ADP and bursting even when their apical dendrites are cut (Yue et al. 2005; Golomb et al. 2006). The ADP there is caused by the slow deactivation of somatic persistent $Na^+$ current.

Slow ADPs can also be generated by a nonlinear interplay of fast currents responsible for spiking, rather than by slow currents or dendritic spikes. One obvious example is the damped oscillation of membrane potential of the $I_{Na,p}+I_K$-model in Fig.7.53 immediately after the spike, with the trough and the peak corresponding to an AHP and an ADP, respectively. Note that the duration of the ADP is ten times the duration of the spike even though the model does not have any slow currents. Such a long-lasting effect appears because the trajectory follows the separatrix, comes close to the saddle point, and spends some time there before returning to the stable resting state.

An example in Fig.7.54 shows the membrane potential of a model neuron slowly passing through a saddle-node on invariant circle bifurcation. Because the vector field is small at the bifurcation, which takes place around $t = 70$ ms, the membrane potential is slowly increasing along the limit cycle and then slowly decreasing along the locus of stable node equilibria, thereby producing a slow ADP. In chapter 9 we will show that such ADPs exist in 4 out of 16 basic types of bursting neurons, including thalamocortical relay neurons and $R_{15}$ bursting cells in the abdominal ganglion of the mollusk *Aplysia*.

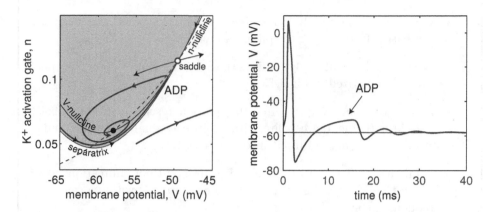

Figure 7.53: A long afterdepolarization (ADP) in the $I_{Na,p}+I_K$-model without any slow currents. Parameters are as in Fig.6.52.

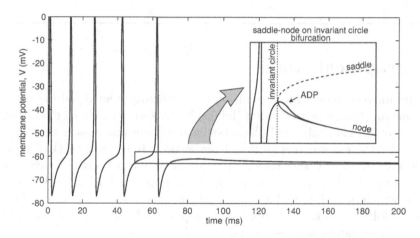

Figure 7.54: Afterdepolarization in the $I_{Na,p}+I_K$-model passing slowly through saddle-node on invariant circle bifurcation, as the magnitude of the injected current ramps down.

## Review of Important Concepts

- A neuron is excitable because, as a dynamical system, it is near a bifurcation from resting to spiking activity.

- The type of bifurcation determines the neuron's computational properties, summarized in Fig.7.15.

- Saddle-node *on* invariant circle bifurcation results in Class 1 excitability: the neuron can fire with arbitrarily small frequency and encode the strength of input into the firing rate.

- Saddle-node *off* invariant circle and Andronov-Hopf bifurcations result in Class 2 excitability: the neuron can fire only within a certain frequency range.

- Neurons near saddle-node bifurcation are integrators: they prefer high-frequency excitatory input, have well-defined thresholds, and fire all-or-none spikes with some latencies.

- Neurons near Andronov-Hopf bifurcation are resonators: they have oscillatory potentials, prefer resonant-frequency input, and can easily fire postinhibitory spikes.

## Bibliographical Notes

There is no universally accepted definition of excitability. Our definition is consistent with the one involving $\varepsilon$-pseudo orbits (Izhikevich 2000a). FitzHugh (1955, 1960, 1976) pioneered geometrical analyses of phase portraits of neuronal models with the view to understanding their neurocomputational properties. It is amazing that such important neurocomputational properties as all-or-none action potentials, firing thresholds, and integration of EPSPs are still introduced and illustrated using the Hodgkin-Huxley model, which according to FitzHugh, cannot have these properties. Throughout, this chapter follows Izhikevich (2000a) to compare and contrast neurocomputational properties of integrators and resonators.

The frozen noise experiment in Fig.7.24 was pioneered by Bryant and Segundo (1976), but due to an interesting quirk of history, it is better known at present as the Mainen-Sejnowski (1995) experiment (despite the fact that the latter paper refers to the former). Postinhibitory facilitation was pointed out by Luk and Aihara (2000) and later by Izhikevich (2001). John Rinzel suggested calling it "postinhibitory exaltation" (in a similar vein; the phenomenon in Fig.7.49b may be called "post-excitatory hesitation").

Richardson et al. (2003) pointed out that frequency preference and resonance may occur without subthreshold oscillations when the system is near the transition from an integrator to a resonator.

The Hodgkin classification of neuronal excitability can be used to classify any rhythmic system, even contractions of the uterus during labor. Typically, the contractions start with low frequency that gradually increases – Class 1 excitability. My wife had to have labor induced pharmacologically, a typical medical intervention when the baby is overdue. The contraction monitor showed a sinusoidal signal with constant period, around 2 minutes, but slowly growing amplitude – Class 2 excitability via supercritical Andronov-Hopf bifurcation! Since my wife has an advanced degree in applied mathematics, I waited for a 1-minute period of quiescence between the contractions and managed to explain to her the basic relationship between bifurcations and excitability. Five years later, induced delivery of our second daughter resulted in the same supercritical Andronov-Hopf bifurcation. I recalled this for my wife and explained it to the obstetrician minutes after the delivery.

# Exercises

1. When can the FitzHugh-Nagumo model (4.11, 4.12) exhibit inhibition-induced spiking, such as in Fig.7.32?

2. (Canards) Numerically investigate the quasi-threshold in the FitzHugh-Nagumo model (4.11, 4.12). How is it related to the canard (French duck; see Eckhaus 1983) limit cycles discussed in section 6.3.4?

3. (Noise-induced oscillations) Consider the system

$$\dot{z} = (-\varepsilon + \mathrm{i}\omega)z + \varepsilon I(t) , \qquad z \in \mathbb{C} \tag{7.3}$$

which has a stable focus equilibrium $z = 0$ and is subject to a weak noisy input $\varepsilon I(t)$. Show that the system exhibits sustained noisy oscillations with an average amplitude $|I^*(\omega)|$, where

$$I^*(\omega) = \lim_{T \to \infty} \frac{1}{T} \int_0^T e^{-\mathrm{i}\omega t} I(t) \, dt$$

is the Fourier coefficient of $I(t)$ corresponding to the frequency $\omega$.

4. (Frequency preference) Show that a system exhibiting damped oscillation with frequency $\omega$ is sensitive to an input having frequency $\omega$ in its power spectrum. (Hint: use exercise 3.)

5. (Rush and Rinzel 1995) Use the phase portrait of the reduced Hodgkin-Huxley model in Fig.5.21 to explain some small but noticeable latencies in Fig.7.26.

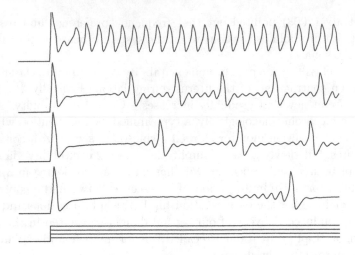

Figure 7.55: exercise 6: Zero frequency firing near subcritical Andronov-Hopf bifurcation in the $I_{\text{Na,p}} + I_{\text{K}}$-model with parameters as in Fig.6.16 and a high-threshold slow K$^+$ current ($g_{\text{K,slow}} = 25$, $\tau_{\text{K,slow}} = 10$ ms, $n_{\infty,\text{slow}}(V)$ has $V_{1/2} = -10$ mV and $k = 5$ mV.)

6. The neuronal model in Fig.7.55 has a high-threshold slow persistent K$^+$ current. Its resting state undergoes a subcritical Andronov-Hopf bifurcation, yet it can fire low-frequency spikes, and hence exhibits Class 1 excitability. Explain. (Hint: Show numerically that the model is near a certain codimension-2 bifurcation involving a homoclinic orbit.)

7. Show that the resting state of a Class 3 excitable conductance-based model is near an Andronov-Hopf bifurcation if some other variable, not $I$, is used as a bifurcation parameter.

# Chapter 8

# Simple Models

The advantage of using conductance-based models, such as the $I_{Na}+I_K$-model, is that each variable and parameter has a well-defined biophysical meaning. In particular, they can be measured experimentally. The drawback is that the measurement procedures may not be accurate: the parameters are usually measured in different neurons, averaged, and then fine-tuned (a fancy term meaning "to make arbitrary choices"). As a result, the model does not have the behavior that one sees in experiments. And even if it "looks" right, there is no guarantee that the model is accurate from the dynamical systems point of view, that is, it exhibits the same kind of bifurcations as the type of neuron under consideration.

Sometimes we do not need or cannot afford to have a biophysically detailed conductance-based model. Instead, we want a simple model that faithfully reproduces all the neurocomputational features of the neuron. In this chapter we review salient features of cortical, thalamic, hippocampal, and other neurons, and we present simple models that capture the essence of their behavior from the dynamical systems point of view.

## 8.1 Simplest Models

Let us start with reviewing the simplest possible models of neurons. As one can guess from their names, the integrate-and-fire and resonate-and-fire neurons capture the essence of integrators and resonators, respectively. The models are similar in many respects: both are described by linear differential equations, both have a hard firing threshold and a reset, and both have a unique stable equilibrium at rest. The only difference is that the equilibrium is a node in the integrate-and-fire case, but a focus in the resonate-and-fire case. One can model the former using only one equation, and the latter using only two equations, though multi-dimensional extensions are straightforward. Both models are useful from the analytical point of view, that is, to prove theorems.

Many scientists, including myself, refer to these neural models as "spiking models". The models have a threshold, but they lack any spike generation mechanism, that is, they cannot produce a brief regenerative depolarization of membrane potential corre-

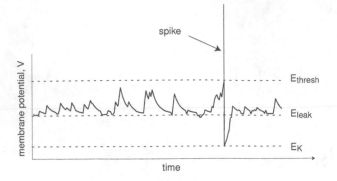

Figure 8.1: Leaky integrate-and-fire neuron with noisy input. The spike is added manually for aesthetic purposes and to fool the reader into believing that this is a spiking neuron.

sponding to the spike upstroke. Therefore, they are not *spiking models*; the spikes in figures 8.1 and 8.2, as well as in hundreds of scientific papers devoted to these models, are drawn by hand. The quadratic integrate-and-fire model is the simplest truly spiking model.

## 8.1.1   Integrate-and-Fire

The leaky integrate-and-fire model (Lapicque 1907; Stein 1967; Tuckwell 1988) is an idealization of a neuron having Ohmic leakage current and a number of voltage-gated currents that are completely deactivated at rest. Subthreshold behavior of such a neuron can be described by the linear differential equation

$$C\dot{V} = I - \overbrace{g_{\text{leak}}(V - E_{\text{leak}})}^{\text{Ohmic leakage}},$$

where all parameters have the same biophysical meanings as in the previous chapters. When the membrane potential $V$ reaches the threshold value $E_{\text{thresh}}$, the voltage-sensitive currents instantaneously activate, the neuron is said to fire an action potential, and $V$ is reset to $E_{\text{K}}$, as in Fig.8.1. After appropriate rescaling, the leaky integrate-and-fire model can be written in the form

$$\dot{v} = b - v\,, \qquad \text{if } v = 1, \text{ then } v \leftarrow 0, \tag{8.1}$$

where the resting state is $v = b$, the threshold value is $v = 1$, and the reset value is $v = 0$. Apparently the neuron is excitable when $b < 1$ and fires a periodic spike train when $b > 1$ with period $T = -\ln(1 - 1/b)$. (The reader should verify this.)

The integrate-and-fire neuron illustrates a number of important neurocomputational properties:

- *All-or-none spikes*. Since the shape of the spike is not simulated, all spikes are implicitly assumed to be identical in size and duration.

- *Well-defined threshold*. A stereotypical spike is fired as soon as $V = E_{\text{thresh}}$, leaving no room for any ambiguity (see, however, exercise 1).

- *Relative refractory period.* When $E_K < E_{leak}$, the neuron is less excitable immediately after the spike.

- *Distinction between excitation and inhibition.* Excitatory inputs ($I > 0$) bring the membrane potential closer to the threshold, and hence facilitate firing, while inhibitory inputs ($I < 0$) do the opposite.

- *Class 1 excitability.* The neuron can continuously encode the strength of an input into the frequency of spiking.

In summary, the neuron seems to be a good model for an integrator.

However, a closer look reveals that the integrate-and-fire neuron has flaws. The transition from resting to repetitive spiking occurs neither via saddle-node nor via Andronov-Hopf bifurcation, but via some other weird type of bifurcation that can be observed only in piecewise continuous systems. As a result, the F-I curve has logarithmic scaling and not the expected square-root scaling of a typical Class 1 excitable system (see, however, exercise 19 in chapter 6). The integrate-and-fire model cannot have spike latency to a transient input because superthreshold stimuli evoke immediate spikes without any delays (compare with Fig.8.8(I)). In addition, the model has some weird mathematical properties, such as non-uniqueness of solutions, as we show in exercise 1. Finally, the integrate-and-fire model is not a spiking model. Technically, it did not fire a spike in Fig.8.1, it was only "said to fire a spike", which was manually added afterward to fool the reader.

Despite all these drawbacks, the integrate-and-fire model is an acceptable sacrifice for a mathematician who wants to prove theorems and derive analytical expressions. However, using this model might be a waste of time for a computational neuroscientist who wants to simulate large-scale networks. At the end of this section we present alternative models that are as computationally efficient as the integrate-and-fire neuron, yet as biophysically plausible as Hodgkin-Huxley-type models.

## 8.1.2 Resonate-and-Fire

The resonate-and-fire model is a two-dimensional extension of the integrate-and-fire model that incorporates an additional low-threshold persistent $K^+$ current or h-current, or any other resonant current that is partially activated at rest. Let $W$ denote the magnitude of such a current. In the linear approximation, the conductance-based equations describing neuronal dynamics can be written in the form

$$\begin{aligned} C\dot{V} &= I - g_{leak}(V - E_{leak}) - W \ , \\ \dot{W} &= (V - V_{1/2})/k - W \ . \end{aligned}$$

known as the Young (1937) model (see also equation 2-1 in FitzHugh 1969). Whenever the membrane potential reaches the threshold value, $V_{thresh}$, the neuron is said to fire a spike. Young did not specify what happens after the spike. The resonate-and-fire

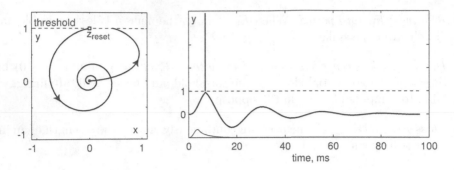

Figure 8.2: Resonate-and-fire model with $b = -0.05$, $\omega = 0.25$, and $z_{\text{reset}} = \text{i}$. The spike was added manually.

model is the Young model with the following resetting: if $V \geq V_{\text{thresh}}$, then $V \leftarrow V_{\text{reset}}$ and $W \leftarrow W_{\text{reset}}$, where $V_{\text{rest}}$ and $W_{\text{reset}}$ are some parameters.

When the resting state is a stable focus, the model can be recast in complex coordinates as

$$\dot{z} = (b + \text{i}\omega)z + I \ ,$$

where $b + \text{i}\omega \in \mathbb{C}$ is the complex eigenvalue of the resting state, and $z = x + \text{i}y \in \mathbb{C}$ is the complex-valued variable describing damped oscillations with frequency $\omega$ around the resting state. The real part, $x$, is a current-like variable. It describes the dynamics of the resonant current and synaptic currents. The imaginary part, $y$, is a voltage-like variable. The neuron is said to fire a spike when $y$ reaches the threshold $y = 1$. Thus, the threshold is a horizontal line on the complex plane that passes through $\text{i} \in \mathbb{C}$, as in Fig.8.2, though other choices are also possible. After firing the spike, the variable $z$ is reset to $z_{\text{reset}}$.

The resonate-and-fire model illustrates the most important features of resonators: damped oscillations, frequency preference, postinhibitory (rebound) spikes, and Class 2 excitability. It cannot have sustained subthreshold oscillations of membrane potential.

Integrate-and-fire and resonate-and-fire neurons do not contradict, but complement, each other. Both are linear, and hence are useful when we prove theorems and derive analytical expressions. They have the same flaws limiting their applicability, which were discussed earlier. In contrast, two simple models described below are difficult to treat analytically, but because of their universality they should be the models of choice when large-scale simulations are concerned.

### 8.1.3   Quadratic Integrate-and-Fire

Replacing $-v$ with $+v^2$ in (8.1) results in the *quadratic integrate-and-fire* model

$$\dot{v} = b + v^2 \ , \qquad \text{if } v = v_{\text{peak}}, \text{ then } v \leftarrow v_{\text{reset}}, \tag{8.2}$$

which we considered in section 3.3.8. Here $v_{\text{peak}}$ is not a threshold, but the peak (cut off) of a spike, as we explain below. It is useful to use $v_{\text{peak}} = +\infty$ in analytical studies.

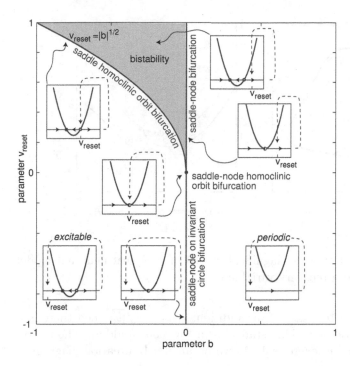

Figure 8.3: Bifurcation diagram of the quadratic integrate-and-fire neuron (8.2).

In simulations, the peak value is assumed to be large but finite, so it can be normalized to $v_{\text{peak}} = 1$.

Note that $\dot{v} = b + v^2$ is a topological normal form for the saddle-node bifurcation. That is, it describes dynamics of any Hodgkin-Huxley-type system near that bifurcation, as we discuss in chapter 3 and 6. There we derived the normal form (6.3) for the $I_{\text{Na,p}} + I_{\text{K}}$-model and showed that the two systems agree quantitatively in a reasonably broad voltage range. By resetting $v$ to $v_{\text{reset}}$, the quadratic integrate-and-fire model captures the essence of recurrence when the saddle-node bifurcation is on an invariant circle.

When $b > 0$, the right-hand side of the model is strictly positive, and the neuron fires a periodic train of action potentials. Indeed, $v$ increases, reaches the peak, resets to $v_{\text{reset}}$, and then increases again, as we show in Fig.3.35 (top). In exercise 3 we prove that the period of such spiking activity is

$$T = \frac{1}{\sqrt{b}} \left( \text{atan} \frac{v_{\text{peak}}}{\sqrt{b}} - \text{atan} \frac{v_{\text{reset}}}{\sqrt{b}} \right) < \frac{\pi}{\sqrt{b}},$$

so that the frequency scales as $\sqrt{b}$, as in Class 1 excitable systems.

When $b < 0$, the parabola $b + v^2$ has two zeroes, $\pm\sqrt{|b|}$. One corresponds to the stable node equilibrium (resting state), and the other corresponds to the unstable node (threshold state); see exercise 2. Subthreshold perturbations are those that keep $v$ below the unstable node. Superthreshold perturbations are those that push $v$ beyond the unstable node, resulting in the initiation of an action potential, reaching the peak

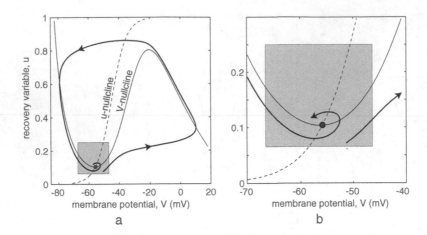

Figure 8.4: Phase portrait (a) and its magnification (b) of a typical neuronal model having voltage variable $V$ and a recovery variable $u$.

value $v_{\text{peak}}$, and then resetting to $v_{\text{reset}}$. If, in addition, $v_{\text{reset}} > \sqrt{|b|}$, then there is a coexistence of resting and periodic spiking states, as in Fig.3.35 (middle). The period of the spiking state is provided in exercise 4. A two-parameter bifurcation diagram of (8.2) is depicted in Fig.8.3.

Unlike its linear predecessor, the quadratic integrate-and-fire neuron is a genuine integrator. It exhibits saddle-node bifurcation; it has a soft (dynamic) threshold; and it generates spikes with latencies, as many mammalian cells do. Besides, the model is canonical in the sense that the entire class of neuronal models near saddle-node on invariant circle bifurcation can be transformed into this model by a piecewise continuous change of variables (see section 8.1.5 and the Ermentrout-Kopell theorem in Hoppensteadt and Izhikevich 1997). In conclusion, the quadratic, and not the leaky, integrate-and-fire neuron should be used in simulations of large-scale networks of integrators. A generalization of this model is discussed next.

## 8.1.4   Simple Model of Choice

A striking similarity among many spiking models, discussed in chapter 5, is that they can be reduced to two-dimensional systems having a fast voltage variable and a slower "recovery" variable, which may describe activation of the $K^+$ current or inactivation of the $Na^+$ current or their combination. Typically, the fast variable has an N-shaped nullcline and the slower variable has a sigmoid-shaped nullcline. The resting state in such models is the intersection of the nullclines near the left knee, as we illustrate in Fig.8.4a. There, $V$ and $u$ denote the fast and the slow variable, respectively. In chapter 7 we showed that many computational properties of biological neurons can be explained by considering dynamics at the left knee.

In section 5.2.4 we derive a simple model that captures the subthreshold behavior

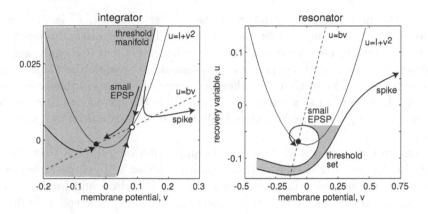

Figure 8.5: The simple model (8.3, 8.4) can be an integrator or a resonator. Compare with Fig.7.27.

in a small neighborhood of the left knee confined to the shaded square in Fig.8.4 and the initial segment of the upstroke of an action potential. In many cases, especially involving large-scale simulations of spiking models, the shape of the action potential is less important than the subthreshold dynamics leading to this action potential. Thus, retaining detailed information about the left knee and its neighborhood and simplifying the vector field outside the neighborhood is justified.

The simple model

$$\dot{v} = I + v^2 - u \qquad \text{if } v \geq 1, \text{ then} \qquad (8.3)$$
$$\dot{u} = a(bv - u) \qquad v \leftarrow c, \, u \leftarrow u + d \qquad (8.4)$$

has only four dimensionless parameters. Depending on the values of $a$ and $b$, it can be an integrator or a resonator, as we illustrate in Fig.8.5. The parameters $c$ and $d$ do not affect steady-state subthreshold behavior. Instead, they take into account the action of high-threshold voltage-gated currents activated during the spike, and affect only the after-spike transient behavior. If there are many currents with diverse time scales, then $u, a, b$, and $d$ are vectors, and (8.3) contains $\sum u$ instead of $u$.

The simple model may be treated as a quadratic integrate-and-fire neuron with adaptation in the simplest case $b = 0$. When $b < 0$, the model can be treated as a quadratic integrate-and-fire neuron with a passive dendritic compartment (see exercise 10). When $b > 0$, the connection to the quadratic integrate-and-fire neuron is lost, and the simple model represents a novel class of spiking models.

In the rest of this chapter we tune the simple model to reproduce spiking and bursting behavior of many known types of neurons. It is convenient to use it in the form

$$C\dot{v} = k(v - v_r)(v - v_t) - u + I \qquad \text{if } v \geq v_{\text{peak}}, \text{ then} \qquad (8.5)$$
$$\dot{u} = a\{b(v - v_r) - u\} \qquad v \leftarrow c, \, u \leftarrow u + d \qquad (8.6)$$

where $v$ is the membrane potential, $u$ is the recovery current, $C$ is the membrane capacitance, $v_r$ is the resting membrane potential, and $v_t$ is the instantaneous threshold potential. Though the model seems to have ten parameters, but it is equivalent to (8.3, 8.4) and hence has only four independent parameters. As we described in section 5.2.4, the parameters $k$ and $b$ can be found when one knows the neuron's rheobase and input resistance. The sum of all slow currents that modulate the spike generation mechanism is combined in the phenomenological variable $u$ with outward currents taken with the plus sign.

The sign of $b$ determines whether $u$ is an amplifying ($b < 0$) or a resonant ($b > 0$) variable. In the latter case, the neuron sags in response to hyperpolarized pulses of current, peaks in response to depolarized subthreshold pulses, and produces rebound (postinhibitory) responses. The recovery time constant is $a$. The spike cutoff value is $v_{peak}$, and the voltage reset value is $c$. The parameter $d$ describes the total amount of outward minus inward currents activated during the spike and affecting the after-spike behavior. All these parameters can easily be fitted to any particular neuron type, as we show in subsequent sections.

### Implementation and Phase Portrait

The following MATLAB code simulates the model and produces Fig.8.6a.

```
C=100; vr=-60; vt=-40; k=0.7;      % parameters used for RS
a=0.03; b=-2; c=-50; d=100;        % neocortical pyramidal neurons
vpeak=35;                          % spike cutoff

T=1000; tau=1;                     % time span and step (ms)
n=round(T/tau);                    % number of simulation steps
v=vr*ones(1,n);   u=0*v;           % initial values
I=[zeros(1,0.1*n),70*ones(1,0.9*n)];% pulse of input DC current

for i=1:n-1                        % forward Euler method
    v(i+1)=v(i)+tau*(k*(v(i)-vr)*(v(i)-vt)-u(i)+I(i))/C;
    u(i+1)=u(i)+tau*a*(b*(v(i)-vr)-u(i));
    if v(i+1)>=vpeak               % a spike is fired!
        v(i)=vpeak;                % padding the spike amplitude
        v(i+1)=c;                  % membrane voltage reset
        u(i+1)=u(i+1)+d;           % recovery variable update
    end;
end;
plot(tau*(1:n), v);                % plot the result
```

Note that the spikes were padded to $v_{peak}$ to avoid amplitude jitter associated with the finite simulation time step `tau=1` ms. In Fig.8.6b we magnify the simulated voltage trace and compare it with a recording of a neocortical pyramidal neuron (dashed curve). There are two discrepancies, marked by arrows: In the first, the pyramidal neuron has (1) a sharper spike upstroke and (2) a smoother spike downstroke. The first discrepancy

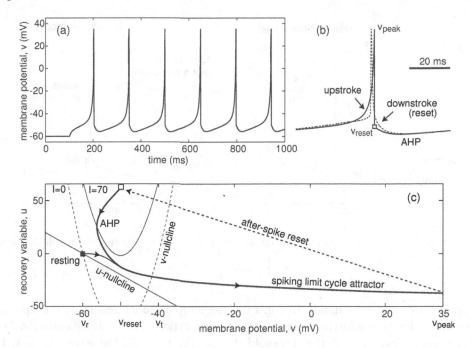

Figure 8.6: (a) Output of the MATLAB code simulating the simple model (8.5, 8.6). (b) Comparison of the simulated (solid curve) and experimental (dashed curve) voltage traces shows two major discrepancies, marked by arrows. (c) Phase portrait of the model.

can be removed by assuming that the coefficient $k$ of the square polynomial in (8.5) is voltage-dependent (e.g., $k = 0.7$ for $v \leq v_t$ and $k = 7$ for $v > v_t$), or by using the modification of the simple model presented in exercise 13 and exercise 17. The second discrepancy results from the instantaneous after-spike resetting, and it less important because it does not affect the decision whether or when to fire. However, the slope of the downstroke may become important in studies of gap-junction-coupled spiking neurons.

The phase portrait of the simple model is depicted in Fig.8.6c. Injection of the step of DC current $I = 70$ pA shifts the $v$-nullcline (square parabola) upward and makes the resting state, denoted by a black square, disappear. The trajectory approaches the spiking limit cycle attractor, and when it crosses the cutoff vertical line $v_{peak} = 35$ mV, it is reset to the white square, resulting in periodic spiking behavior. Note the slow afterhyperpolarization (AHP) following the reset that is due to the dynamics of the recovery variable $u$. Depending on the parameters, the model can have other types of phase portraits, spiking, and bursting behavior, as we demonstrate later.

In Fig.8.7 we illustrate the difference between the integrate-and-fire neuron and the simple model. The integrate-and-fire model is said to fire spikes when the membrane potential reaches a preset threshold value. The potential is reset to a new value, and

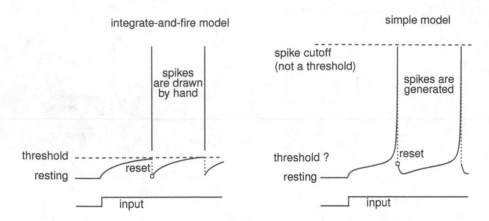

Figure 8.7: Voltage reset in the integrate-and-fire model and in the simple model.

the spikes are drawn by hand. In contrast, the simple model generates the upstroke of the spike due to the intrinsic (regenerative) properties of the voltage equation. The voltage reset occurs not at the threshold, but at the peak, of the spike. In fact, the firing threshold in the simple model *is not a parameter, but a property* of the bifurcation mechanism of excitability. Depending on the bifurcation of equilibrium, the model may not even have a well-defined threshold, a situation similar to many conductance-based models.

When numerically implementing the voltage reset, whether at the threshold or at the peak of the spike, one needs to be aware of the numerical errors, which translate into the errors of spike timing. These errors are inversely proportional to the slope of the voltage trace (i.e. $\dot{v}$) at the reset value. The slope is small in the integrate-and-fire model, so clever numerical methods are needed to catch the exact moment of threshold crossing (Hansel et al. 1998). In contrast, the slope is nearly infinite in the simple model, hence the error is infinitesimal, and no special methods are needed to identify the peak of the spike.

In Fig.8.8 we used the model to reproduce the 20 of the most fundamental neurocomputational properties of biological neurons. Let us check that the model is the simplest possible system that can exhibit the kind of behavior in the figure. Indeed, it has only one nonlinear term, $v^2$. Removing the term makes the model linear (between the spikes) and equivalent to the resonate-and-fire neuron. Removing the recovery variable $u$ makes the model equivalent to the quadratic integrate-and-fire neuron with all its limitations, such as the inability to burst or to be a resonator. In summary, we found the simplest possible model capable of spiking, bursting, being an integrator or a resonator, and it should be the model of choice in simulations of large-scale networks of spiking neurons.

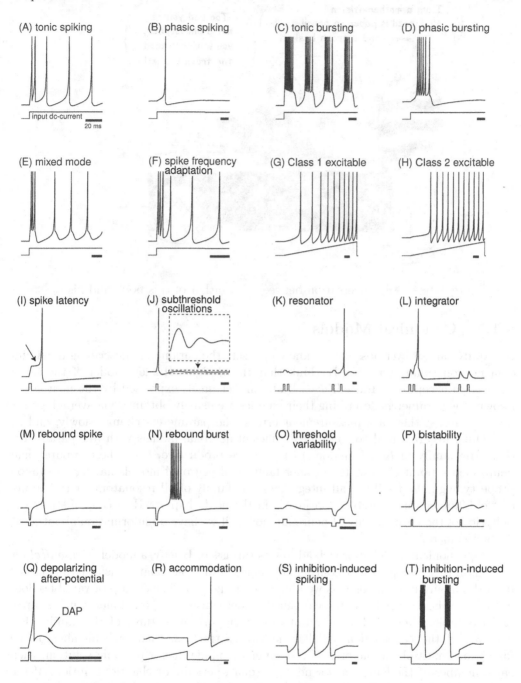

Figure 8.8: Summary of neurocomputational properties exhibited by the simple model; see exercise 11. The figure is reproduced, with permission, from www.izhikevich.com. (An electronic version of the figure, the MATLAB code that generates the voltage responses, and reproduction permissions are available at www.izhikevich.com.)

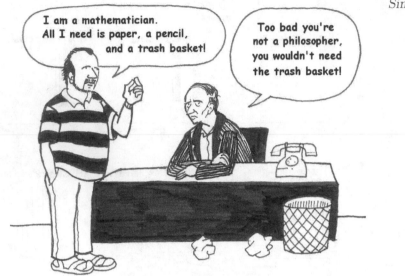

Figure 8.9: A real conversation between the author of this book and his boss.

## 8.1.5  Canonical Models

It is quite rare, if ever possible, to know precisely the parameters describing dynamics of a neuron (many erroneously think that the Hodgkin-Huxley model of the squid axon is an exception). Indeed, even if all ionic channels expressed by the neuron are known, the parameters describing their kinetics are usually obtained via averaging over many neurons; there are measurement errors; the parameters change slowly, and so on. Thus, we are forced to consider families of neuronal models with free parameters (e.g. the family of $I_{Na}+I_K$-models). It is more productive, from the computational neuroscience point of view, to consider families of neuronal models having a common property, e.g., the family of all integrators, the family of all resonators, or the family of "fold/homoclinic" bursters considered in the next chapter. How can we study the behavior of the entire family of neuronal models if we have no information about most of its members?

The canonical model approach addresses this issue. Briefly, a model is *canonical* for a family if there is a piecewise continuous change of variables that transforms any model from the family into this one, as we illustrate in Fig.8.10. The change of variables does not have to be invertible, so the canonical model is usually lower-dimensional, simple, and tractable. Nevertheless, it retains many important features of the family. For example, if the canonical model has multiple attractors, then each member of the family has multiple attractors. If the canonical model has a periodic solution, then each member of the family has a periodic (quasi-periodic or chaotic) solution. If the canonical model can burst, then each member of the family can burst. The advantage of this approach is that we can study universal neurocomputational properties that are shared by all members of the family because all such members can be put into the canonical form by a change of variables. Moreover, we need not actually present such

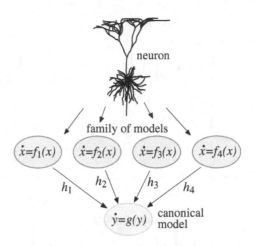

Figure 8.10: Dynamical system $\dot{y} = g(y)$ is a canonical model for the family $\{f_1, f_2, f_3, f_4\}$ of neural models $\dot{x} = f(x)$ because each such model can be transformed into the form $\dot{y} = g(y)$ by the piecewise continuous change of variables $h_i$.

a change of variables explicitly, so derivation of canonical models is possible even when the family is so broad that most of its members are given implicitly (e.g., the family of "all resonators").

The process of deriving canonical models is more an art than a science, since a general algorithm for doing this is not known. However, much success has been achieved in some important cases. The canonical model for a system near an equilibrium is the topological normal form at the equilibrium (Kuznetsov 1995). Such a canonical model is local, but it can be extended to describe global dynamics. For example, the quadratic integrate-and-fire model with a fixed $v_{\text{reset}} < 0$ is a global canonical model for all Class 1 excitable systems, that is, systems near saddle-node on invariant circle bifurcation. The same model with variable $v_{\text{reset}}$ is a global canonical model for all systems near saddle-node homoclinic orbit bifurcation (considered in section 6.3.6). The phase model $\dot{\vartheta} = 1$ derived in chapter 10 is a global canonical model for the family of nonlinear oscillators having exponentially stable limit cycle attractors. Other examples of canonical models for spiking and bursting can be found in subsequent chapters of this book.

The vector-field of excitable conductance-based models in the subthreshold region and in the region corresponding to the upstroke of the spike can be converted into the simple form (8.3, 8.4), possibly with $u$ being a vector. Therefore, the simple model (8.3, 8.4) is a *local* canonical model for the spike generation mechanism and the spike upstroke of Hodgkin-Huxley-type neuronal models. It is not a global canonical model because it ignores the spike downstroke. Nevertheless, it describes remarkably well the spiking and bursting dynamics of many biological neurons, as we demonstrate next.

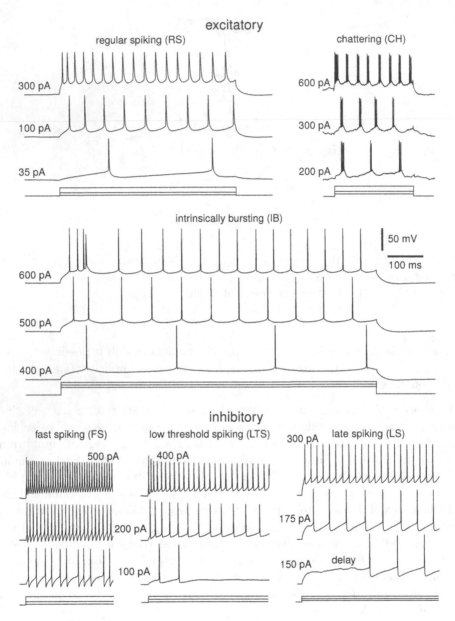

Figure 8.11: The six most fundamental classes of firing patterns of neocortical neurons in response to pulses of depolarizing DC current. RS and IB are in vitro recordings of pyramidal neurons of layer 5 of primary visual cortex of a rat; CH was recorded in vivo in cat visual cortex (area 17; data provided by D. McCormick). FS was recorded in vitro in rat primary visual cortex, LTS was recorded in vitro in layer 4 or 6 of rat barrel cortex (data provided by B. Connors). LS was recorded in layer 1 of rat's visual cortex (data provided by S. Hestrin). All recordings are plotted on the same voltage and time scale, and the data are available at www.izhikevich.com.

# 8.2 Cortex

In this section we consider the six most fundamental classes of firing patterns observed in the mammalian neocortex and depicted in Fig.8.11 (Connors and Gutnick 1990; Gray and McCormick 1996; Gibson et al. 1999). Though most biologists agree with the classification in the figure, many would point out that it is greatly oversimplified (Markram et al. 2004), that the distinction between the classes is not sharp, that there are subclasses within each class (Nowak et al. 2003; Toledo-Rodriguez et al. 2004), and that neurons can change their firing class depending on the state of the brain (Steriade 2004).

- (RS) Regular spiking neurons fire tonic spikes with adapting (decreasing) frequency in response to injected pulses of DC current. Most of them have Class 1 excitability in the sense that the interspike frequency vanishes when the amplitude of the injected current decreases. Morphologically, these neurons are spiny stellate cells in layer 4 and pyramidal cells in layers 2, 3, 5, and 6.

- (IB) Intrinsically bursting neurons generate a burst of spikes at the beginning of a strong depolarizing pulse of current, then switch to tonic spiking mode. They are excitatory pyramidal neurons found in all cortical layers, but are most abundant in layer 5.

- (CH) Chattering neurons fire high-frequency bursts of spikes with relatively short interburst periods; hence another name, FRB (fast rhythmic bursting). Output of such a cell fed to the loudspeaker "sounds a lot like a helicopter – cha, cha, cha – real fast", according to Gray and McCormick (1996). CH neurons were found in visual cortex of adult cats, and morphologically they are spiny stellate or pyramidal neurons of layers 2 - 4, mainly layer 3.

- (FS) Fast spiking interneurons fire high-frequency tonic spikes with relatively constant period. They exhibit Class 2 excitability (Tateno et al. 2004). When the magnitude of the injected current decreases below a certain critical value, they fire irregular spikes, switching randomly between resting and spiking states. Morphologically, FS neurons are sparsely spiny or aspiny nonpyramidal cells (basket or chandelier; see Kawaguchi and Kubota 1997) providing local inhibition along the horizontal (intra-laminar) direction of the neocortex (Bacci et al. 2003).

- (LTS) Low-threshold spiking neurons fire tonic spikes with pronounced spike frequency adaptation and rebound (postinhibitory) spikes, often called "low-threshold spikes" by biologists (hence the name). They seem to be able to fire low-frequency spike trains, though their excitability class has not yet been determined. Morphologically, LTS neurons are nonpyramidal interneurons providing local inhibition along the vertical (inter-laminar) direction of the neocortex (Bacci et al. 2003).

- (LS)  Late spiking neurons exhibit voltage ramp in response to injected DC
  current near the rheobase, resulting in delayed spiking with latencies as long
  as 1 sec.  There is a pronounced subthreshold oscillation during the ramp, but
  the discharge frequency is far less than that of FS neurons.  Morphologically,
  LS neurons are nonpyramidal interneurons (neurogliaform; see Kawaguchi and
  Kubota 1997) found in all layers of neocortex (Kawaguchi 1995), especially in
  layer 1 (Chu et al. 2003).

Our goal is to use the simple model (8.5, 8.6) presented in section 8.1.4 to reproduce
each of the firing types. We want to capture the dynamic mechanism of spike generation
of each neuron, so that the model reproduces the correct responses to many types of
the inputs, and not only to the pulses of DC current.  We strive to have not only
qualitative but also quantitative agreement with the published data on neurons' resting
potential, input resistance, rheobase, F-I behavior, the shape of the upstroke of the
action potential, and so on, though this is impossible in many cases, mostly because
the data are contradictory. To fine-tune the model, we use recordings of real neurons.
We consider the tuning successful when the quantitative difference between simulated
and recorded responses is smaller than the difference between the responses of two
"sister" neurons recorded in the same slice. We do not want to claim that the simple
model explains the mechanism of generation of any of the firing patterns recorded in
real neurons (simply because the mechanism is usually not known). Although in many
instances we must resist the temptation to use the Wolfram (2002) new-kind-of-science
criterion: "If it looks the same, it must be the same".

## 8.2.1   Regular Spiking (RS) Neurons

Regular spiking neurons are the major class of excitatory neurons in the neocortex.
Many are Class 1 excitable, as we show in Fig.7.3, using in vitro recordings of a layer
5 pyramidal cell of rat primary visual cortex (see also Tateno et al. 2004). RS neurons
have a transient K$^+$ current $I_A$, whose slow inactivation delays the onset of the first
spike and increases the interspike period, and a persistent K$^+$ current $I_M$, which is
believed to be responsible for the spike frequency adaptation seen in Fig.7.43. Let us
use the simple model (8.5, 8.6) to capture qualitative and some quantitative features
of typical RS neurons.

We assume that the resting membrane potential is $v_r = -60$ mV and the instantaneous threshold potential is $v_t = -40$ mV; that is, instantaneous depolarizations above
$-40$ mV cause the neuron to fire, as in Fig.3.15. Assuming that the rheobase is 50 pA
and the input resistance is 80 M$\Omega$, we find $k = 0.7$ and $b = -2$. We take the membrane
capacitance $C = 100$ pF, which yields a membrane time constant of 8 ms.

Since $b < 0$, depolarizations of $v$ decrease $u$ as if the major slow current is the
inactivating K$^+$ current $I_A$. The inactivation time constant of $I_A$ is around 30 ms in
the subthreshold voltage range; hence one takes $a = 0.03 \approx 1/30$. The membrane
potential of a typical RS neuron reaches the peak value $v_{peak} = +35$ mV during a
spike (the precise value has little effect on dynamics) and then repolarizes to $c = -50$

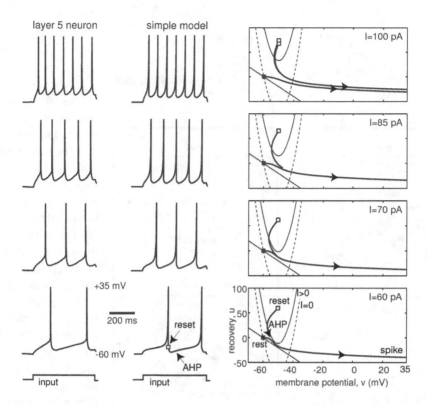

Figure 8.12: Comparison of in vitro recordings of a regular spiking (RS) pyramidal neuron with simulations of the simple model $100\dot{v} = 0.7(v + 60)(v + 40) - u + I$, $\dot{u} = 0.03\{-2(v + 60) - u\}$, if $v \geq +35$, then $v \leftarrow -50$, $u \leftarrow u + 100$.

mV or below, depending on the firing frequency. The parameter $d$ describes the total amount of outward minus inward currents activated during the spike and affecting the after-spike behavior. Trying different values, we find that $d = 100$ gives a reasonable F-I relationship, at least in the low-frequency range.

As follows from exercise 10, one can also interpret $u$ as the membrane potential of a passive dendritic compartment, taken with the minus sign. Thus, when $b < 0$, the variable $u$ represents the combined action of slow inactivation of $I_A$ and slow charging of the dendritic tree. Both processes slow the frequency of somatic spiking.

Note that we round up all the parameters, that is, we use $d = 100$ and not 93.27. Nevertheless, the simulated voltage responses in Fig.8.12 agree quantitatively with the in vitro recordings of the layer 5 pyramidal neuron used in Fig.7.3. Tweaking the parameters, considering multidimensional $u$, or adding multiple dendritic compartments, one can definitely improve the quantitative correspondence between the model and the in vitro data of that particular neuron, but this is not our goal here. Instead, we want to understand the qualitative dynamics of RS neurons, using the geometry of their phase portraits.

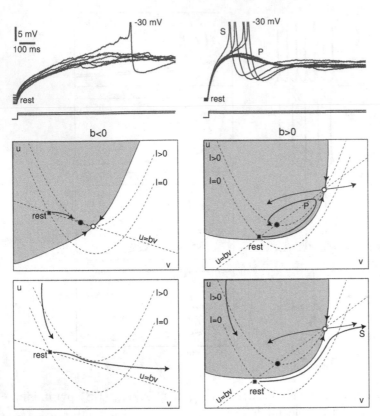

Figure 8.13: Two types of qualitative behavior of RS neurons. Some exhibit monotone responses to weak injected currents (case $b < 0$); others exhibit non-monotone over-shooting responses (case $b > 0$). Shown are in vitro recordings of two RS neurons from the same slice of rat primary visual cortex while an automated procedure was trying to determine the neurons' rheobase. Phase portraits are drawn by hand and illustrate a possible dynamic mechanism of the phenomenon.

## Phase Plane Analysis

Figure 8.13 shows recordings of two pyramidal RS neurons from the same slice while an automated procedure injects pulses of DC current to determine their rheobase. The neuron on the left exhibits monotonically increasing (ramping) or decreasing responses of membrane potential to weak input pulses, long latencies of the first spike, and no rebound spikes, whereas the neuron on the right exhibits non-monotone overshooting responses to positive pulses, sags and rebound spikes to negative pulses (as in Fig.7.48), relatively short latencies of the first spike, and other resonance phenomena. The even more extreme example in Fig.7.42 shows a pyramidal neuron executing a subthreshold oscillation before switching to a tonic spiking mode.

The difference between the types in Fig.8.13 can be explained by the sign of the parameter $b$ in the simple model (8.5, 8.6), which depends on the relative contributions of amplifying and resonant slow currents and gating variables. When $b < 0$ (or $b \approx 0$; e.g., $b = 0.5$ in Fig.8.14), the neuron is a pure integrator near saddle-node on invariant circle bifurcation. Greater values of $b > 0$ put the model near the transition from an integrator to a resonator the via codimension-2 Bogdanov-Takens bifurcation studied in section 6.3.3 and 7.2.11.

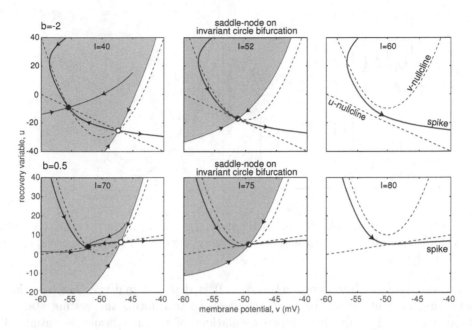

Figure 8.14: Saddle-node on invariant circle bifurcations in the RS neuron model as the magnitude of the injected current $I$ increases.

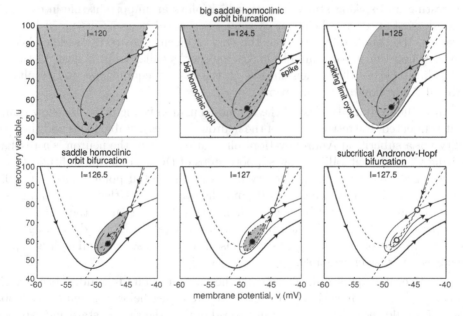

Figure 8.15: The sequence of bifurcations of the RS model neuron (8.5, 8.6) in resonator regime. Parameters are as in Fig.8.12 and $b = 5$; see also Fig.6.40.

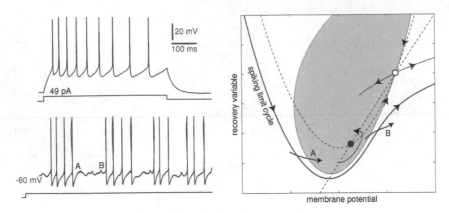

Figure 8.16: Stuttering behavior of an RS neuron. (Data provided by Dr. Klaus M. Stiefel: P28-36 adult mouse, coronal slices, 300$\mu$m, layer II/III pyramid, visual cortex.)

The sequence of bifurcations when $b > 0$ is depicted in Fig.8.15. Injection of depolarizing current below the neuron's rheobase transforms the resting state into a stable focus and results in damped oscillations of the membrane potential. The attraction domain of the focus (shaded region in the figure) is bounded by the stable manifold of the saddle. As $I$ increases, the stable manifold makes a loop and becomes a big homoclinic orbit giving birth to a spiking limit cycle attractor. When $I = 125$, stable resting and spiking states coexist, which plays an important role in explaining the paradoxical stuttering behavior of some neocortical neurons discussed later. As $I$ increases, the saddle quantity (i.e., the sum of eigenvalues of the saddle) becomes positive. When the stable manifold makes another, smaller loop, it gives birth to an unstable limit cycle, which then shrinks to the resting equilibrium and results in a subcritical Andronov-Hopf bifurcation.

What is the excitability class of the RS model neuron in Fig.8.15? If a slow ramp of current is injected, the resting state of the neuron becomes a stable focus and then loses stability via a subcritical Andronov-Hopf bifurcation. Hence the neuron is a resonator exhibiting Class 2 excitability. Now suppose steps of DC current of amplitude $I = 125$ pA or less are injected. The trajectory starts at the initial point $(v, u) = (-60, 0)$, which is the resting state when $I = 0$, and then approaches the spiking limit cycle. Because the limit cycle was born via a homoclinic bifurcation to the saddle, it has a large period, and hence the neuron is Class 1 excitable. Thus, depending on the nature of stimulation, that is, ramps vs. pulses, we can observe small or large spiking frequencies, at least in principle.

In practice, it is quite difficult to catch homoclinic orbits to saddles because they are sensitive to noise. Injection of a constant current just below the neuron's rheobase in Fig.8.15 would result in random transitions between the resting state and a periodic spiking state. Indeed, the two attractors coexist and are near each other, so weak membrane noise can push the trajectory in and out of the shaded region, resulting

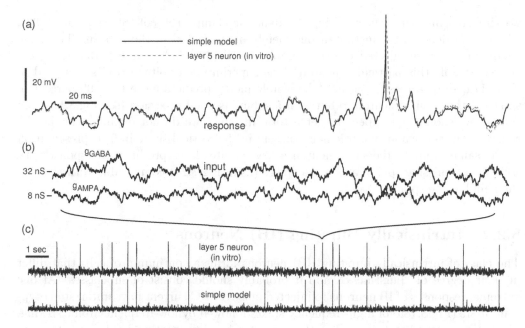

Figure 8.17: (a) Comparison of responses of a rat motor cortex layer 5 pyramidal neuron of RS type and the simple model (8.5, 8.6) to in vivo-like stochastic input (8.7) with the random conductances in (b). Part (a) is a magnification of a small region in (c). Shown are simulations of $30\dot{v} = 3(v+55)(v+42)-u+I(t)$, $\dot{u} = 0.01\{-0.25(v+55)-u\}$, if $v \geq +10$, then $v \leftarrow -40$, $u \leftarrow u + 90$. (Data provided by Niraj S. Desai and Betsy C. Walcott.)

in a stuttering spiking (illustrated in Fig.8.16) mingled with subthreshold oscillations. Such behavior is also exhibited by FS interneurons, studied later in this section.

## In Vivo-like Conditions

In Fig.8.17a (dashed curve) we show the response of in vitro recorded layer 5 pyramidal neuron of rat motor cortex to fluctuating in vivo-like input. First, random excitatory and inhibitory conductances, $g_{\mathrm{AMPA}}(t)$ and $g_{\mathrm{GABA}}(t)$ (Fig.8.17b), were generated using the Ornstein-Uhlenbeck stochastic process (Uhlenbeck and Ornstein 1930), which was originally developed to describe Brownian motion, but can equally well describe in vivo-like fluctuating synaptic conductances produced by random firings (Destexhe et al. 2001). Let $E_{\mathrm{AMPA}} = 0$ mV and $E_{\mathrm{GABA}} = -65$ mV denote the reverse potentials of excitatory and inhibitory synapses, respectively. The corresponding current

$$I(t) = \overbrace{g_{\mathrm{AMPA}}(t)(E_{\mathrm{AMPA}} - V(t))}^{\text{excitatory input}} + \overbrace{g_{\mathrm{GABA}}(t)(E_{\mathrm{GABA}} - V(t))}^{\text{inhibitory input}}, \qquad (8.7)$$

was injected into the neuron, using the dynamic clamp protocol (Sharp et al. 1993), where $V(t)$ denotes the instantaneous membrane potential of the neuron. The same conductances were injected into the simple model (8.5, 8.6), whose parameters were adjusted to fit this particular neuron. The superimposed voltage traces, depicted in Fig.8.17a, show a reasonable fit. The simple model predicts more than 90 percent of spikes of the in vitro neuron, often with a submillisecond precision (see Fig.8.17c). Of course, we should not expect to get a total fit, since we do not explicitly model the sources of intrinsic and synaptic noise present in the cortical slice. In fact, presentation of the same input to the same neuron a few minutes later produces a response with spike jitter, missing spikes, and extra spikes (as in Fig.7.24) comparable with those in the simulated response.

## 8.2.2   Intrinsically Bursting (IB) Neurons

The class of intrinsically bursting (IB) neurons forms a continuum of cells that differ in their degree of "burstiness", and it probably should consist of subclasses. At one extreme, responses of IB neurons to injected pulses of DC current have initial stereotypical bursts (Fig.8.18a) of high-frequency spikes followed by low-frequency tonic spiking. Many IB neurons burst even when the current is barely superthreshold and not strong enough to elicit a sustained response (as in Fig.8.21, bottom traces). At the other extreme, bursts can be seen only in response to sufficiently strong current, as in Fig.8.11 or Fig.9.1b. Weaker stimulation elicits regular spiking responses. In comparison with typical RS neurons, the regular spiking response of IB neurons has lower firing frequency and higher rheobase (threshold) current, and exhibits shorter latency to the first spike and noticeable afterdepolarizations (ADPs) (Compare RS and IB cells in Fig.8.11.)

Magnifications of the responses of two IB neurons in Fig.8.18b and 8.18c show that the interspike intervals within the burst may be increasing or decreasing, possibly reflecting different ionic mechanisms of burst generation and termination. In any case, the initial high-frequency spiking is caused by the excess of the inward current or the deficit of the outward current needed to repolarize the membrane potential below the threshold. As a result, many spikes are needed to build up outward current to terminate the high-frequency burst. After the neuron recovers, it fires low-frequency tonic spikes because there is a residual outward current (or residual inactivation of inward current) that prevents the occurrence of another burst. Many IB neurons can fire two or more bursts before they switch into tonic spiking mode, as in Fig.8.18a. Below, we present two models of IB neurons, one relying on the interplay of voltage-gated currents, and the other relying on the interplay of fast somatic and slow dendritic spikes.

Let us use the available data on the IB neuron in Fig.8.11 to build a simple one-compartment model (8.5, 8.6) exhibiting IB firing patterns. The neuron has a resting state at $v_r = -75$ mV and an instantaneous threshold at $v_t = -45$ mV. Its rheobase is 350 pA, and the input resistance is around 30 M$\Omega$, resulting in $k = 1.2$ and $b = 5$. The peak of the spike is at $+50$ mV, and the after-spike resetting point is around

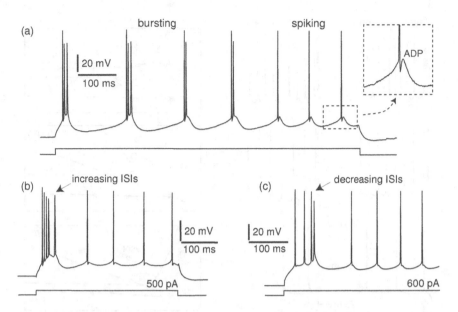

Figure 8.18: (a) bursting and spiking in an IB neuron (layer 5 of somatosensory cortex of a four week old rat at 35°C; (data provided by Greg Stuart and Maarten Kole). Note the afterdepolarization (ADP). (b) IB neuron of a cat (modified from figure 2 of Timofeev et al. 2000). (c) pyramidal neuron of rat visual cortex. Note that IB neurons may exhibit bursts with increasing or decreasing inter-spike intervals (ISIs).

$c = -56$ mV. The parameters $a = 0.01$ and $d = 130$ give a reasonable fit of the neuron's current-frequency relationship.

The phase portraits in Fig.8.19 explain the mechanism of firing of IB patterns in the simple model. When $I = 0$, the model has an equilibrium at $-75$ mV, which is the intersection of the $v$-nullcline (dashed parabola) and the $u$-nullcline (straight line). Injection of a depolarizing current moves the $v$-nullcline upward. The pulse of current of magnitude $I = 300$ pA is below the neuron's rheobase, so the trajectory moves from the old resting state (black square) to the new one (black circle). Since $b > 0$, the trajectory overshoots the new equilibrium. The pulse of magnitude $I = 370$ pA is barely above the rheobase, so the model exhibits low-frequency tonic firing with some spike frequency adaptation. Elevating the fast nullcline by injecting $I = 500$ pA transforms the first spike into a doublet. Indeed, the after-the-first-spike resetting point (white square marked "1") is below the parabola, so the second spike is fired immediately. Similarly, injection of an even stronger current of magnitude $I = 550$ pA transforms the doublet into a burst of three spikes, each raising the after-spike resetting point. Once the resetting point is inside the parabola, the neuron is in tonic spiking mode.

Figure 8.20a shows simultaneous recording of somatic and dendritic membrane potentials of a layer 5 pyramidal neuron. The somatic spike backpropagates into the

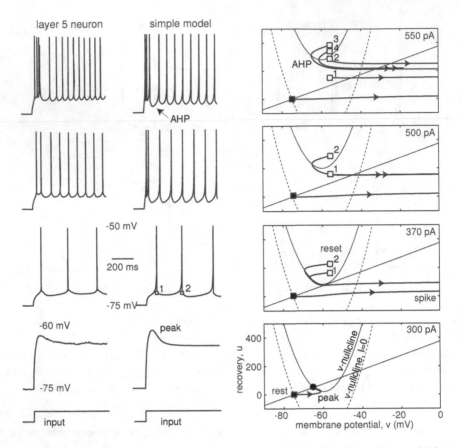

Figure 8.19: Comparison of in vitro recordings of an intrinsically bursting (IB) neuron with the simple model $150\dot{v} = 1.2(v + 75)(v + 45) - u + I$, $\dot{u} = 0.01\{5(v + 75) - u\}$, if $v \geq +50$, then $v \leftarrow -56$, $u \leftarrow u + 130$. White squares denote the reset points, numbered according to the spike number.

dendrite, activates voltage-gated dendritic $Na^+$ and $Ca^{2+}$ currents (Stuart et al. 1999; Hausser et al. 2000), and results in a slower dendritic spike (clearly seen in the figure). The slow dendritic spike depolarizes the soma, resulting in an ADP, which is typical in many IB cells. Depending on the strength of the injected dc current and the state of the neuron, the ADP can be large enough to cause another somatic spike, as illustrated in Fig.7.52. The somatic spike may initiate another dendritic spike, and so on, resulting in a burst in Fig.8.20b. This mechanism is known as the dendritic-somatic Ping-Pong (Wang 1999), and it occurs in the Pinsky-Rinzel (1994) model of the hippocampal CA3 neuron, the sensory neuron of weakly electric fish (Doiron et al. 2002), and in chattering neurons considered below.

Let us build a two-compartment simple model that simulates the somatic and dendritic spike generation of IB neurons. Since we do not know the rheobase, input

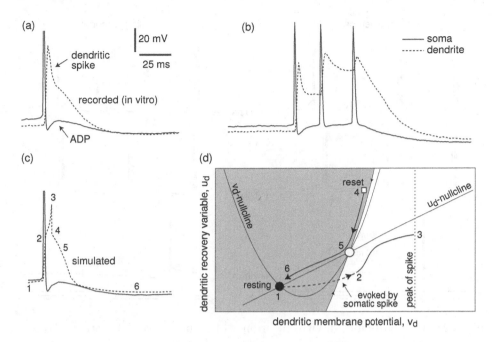

Figure 8.20: Somatic and dendritic spike (a) and burst (b) in an IB neuron. The dendritic spike in (a) is simulated in (c), using the simple model described in Fig.8.20. The phase portrait (d) describes the geometry of the dendritic spike generation mechanism. Recordings are from layer 5 of the somatosensory cortex of a four-week-old rat at 35°C; the dendritic electrode is 0.43mm from the soma. (Data provided by Greg Stuart and Maarten Kole.)

resistance, and resting and instantaneous threshold potentials of the dendritic tree of IB neurons, we cannot determine parameters of the dendritic compartment. Instead, we feed the somatic recording $V(t)$ in Fig.8.20a into the model dendritic compartment and fine-tune the parameters so that the simulated dendritic spike in Fig.8.20c "looks like" the recorded one in Fig.8.20a.

The phase portrait in Fig.8.20d explains the peculiarities of the shape of the simulated dendritic spike. The recorded somatic spike quickly depolarizes the dendritic membrane potential from point 1 to point 2, and starts the regenerative process – the upstroke of a spike. Upon reaching the peak of the spike (3), the dendritic membrane potential and the recovery variable are reset by the action of fast voltage-gated $K^+$ currents, which are not modeled here explicitly. The reset point (4) is near the stable manifold of the saddle, so the membrane potential slowly repolarizes (5) and returns to the resting state (6).

In Fig.8.21 we put the somatic and dendritic compartments together, adjust some of the parameters, and simulate the response of the IB neuron to pulses of current of various amplitudes. Note that the model correctly reproduces the transient burst of

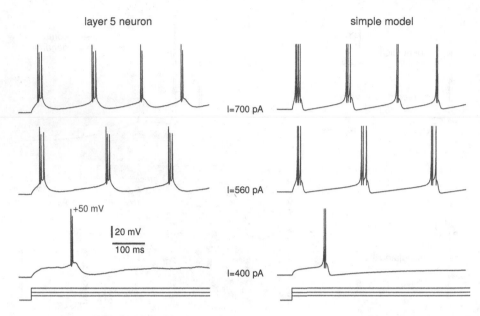

Figure 8.21: Comparison of in vitro recordings of an intrinsically bursting (IB) neuron (layer 5 of somatosensory cortex of a four-week-old rat at 35°C; data provided by Greg Stuart and Maarten Kole) with the two-compartment simple model. Soma: $150\dot{v} = 3(v + 70)(v + 45) + 50(v_d - v) - u + I$, $\dot{u} = 0.01\{5(v + 70) - u\}$, if $v \geq +50$, then $v \leftarrow -52$, $u \leftarrow u + 240$. Active dendrite: $30\dot{v}_d = (v_d + 50)^2 + 20(v - v_d) - u_d$, $\dot{u}_d = 3\{15(v_d + 50) - u_d\}$, if $v_d \geq +20$, then $v_d \leftarrow -20$, $u_d \leftarrow u_d + 500$.

two closely spaced spikes when stimulation is weak, and the rhythmic bursting with decreasing number of spikes per burst when stimulation is strong. Using this approach, one can build models of pyramidal neurons having multiple dendritic compartments, as we do next.

## 8.2.3   Multi-Compartment Dendritic Tree

In Fig.8.22 we simulate an IB pyramidal neuron having 47 compartments (Fig.8.22a, b), each described by a simple model with parameters provided in the caption of the figure. Our goal is to illustrate a number of interesting phenomena that occur in neuronal models having active dendrites, that is, dendrites capable of generating action potentials.

In Fig.8.22c we inject a current into compartment 4 on the apical dendrite to evoke an excitatory postsynaptic potential (EPSP) of 4 mV, which is subthreshold for the spike generation mechanism. This depolarization produces a current that passively spreads to neighboring compartments, and eventually into the somatic compartment. However, the somatic EPSP is much weaker, only 1 mV, reflecting the distance-dependent attenuation of dendritic synaptic inputs. Note also that somatic

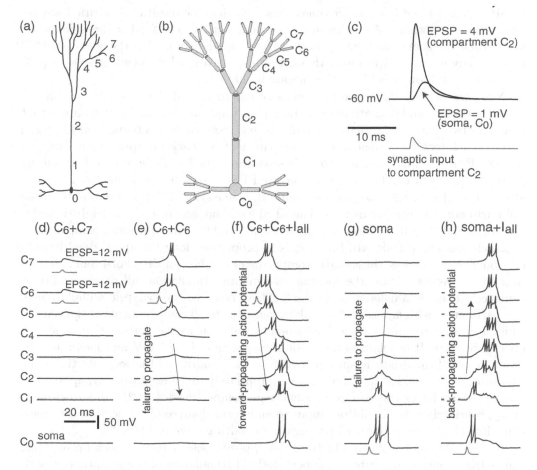

Figure 8.22: (a) Hand drawing and (b) a 47-compartment representation of a layer 5 pyramidal neuron. (c) Injection of current (simulating excitatory synaptic input) into compartment 2 evokes a large excitatory postsynaptic potential (EPSP) in that compartment, but a much smaller EPSP in the somatic compartment. (d) Synaptic inputs to compartments 6 and 7 result in large EPSPs there, but no dendritic spike. (e) The same synaptic inputs into compartment 6 result in a dendritic spike, which fails to propagate forward to the soma. (f) The same input combined with background excitation $I_{\text{all}} = 60$ pA to all compartments results in forward-propagating dendritic spikes. (g) Strong synaptic input to the soma results in a spike that fails to propagate into the dendritic tree. (h) The same input combined with injection of $I_{\text{all}} = 70$ pA to all compartments (to simulate in vivo tonic background input) promotes back-propagation of spike into the dendritic tree. Each compartment is simulated by the simple model $100\dot{v} = 3(v + 60)(v + 50) - u + I$, $\dot{u} = 0.01\{5(v + 60) - u\}$. Soma: if $v \geq +50$, then $v \leftarrow -55$, $u \leftarrow u + 500$. Dendrites: if $v \geq +10$, then $v \leftarrow -35$, $u \leftarrow u + 1000$. The conductance between any two adjacent compartments is 70 nS.

EPSP is delayed and has a wider time course, which is the result of dendritic low-pass filtering, or smoothing, of subthreshold neuronal signals. The farther the stimulation site is from the soma, the weaker, more delayed, and longer lasting the somatic EPSP is. For many years, dendrites were thought to be passive conductors whose sole purpose is to collect and low-pass filter the synaptic input.

Now, we explore the active properties of dendrites and their dependence on the location, timing, and strength of synaptic input. First, we stimulate two synapses that innervate two sister dendritic compartments, e.g., compartments 6 and 7 in Fig.8.22d that could interact via their mother compartment 5. Each synaptic input evokes a strong EPSP of 12 mV, but due to their separation, the EPSPs do not add up and no dendritic spike is fired. The resulting somatic EPSP is only 0.15 mV due to the passive attenuation. In Fig.8.22e we provide exactly the same synaptic input, but into the same compartment, i.e., compartment 6. The EPSPs add up, and result in a dendritic spike, which propagates into the mother compartment 5 and then into the sister compartment 7 (which was not stimulated), but it fails to propagate along the apical dendrite into the soma. Nevertheless, the somatic compartment exhibits an EPSP of 1.5 mV, hardly seen in the figure. Thus, the location of synaptic stimulation, all other conditions being equal, made a difference. In Fig.8.22f we combine the synaptic stimulation to compartment 6 with injection of a weak current, $I_{all}$, to all compartments of the neuron. This current represents a tonic background excitation to the neuron that is always present in vivo. It depolarizes the membrane potential by 2.5 mV and facilitates the propagation of the dendritic spike along the apical dendrite all the way into the soma. The same effect could be achieved by an appropriately timed excitatory synaptic input arriving at an intermediate compartment, e.g., compartment 3 or 2. Not surprisingly, an appropriately timed inhibitory input to an intermediate compartment on the apical dendrite could stop the forward-propagating dendritic spike in Fig.8.22f.

In Fig.8.22g and 8.22h we illustrate the opposite phenomenon – back-propagating spikes from soma to dendrites. A superthreshold stimulation of the somatic compartment evokes a burst of three spikes, which fails to propagate along the apical dendrites by itself, but can propagate if combined with a tonic depolarization of the dendritic tree.

We see that dendritic trees can do more than just averaging and low-pass filtering of distributed synaptic inputs. Separate parts of the tree can perform independent local signal processing and even fire dendritic spikes. Depending on the synaptic inputs to other parts of the tree, the spikes can be localized or they can forward-propagate into the soma, causing the cell to fire. Spikes at the soma can backpropagate into the dendrites, triggering spike-time-dependent processes such as synaptic plasticity.

## 8.2.4   Chattering (CH) Neurons

Chattering neurons, also known as fast rhythmic bursting (FRB) neurons, generate high-frequency repetitive bursts in response to injected depolarizing currents. The magnitude of the DC current determines the interburst period, which could be as long

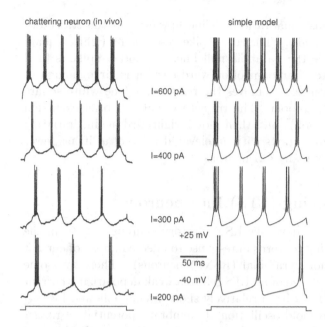

chattering neuron (in vivo)          simple model

I=600 pA

I=400 pA

I=300 pA

+25 mV

50 ms

-40 mV

I=200 pA

Figure 8.23: Comparison of in vivo recordings from cat primary visual cortex with simulations of the simple model $50\dot{v} = 1.5(v+60)(v+40) - u + I$, $\dot{u} = 0.03\{(v+60) - u\}$, if $v \geq +25$, then $v \leftarrow -40$, $u \leftarrow u + 150$. (Data provided by D. McCormick.)

as 100 ms or as short as 15 ms, and the number of spikes within each burst, typically two to five, as we illustrate in Fig.8.23, using in vivo recordings of a pyramidal neuron of cat visual cortex.

An RS model neuron, as shown in Fig.8.12, can easily be transformed into a CH neuron by increasing the after-spike reset voltage to $c = -40$ mV, mimicking decreased K$^+$ and increased Na$^+$ currents activated during each spike. The phase portrait in Fig.8.24 explains the mechanism of chattering of the simple model (8.5, 8.6). A step

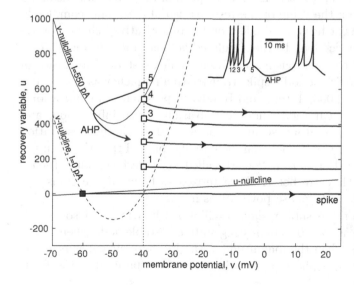

Figure 8.24: Phase portrait of the simple model in Fig.8.23 exhibiting CH firing pattern.

of depolarizing current shifts the fast quadratic nullcline upward and the trajectory quickly moves rightward to fire a spike. The after-spike reset point (white square marked "1" in the figure) is outside the parabola nullcline, so another spike is fired immediately, and so on, until the total amount of outward current is large enough to stop the burst; that is, until the variable $u$ moves the reset point (the white square marked "5") inside the quadratic parabola. The trajectory makes a brief excursion to the left knee (afterhyperpolarization) and then moves rightward again, initiating another burst. Since the second burst starts with an elevated value of $u$, it has fewer spikes – a phenomenon exhibited by many CH neurons.

## 8.2.5   Low-Threshold Spiking (LTS) Interneurons

Low-threshold spiking interneurons behave like RS excitatory neurons ($b > 0$) in the sense that they exhibit regular spiking patterns in response to injected pulses of current (some call them regular spiking non-pyramidal (RSNP) neurons). There are some subtle differences, however. The response of an LTS cell to a weak depolarizing current consists of a phasic spike or a doublet with a relatively short latency followed by low-frequency (less than 10 Hz) subthreshold oscillation of membrane potential. Stronger pulses elicit tonic spikes with slow frequency adaptation, decreasing amplitudes, and decreasing after-hyperpolarizations, as one can see in Fig.8.11.

LTS neurons have more depolarized resting potentials, lower threshold potentials, and lower input resistances than RS neurons. To match the in vitro firing patterns of the LTS interneuron of rat barrel cortex in Fig.8.25, we take the simple model of the RS neuron and adjust the resting and instantaneous threshold potentials $v_r = -56$ mV and $v_t = -42$ mV, and the values $p = 1$ and $b = 8$, resulting in the rheobase current of 120 pA and the input resistance of 50 MΩ. To model the decreasing nature of the spike and AHP amplitudes, we assume that the peak of the spike and the after-spike resetting point depend on the value of the recovery variable $u$. This completely unnecessary cosmetic adjustment has a mild effect on the quantitative behavior of the model but gives a more "realistic" look to the simulated voltage traces in Fig.8.25.

The class of excitability of LTS neurons has not been studied systematically, though the neurons seem to be able to fire periodic spike trains with a frequency as low as that of RS neurons (Beierlein et al. 2003; Tateno and Robinson, personal communication). The conjecture that they are near saddle-node on invariant circle bifurcation, and hence are Class 1 excitable integrators, seems to be at odds with the observation that their membrane potential exhibits slow damped oscillation and that they can fire postinhibitory rebound spikes (Bacci et al. 2003a), called low-threshold spikes (hence the name – LTS neurons). They are better characterized as being at the transition from integrators to resonators, with phase portraits as in Fig.8.15.

A possible explanation for the subthreshold oscillations in LTS (and some RS) neurons is given in Fig.8.13, case $b > 0$. The resting state is a stable node when $I = 0$, but it becomes a stable focus when the magnitude of the injected current is near the neuron's rheobase. After firing a phasic spike, the trajectory spirals into the focus

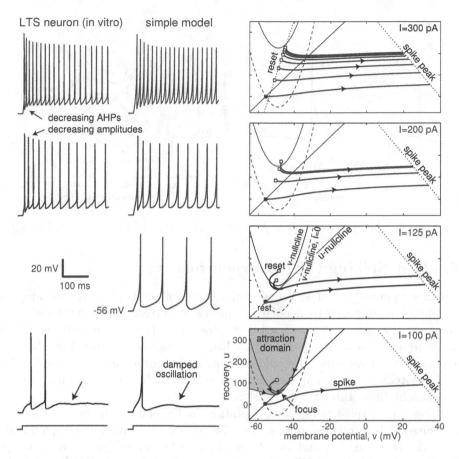

Figure 8.25: Comparison of in vitro recordings of a low threshold spiking (LTS) interneuron (rat barrel cortex; data provided by B. Connors) with simulations of the simple model $100\dot{v} = (v + 56)(v + 42) - u + I$, $\dot{u} = 0.03\{8(v + 56) - u\}$, if $v \geq 40 - 0.1u$, then $v \leftarrow -53 + 0.04u$, $u \leftarrow \min\{u + 20, 670\}$.

exhibiting damped oscillation. Its frequency is the imaginary part of the complex-conjugate eigenvalues of the equilibrium, and it is small because the system is near Bogdanov-Takens bifurcation.

A possible explanation for the rebound spike in LTS (or some RS) neurons is given in Fig.8.26. The shaded region is the attraction domain of the resting state (black circle), which is bounded by the stable manifold of the saddle (white circle). A sufficiently strong hyperpolarizing pulse moves the trajectory to the new, hyperpolarized equilibrium (black square), which is outside the attraction domain. Upon release from the hyperpolarization, the trajectory fires a phasic spike and then returns to the resting state. Some LTS interneurons fire bursts of spikes, and for that reason are called burst-spiking non-pyramidal (BSNP) neurons.

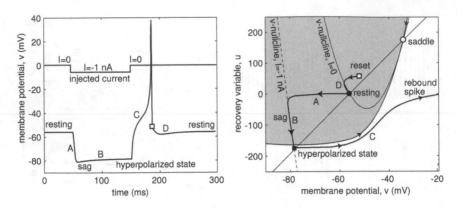

Figure 8.26: The mechanism of sag and rebound spike of the model in Fig.8.25.

## 8.2.6  Fast Spiking (FS) Interneurons

Fast spiking neurons fire "fast" tonic spike trains of relatively constant amplitude and frequency in response to depolarized pulses of current. In a systematic study, Tateno et al. (2004) have shown that FS neurons have Class 2 excitability in the sense that their frequency-current (F-I) relation has a discontinuity around 20 Hz. When stimulated with barely superthreshold current, such neurons exhibit irregular firing, randomly switching between spiking and fast subthreshold oscillatory mode (Kubota and Kawaguchi 1999; Tateno et al. 2004).

The absence of spike frequency adaptation in FS neurons is mostly due to the fast $K^+$ current that activates during the spike, produces deep AHP, completely deinactivates the $Na^+$ current, and thereby facilitates the generation of the next spike. Blocking the $K^+$ current by TEA (Erisir et al. 1999) removes AHP, leaves residual inactivation of the $Na^+$ current, and slows the spiking, essentially transforming the FS firing pattern into LTS.

The existence of fast subthreshold oscillations of membrane potential suggests that the resting state of the FS neurons is near the Andronov-Hopf bifurcation. Stuttering behavior at the threshold currents points to the coexistence of resting and spiking states, as in Fig.8.16, and suggests that the bifurcation is of the subcritical type. However, FS neurons do not fire postinhibitory (rebound) spikes – the feature used to distinguish them experimentally from LTS types. Thus, we cannot use the simple model (8.5, 8.6) in its present form to simulate FS neurons because the model with linear slow nullcline would fire rebound spikes according to the mechanism depicted in Fig.8.26. In addition, the simple model has a non-monotone I-V relation, whereas FS neurons have a monotone relation.

The absence of rebound responses in FS neurons means that the phenomenological recovery variable (activation of the fast $K^+$ current) does not decrease significantly below the resting value when the membrane potential is hyperpolarized. That is, the slow $u$-nullcline becomes horizontal in the hyperpolarized voltage range. Accordingly,

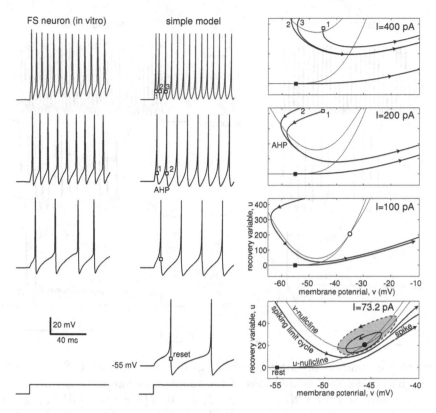

Figure 8.27: Comparison of in vitro recordings of a fast spiking (FS) interneuron of layer 5 rat visual cortex with simulations of the simple model $20\dot{v} = (v+55)(v+40) - u + I$, $\dot{u} = 0.2\{U(v) - u\}$, if $v \geq 25$, then $v \leftarrow -45$ mV. Slow nonlinear nullcline $U(v) = 0$ when $v < v_\mathrm{b}$ and $U(v) = 0.025(v - v_\mathrm{b})^3$ when $v \geq v_\mathrm{b}$ with $v_\mathrm{b} = -55$ mV. Shaded area denotes the attraction domain of the resting state.

we simulate the FS neuron in Fig.8.27, using the simple model (8.5) with nonlinear $u$-nullcline.

The phase portraits and bifurcation diagram of the FS neuron model are qualitatively similar to the fast subsystem of a "subHopf/fold cycle" burster: injection of DC current $I$ creates a stable and an unstable limit cycle via fold limit cycle bifurcation. The frequency of the newborn stable cycle is around 20 Hz; hence the discontinuity of the F-I curve and Class 2 excitability. There is a bistability of resting and spiking states, as in Fig.8.27 (bottom right), so that noise can switch the state of the neuron back and forth, and result in irregular stuttering spiking with subthreshold oscillations in the $10 - 40$ Hz range between the spike trains. Further increase of $I$ shrinks the amplitude of the unstable limit cycle, results in the subcritical Andronov-Hopf bifurcation of the resting state, removes the coexistence of attractors, and leaves only the tonic spiking mode.

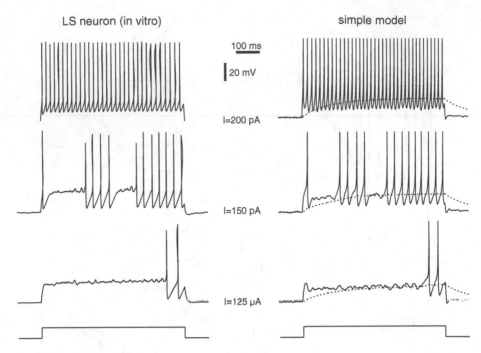

Figure 8.28: Comparison of in vitro recordings of a late spiking (LS) interneuron of layer 1 rat neocortex with simulations of the simple two-compartment model. Soma: $20\dot{v} = 0.3(v+66)(v+40) + 1.2(v_d - v) - u + I$, $\dot{u} = 0.17\{5(v+66) - u\}$, if $v \geq 30$, then $v \leftarrow -45$, $u \leftarrow u + 100$. Passive dendrite (dotted curve): $\dot{v}_d = 0.01(v - v_d)$. Weak noise was added to simulations to unmask the subthreshold oscillations. (Recordings were provided by Zhiguo Chu, Mario Galarreta, and Shaul Hestrin; traces $I = 125$ and $I = 150$ are from one cell; trace $I = 200$ is from another cell.)

## 8.2.7   Late Spiking (LS) Interneurons

When stimulated with long pulses of DC current, late spiking neurons exhibit a long voltage ramp, barely seen in Fig.8.28 (bottom), and then switch into a tonic firing mode. A stronger stimulation may evoke an immediate (transient) spike followed by a long ramp and a long latency to the second spike. There are pronounced fast subthreshold oscillations during the voltage ramp, indicating the existence of at least two time scales: (1) fast oscillations resulting from the interplay of amplifying and resonant currents, and (2) slow ramp resulting from the slow kinetic of an amplifying variable, such as slow inactivation of an outward current (e.g., the K$^+$ A-current) or slow activation of an inward current, or both. In addition, the ramp could result from the slow charging of the dendritic compartment of the neuron.

The exact mechanism responsible for the slow ramp in LS neurons is not known at present. Fortunately, we do not need to know the mechanism in order to simulate LS neurons using the simple model approach. Indeed, simple models with passive dendrites are equivalent to simple models with linear amplifying currents. For example, the model in Fig.8.28 consists of a two-dimensional system $(v, u)$ responsible for the spike generation mechanism at the soma and a linear equation for the passive dendritic compartment $v_d$.

When stimulated with the threshold current (i.e., just above the neuronal rheobase), LS neurons often exhibit the stuttering behavior seen in Fig.8.28 (middle). Subthreshold oscillations, voltage ramps, and stuttering are consistent with the following geometrical picture. Abrupt onset of stimulation evokes a transient spike followed by brief hyperpolarization and then sustained depolarization. While depolarized, the fast subsystem affects the slow subsystem, e.g., slowly charges the dendritic tree or slowly inactivates the $K^+$ current. In any case, there is a slow decrease of the outward current or, equivalently, a slow increase of the inward current that drives the fast subsystem through the subcritical Andronov-Hopf bifurcation. Because of the coexistence of resting and spiking states near the bifurcation, the neuron can be switched from one state to the other by the membrane noise. Once the bifurcation is passed, the neuron is in the tonic spiking mode. Overall, LS neurons can be thought of as being FS neurons with a slow subsystem that damps any abrupt changes, delays the onset of spiking, and slows the frequency of spiking.

## 8.2.8 Diversity of Inhibitory Interneurons

In contrast to excitatory neocortical pyramidal neurons, which have stereotypical morphological and electrophysiological classes (RS, IB, CH), inhibitory neocortical interneurons have wildly diverse classes with various firing patterns that cannot be classified as FS, LTS, or LS. Markram et al. (2004) reviewed recent results on the relationship between electrophysiology, pharmacology, immunohistochemistry, and gene expression patterns of inhibitory interneurons. An extreme interpretation of their findings is that there is a continuum of different classes of interneurons rather than a set of three classes.

Figure 8.29 summarizes five of the most ubiquitous groups in the continuum:

- (NAC) Non-accommodating interneurons fire repetitively without frequency adaptation in response to a wide range of sustained somatic current injections. Many FS and LS neurons are of this type.

- (AC) Accommodating interneurons fire repetitively with frequency adaptation and therefore do not reach the high firing rates of NAC neurons. Some FS and LS cells, but mostly LTS cells, are of this type.

- (STUT) Stuttering interneurons fire high-frequency clusters of regular spikes intermingled with unpredictable periods of quiescence. Some FS and LS cells exhibit this firing type.

- (BST) Bursting interneurons fire a cluster of three to five spikes riding on a slow depolarizing wave, followed by a strong slow AHP.

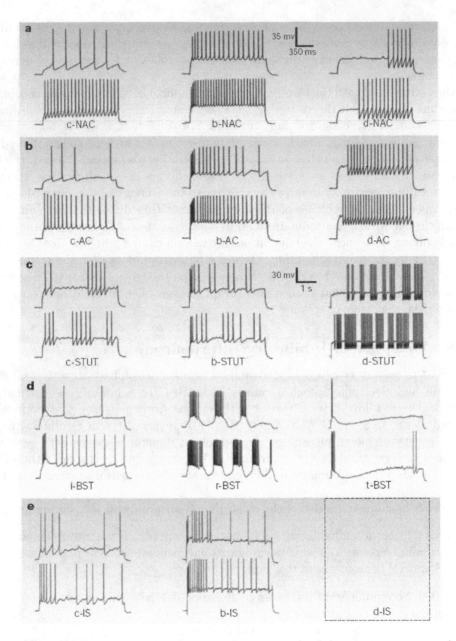

Figure 8.29: An alternative classification of neocortical inhibitory interneurons (modified from Markram et al. 2004). Five major classes: non-accommodating (NAC), accommodating (AC), stuttering (STUT), bursting (BST), and irregular spiking (IS). Most classes contain subclasses: delay (d), classic (c), and burst (b). For bursting interneurons, the three types are repetitive (r), initial (i), and transient (t). Subclass d-IS is not provided in the original picture by Markram et al.

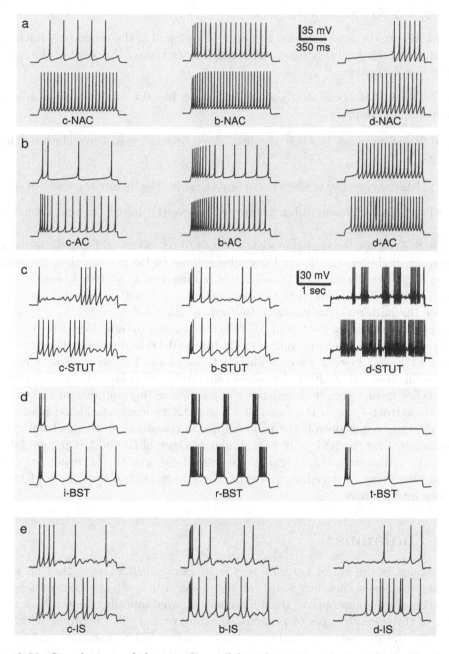

Figure 8.30: Simulations of the simple model with various parameters can reproduce all firing patterns of neocortical inhibitory interneurons in Fig.8.29.

- (IS) Irregular spiking interneurons fire single spikes randomly with pronounced frequency accommodation.

NAC and AC are the most common response types found in the neocortex. Each group can be divided into three subgroups depending on the type of the onset of the response to a step depolarization:

- (c) Classical response is when the first spike has the same shape as any other spike in the response.

- (b) Burst response is when the first three or more spikes are clustered into a burst.

- (d) Delayed response is when there is noticeable delay before the onset of spiking.

The BST type has different subdivisions: repetitive (r), initial (i), and transient (t) bursting.

In Fig.8.30 we use the simple model (8.5, 8.6) to reproduce all firing patterns of the interneurons, including the delayed irregular spiking (d-IS) pattern that was omitted from Fig.8.29. We use one-size-fits-all set of parameters: $C = 100$, $k = 1$, $v_r = -60$ mV, and $v_t = -40$ mV. We vary the parameters $a, b, c$, and $d$. We do not strive to reproduce the patterns quantitatively, but only qualitatively.

The parameters for the NAC and AC cells were similar to those for RS neurons, with an additional passive dendritic compartment for the delayed response. The parameters for the STUT and IS cells were similar to those of the LS interneuron, with some minor modifications that affect the initial burstiness and delays. Irregular stuttering in these types results from the coexistence of a stable resting equilibrium and a spiking limit cycle attractor, as in the cases of FS and LS neurons considered above. The level of intrinsic noise controls the probabilities of transitions between the attractors. The parameters for the BST cells were similar to those of IB and CH pyramidal cells. Varying the parameters $a, b, c$, and $d$, we indeed can get all the firing patterns in Fig.8.29, plus many intermediate patterns, thereby creating a continuum of types of inhibitory interneurons.

## 8.3  Thalamus

The thalamus is the major gateway to the neocortex in the sense that no sensory signal, such as vision, hearing, touch, or taste, etc., can reach the neocortex without passing through an appropriate thalamic nucleus. Anatomically, the thalamic system consists of three major types of neurons: thalamocortical (TC) neurons, which relay signals into the neocortex; reticular thalamic nucleus (RTN) neurons; and thalamic interneurons, which provide local reciprocal inhibition (Shepherd 2004). The three types have distinct electrophysiological properties and firing patterns.

There are undoubtedly subtypes within each type of thalamic neurons, but the classification is not as elaborate as the one in the neocortex. This, and the differences

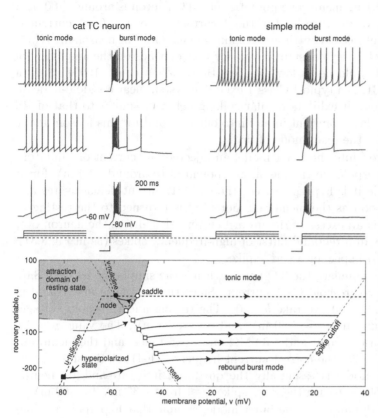

Figure 8.31: Comparison of in vitro recordings of a thalamocortical (TC) cell of cat dorsal lateral geniculate nucleus with simulations of the simple model $200\dot{v} = 1.6(v + 60)(v + 50) - u + I$, $\dot{u} = 0.01\{b(v+65)-u\}$, $b = 15$ if $v \leq -65$ and $b = 0$ otherwise. When $v \geq 35+0.1u$, then $v \leftarrow -60-0.1u$, $u \leftarrow u+10$. Injected current pulses are in 50 pA increments. In burst mode, the cell was hyperpolarized to $-80$ mV prior to injection of a depolarizing pulse of current. (Data provided by C. L. Cox and S. M. Sherman.)

between species, ages, and various thalamic nuclei, explain the contradictory reports of different firing patterns in presumably the same types of thalamic neurons. Below we use the simple model (8.5, 8.6) to simulate a "typical" TC, TRN, and interneuron. The reader should realize, though, that our attempt is as incomplete as the attempt to simulate a "typical" neocortical neuron ignoring the fact that there are RS, IB, CH, FS, and other cells.

## 8.3.1   Thalamocortical (TC) Relay Neurons

Thalamocortical (TC) relay neurons, the type of thalamic neurons that project sensory input to the cortex, have two prominent models of firing, illustrated in Fig.8.31: tonic mode and burst mode. Both modes are ubiquitous in vitro and in vivo, including awake and behaving animals, and both represent different patterns of relay of sensory information into the cortex (Sherman 2001). The transition between the firing modes depends on the degree of inactivation of a low-threshold Ca$^{2+}$ T-current (Jahnsen and Llinas 1984; McCormick and Huguenard 1992), which in turn depends on the holding membrane potential of the TC neuron.

In tonic mode, the resting membrane potential of a TC neuron is around $-60$ mV, which is above the inactivation threshold of the T-current. The slow $Ca^{2+}$ current is inactivated and is not available to contribute to spiking behavior. The neuron fires $Na^+$-$K^+$ tonic spikes with a relatively constant frequency that depends on the amplitude of the injected current and could be as low as a few Hertz (Zhan et al. 1999). Such a cell, illustrated in Fig.8.31, is a typical Class 1 excitable system near a saddle-node on invariant circle bifurcation. It exhibits regular spiking behavior similar to that of RS neocortical neurons. It relays transient inputs into outputs, and for this reason, many refer to the tonic mode as the relay mode of firing.

To switch a TC neuron into the burst mode, an injected DC current or inhibitory synaptic input must hyperpolarize the membrane potential to around $-80$ mV for at least $50 - 100$ ms. While it is hyperpolarized, the $Ca^{2+}$ T-current deinactivates and becomes available. As soon as the membrane potential is returned to the resting or depolarized state, there is an excess of the inward current that drives the neuron over the threshold and results in a rebound burst of high-frequency spikes (as in Fig.8.31), called a low-threshold (LT) spike or a $Ca^{2+}$ spike.

In Fig.8.31 (right) we simulate the TC neuron, using the simple model (8.5, 8.6), and treating $u$ as the low-threshold $Ca^{2+}$ current. Since the current is inactivated in the tonic mode, that is, $u \approx 0$, we take $b = 0$. The resting and threshold voltages of the neuron in the figure are $v_r = -60$ mV and $v_t = -50$ mV. The value $p = 1.6$ results in a 40 pA rheobase current and a 60 M$\Omega$ input resistance, and the membrane capacitance $C = 200$ pF gives the correct current-frequency (F-I) relationship. Thus, in the tonic mode, our model is essentially the quadratic integrate-and-fire neuron $200\dot{v} = 1.6(v + 60)(v + 50) + I$ with the after-spike reset from $+35$ mV to $-60$ mV.

To model slow $Ca^{2+}$ dynamics in the burst mode, assume that hyperpolarizations below the $Ca^{2+}$ inactivation threshold of $-65$ mV decrease $u$, thereby creating inward current. In the linear case, take $\dot{u} = 0.01\{b(v + 65) - u\}$ with $b = 0$ when $v \geq -65$, and $b = 15$ when $v < -65$, resulting in the piecewise linear $u$-nullcline depicted in Fig.8.31 (bottom). Prolonged hyperpolarization below $-65$ mV decreases $u$ and moves the trajectory outside the attraction domain of the resting state (shaded region in the figure). Upon release from the hyperpolarization, the model fires a rebound burst of spikes; the variable $u \to 0$ (inactivation of $Ca^{2+}$), and the trajectory reenters the attraction domain of the resting state. Steps of depolarized current produce rebound bursts followed by tonic spiking with adapting frequency. A better quantitative agreement with TC recordings can be achieved when two slow variables, $u_1$ and $u_2$, are used.

## 8.3.2    Reticular Thalamic Nucleus (RTN) Neurons

Reticular thalamic nucleus (RTN) neurons provide reciprocal inhibition to TC relay neurons. RTN and TC cells are similar in the sense that they have two firing modes, illustrated in Fig.8.32: They fire trains of single spikes following stimulation from resting or depolarized potentials in the tonic mode, as well as rebound bursts upon release from hyperpolarized potentials in the burst mode.

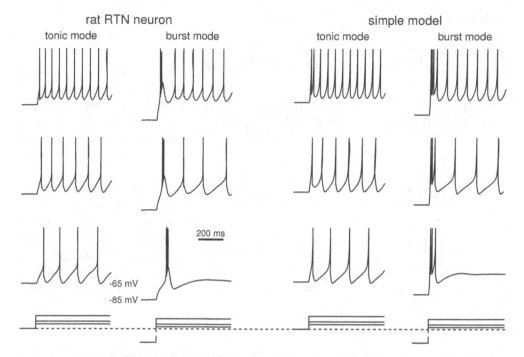

Figure 8.32: Comparison of in vitro recordings of a reticular thalamic nucleus (RTN) neuron of a rat with simulations of the simple model $40\dot{v} = 0.25(v+65)(v+45) - u + I$, $\dot{u} = 0.015\{b(v+65) - u\}$, $b = 10$ if $v \leq -65$ and $b = 2$ otherwise. When $v \geq 0$ (spike cutoff), then $v \leftarrow -55$, $u \leftarrow u + 50$. Injected current pulses are $50, 70$, and $110$ pA. In burst mode, the cell was hyperpolarized to $-80$ mV prior to injection of a depolarizing pulse of current. (Data provided S. H. Lee and C. L. Cox.)

The parameters of the simple model in Fig.8.32 are adjusted to match the in vitro recording of the RTN cell in the figure, and they differ from the parameters of the TC model cell. Nevertheless, the mechanism of rebound bursting of the RTN neuron is the same as that of the TC neuron in Fig.8.31 (bottom). In contrast, the tonic mode of firing is different. Since $b > 0$, the model neuron is near the transition from an integrator to a resonator; it can fire transient spikes followed by slow subthreshold oscillations of membrane potential; it has coexistence of stable resting and spiking states, with the bifurcation diagram similar to the one in Fig.8.15, and it can stutter and produce clustered spikes when stimulated with barely threshold current. Interestingly, similar behavior of TC neurons was reported by Pirchio et al. (1997), Pedroarena and Llinas (1997), and Li et al. (2003). We will return to the issue of subthreshold oscillations and stuttering spiking when we consider stellate cells of entorhinal cortex in section 8.4.4.

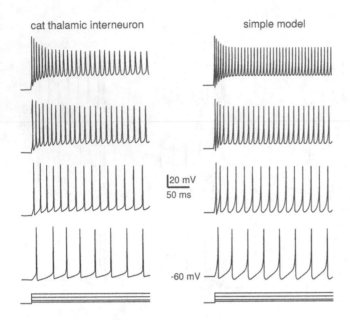

Figure 8.33: Comparison of in vitro recordings of dorsal lateral geniculate nucleus interneuron of a cat with simulations of the simple model $20\dot{v} = 0.5(v + 60)(v + 50) - u + I$, $\dot{u} = 0.05\{7(v + 60) - u\}$. When $v \geq 20 - 0.08u$ (spike cutoff), $v \leftarrow -65 + 0.08u$, $u \leftarrow \min\{u + 50, 530\}$. Injected current pulses are $50, 100, 200$, and $250$ pA. (Data provided by C. L. Cox and S. M. Sherman.)

### 8.3.3   Thalamic Interneurons

In contrast to TC and RTN neurons, thalamic interneurons do not have a prominent burst mode, though they can fire rebound spikes upon release from hyperpolarization (Pape and McCormick 1995). They have action potentials with short duration, and they are able to generate high-frequency trains of spikes reaching 800 Hz, as do cortical FS interneurons. The simple model in Fig.8.33 reproduces all these features. Its phase portrait and bifurcation diagram are similar to those in Fig.8.15, but its dynamics has a much faster time scale.

## 8.4   Other Interesting Cases

The neocortical and thalamic neurons span an impressive range of dynamic behavior. Many neuronal types found in other brain regions have dynamics quite similar to some of the types discussed above, while many do not.

### 8.4.1   Hippocampal CA1 Pyramidal Neurons

Hippocampal pyramidal neurons and interneurons are similar to those of the neocortex, and hence could be simulated using the simple model presented in section 8.2. Let us elaborate, using the pyramidal neurons of the CA1 region of the hippocampus as an example.

Jensen et al. (1994) suggested classifying all CA1 pyramidal neurons according to their propensity to fire bursts of spikes, often called *complex spikes*. The majority (more than 80 percent) of CA1 pyramidal neurons are non-bursting cells, whereas the

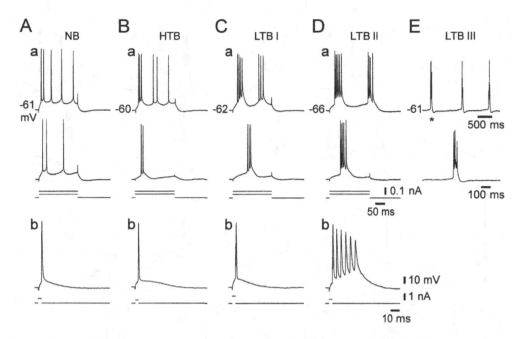

Figure 8.34: Classification of hippocampal CA1 pyramidal neurons. A–E, in vitro recordings from five different pyramidal neurons arranged according to a gradient of increasing propensity to burst. The neurons were stimulated with current pulses of 200 ms duration and amplitude 50 pA and 100 pA (a), or brief (3–5 ms) superthreshold pulses (b). The non-burster (NB) neuron fires tonic spikes in response to long pulses and a single spike in response to brief pulses. The high-threshold burster (HTB) fires bursts only in response to strong long pulses, and single spikes in response to weak or brief pulses. The grade I low-threshold burster (LTB I) generates bursts in response to long pulses of current, but single spikes in response to brief pulses. The grade II LTB (LTB II) fires bursts in response to both long (a) and brief (b) current pulses. The grade III LTB (LTB III), in addition to firing bursts in response to long and brief pulses of current (not shown), also fires spontaneous rhythmic bursts, shown in contracted and expanded time scales. (Reproduced from Su et al. 2001 with permission.)

remaining ones exhibit some form of bursts, which are defined in this context as sets of three or more closely spaced spikes. There are five different classes:

- (NB) Non-bursting cells generate accommodating trains of tonic spikes in response to depolarizing pulses of DC current, and a single spike in response to a brief superthreshold pulse of current, as in Fig.8.34A.

- (HTB) High-threshold bursters fire bursts only in response to strong long pulses of current, but fire single spikes in response to weak or brief pulses of current, as

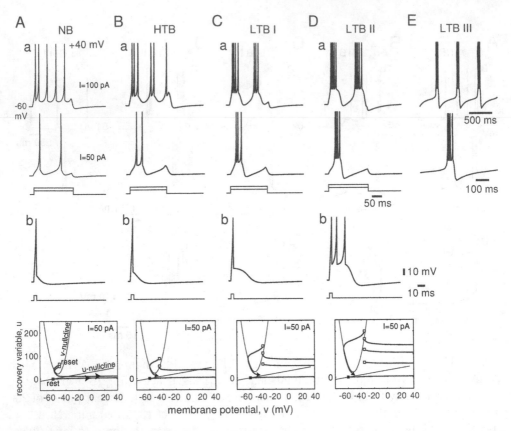

Figure 8.35: Simulations of hippocampal CA1 pyramidal neurons (compare with Fig.8.34) using simple model $50\dot{v} = 0.5(v+60)(v+45)-u+I$, $\dot{u} = 0.02\{0.5(v+60)-u\}$. When $v \geq 40$ (spike cutoff), $v \leftarrow c$ and $u \leftarrow u + d$. Here $c = -50, -45, -40, -35$ mV and $d = 50, 50, 55, 60$ for A–D, respectively. Parameters in E are the same as in D, but $I = 33$ pA.

in Fig.8.34B.

- (LTB I) Grade I low-threshold bursters fire bursts in response to long pulses, but single spikes in response to brief pulses of current, as in Fig.8.34C.

- (LTB II) Grade II low-threshold bursters fire stereotypical bursts in response to brief pulses, as in Fig.8.34D.

- (LTB III) Grade III low-threshold bursters fire rhythmic bursts spontaneously, which are depicted in Fig.8.34E, using two time scales.

NB neurons are equivalent to neocortical pyramidal neurons of the RS type, whereas HTB and LTB I neurons are equivalent to neocortical pyramidal neurons of the IB type. The author is not aware of any systematic studies of the ability of IB neurons to fire stereotypical bursts in response to brief pulses, as in Fig.8.34Db, or to have intrinsic rhythmic activity, as in Fig.8.34E. Therefore, it is not clear whether there are any analogues of LTB grades II and III neurons in the neocortex.

The classification of hippocampal CA1 pyramidal neurons into five different classes does not imply a fundamental difference in the ionic mechanism of spike generation, but only a quantitative difference. This follows from the observation that pharmacological manipulations can gradually and reversibly transform an NB neuron into an LTB III neuron, and vice versa, by elevating the extracellular concentration of K$^+$ (Jensen et al. 1994), reducing extracellular Ca$^{2+}$ (Su et al. 2001), blocking the K$^+$ M-current (Yue and Yaari 2004), or manipulating Ca$^{2+}$ current dynamics in apical dendrites (Magee and Carruth 1999).

In Fig.8.35 we modify the simple model for the neocortical RS neuron to reproduce firing patterns of hippocampal pyramidal cells. To get the continuum of responses from NB to LTB II, fix all the parameters and vary only the after-spike reset parameter $c$ by an increment of 5 mV, and the parameter $d$. These phenomenological parameters describe the effect of high-threshold inward and outward currents activated during each spike and affecting the after-spike behavior. Increasing $c$ corresponds to up-regulating slow $I_{\text{Na,p}}$ or down-regulating slow K$^+$ currents, which leads to transition from NB to LTB III in the CA1 slice (Su et al. 2001) and in the simple model in Fig.8.35. Interestingly, the same procedure results in transitions from RS to IB and possibly to CH classes in neocortical pyramidal neurons (Izhikevich 2003). This is consistent with the observation by Steriade (2004) that many neocortical neurons can change their firing classes in vivo, depending on the state of the brain.

## 8.4.2 Spiny Projection Neurons of Neostriatum and Basal Ganglia

Spiny projection neurons, the major class of neurons in neostriatum and basal ganglia, display a prominent bistable behavior in vivo, shown in Fig.8.36 (Wilson and Groves

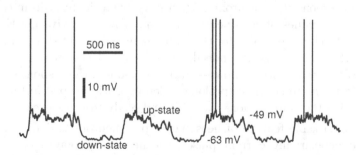

Figure 8.36: Neostriatal spiny neurons have two-state behavior in vivo. (Data provided by Charles Wilson.)

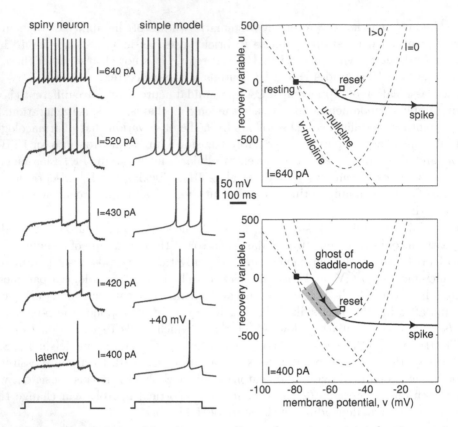

Figure 8.37: Comparison of in vitro recordings of a rat neostriatal spiny projection neuron with simulations of the simple model $50\dot{v} = (v + 80)(v + 25) - u + I$, $\dot{u} = 0.01\{-20(v+80) - u\}$, if $v \geq 40$, then $v \leftarrow -55$, $u \leftarrow u + 150$. (In vitro data provided by C. Wilson.)

1981; Wilson 1993): they shift the membrane potential from hyperpolarized to depolarized states in response to synchronous excitatory synaptic input from cortex and/or thalamus. In vitro studies of such neurons reveal a slowly inactivating $K^+$ A-current, which is believed to be responsible for the maintenance of the up-state and down-state, in addition to the synaptic input. Indeed, the $K^+$ current is completely deinactivated at the hyperpolarized potentials (down-state), and reduces the response of the neuron to any synaptic input. In contrast, prolonged depolarization (up-state) inactivates the current and makes the neuron more excitable and ready to fire spikes.

The most remarkable feature of neostriatal spiny neurons is depicted in Fig.8.37. In response to depolarizing current pulses, the neurons display a prominent slowly depolarizing (ramp) potential, and hence long latency to spike discharge (Nisenbaum et al. 1994). The ramp is mostly due to the slow inactivation of the $K^+$ A-current and slow charging of the dendritic tree. The delay to spike can be as long as 1 sec, but the subsequent spike train has a shorter, relatively constant period that depends on the magnitude of the injected current – a feature consistent with the saddle-node off limit cycle bifurcation.

Let us use the simple model (8.5, 8.6) to simulate the responses of spiny neurons to current pulses. The resting membrane potential of the neuron in Fig.8.37 is around $v_r = -80$ mV, and we set $v_t = -25$ mV, $p = 1$, and $b = -20$ to get 30 M$\Omega$ input resistance and 300 pA rheobase current. We take $a = 0.01$ to reflect the slow inactivation of the K$^+$ A-current in the subthreshold voltage range. The membrane potential in the figure reaches the peak of $+40$ mV during the spike and then resets to $-55$ mV or lower, depending on the firing frequency. The value $d = 150$ provides a reasonable match of the interspike frequencies for all magnitudes of injected current. Note that $b < 0$, so $u$ represents either slow inactivation of $I_A$ or slow charging of the passive dendritic compartment, or both. In any case, it is a slow amplifying variable, which is consistent with the observation that spiny neurons do not "sag" in response to hyperpolarizing current pulses, do not "peak" in response to depolarizing pulses (Nisenbaum et al. 1994), and do not generate rebound (postinhibitory) spikes.

Injection of a depolarizing current shifts the $v$-nullcline of the simple model upward, and the resting state disappears via saddle-node bifurcation. The trajectory slowly moves through the ghost of the bifurcation point (shaded rectangle in the figure), resulting in the long latency to the first spike. The spike resets the trajectory to a point (white square) below the ghost, resulting in significantly smaller delays to subsequent spikes. Because the resetting point is so close to the saddle-node bifurcation point, the simple model, and probably the spiny projection neuron in the figure, are near the codimension-2 saddle-node homoclinic orbit bifurcation discussed in section 6.3.6.

## 8.4.3   Mesencephalic V Neurons of Brainstem

The best examples of resonators with fast subthreshold oscillations, Class 2 excitability, rebound spikes, and so on, are mesencephalic V (mesV) neurons of the brainstem (Wu et al. 2001) and primary sensory neurons of the dorsal root ganglion (Amir et al. 2002; Jian et al. 2004). MesV neurons of the brainstem have monotone I-V curves, whereas the simple model with linear equation for $u$ does not. In Fig.8.38 we use a modification of the simple model to simulate the responses of a mesV neuron (data from Fig.7.3) to pulses of depolarizing current.

The model's phase portrait is qualitatively similar to that of the FS interneurons in Fig.8.27. The resting state is a stable focus, resulting in damped or noise-induced sustained oscillations of the membrane potential. Their amplitude and frequency depend on $I$ and can be larger than 5 mV and 100 Hz, respectively. The focus loses stability via subcritical Andronov-Hopf bifurcation. Because of the coexistence of the resting and spiking states, the mesV neuron can burst, and so can the simple model if noise or a slow resonant variable is added.

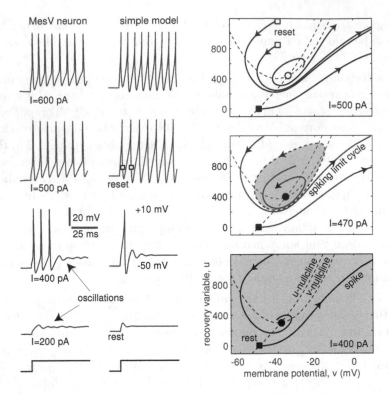

Figure 8.38: Comparison of in vitro recordings of rat brainstem mesV neuron (from Fig.7.3) with simulations of the simple model $25\dot{v} = (v + 50)(v + 30) - u + I$, $\dot{u} = 0.5\{U(v + 50) - u\}$, with cubic slow nullcline $U(x) = 25x + 0.009x^3$. If $v \geq 10$, then $v \leftarrow -40$.

## 8.4.4　Stellate Cells of Entorhinal Cortex

The entorhinal cortex occupies a privileged anatomical position that allows it to gate the main flow of information into and out of the hippocampus. in vitro studies show that stellate cells, a major class of neurons in the entorhinal cortex, exhibit intrinsic subthreshold oscillations with a slow dynamics of the kind shown in Fig.8.39b (Alonso and Llinas 1989; Alonso and Klink 1993; Klink and Alonso 1993; Dickson et al. 2000). The oscillations are generated by the interplay between a persistent Na$^+$ current and an h-current, and they are believed to set the theta rhythmicity in the entorhinal-hippocampal network.

The caption of Fig.8.39 provides parameters of the simple model (8.5, 8.6) that captures the slow oscillatory dynamics of an adult rat entorhinal stellate cell recorded in vitro. The cell sags to injected hyperpolarizing current in Fig.8.39a and then fires a rebound spike upon release from hyperpolarization. From a neurophysiological point of view, the sag and the rebound response are due to the opening of the h-current; from

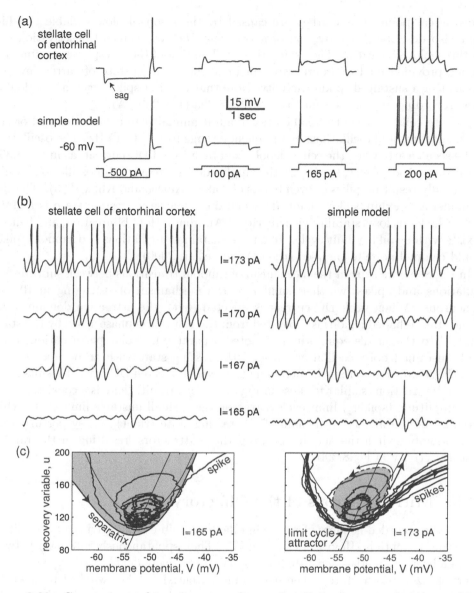

Figure 8.39: Comparison of in vitro recordings of stellate neurons of rat entorhinal cortex with simulations of the simple model $200\dot{v} = 0.75(v + 60)(v + 45) - u + I$, $\dot{u} = 0.01\{15(v + 60) - u\}$, if $v \geq 30$, then $v \leftarrow -50$. (a) Responses to steps of DC current. (b) Subthreshold oscillations and occasional spikes at various levels of injected DC current. (c) Phase portraits corresponding to two levels of injected DC current. Weak noise was added to simulations to unmask subthreshold oscillations. (Data provided by Brian Burton and John A. White. All recordings are from the same neuron, except steps of $-500$ pA and 200 pA were recorded from a different neuron. Spikes are cut at 0 mV.)

a theoretical point of view, they are caused by the resonant slow variable $u$, which could also describe deinactivation of a transient Na$^+$ current and deactivation of a low-threshold K$^+$ current. The geometrical explanation of these responses is similar to the one provided for LTS interneurons in Fig.8.26. Positive steps of current evoke a transient or a sustained spiking activity. Note that the first spike is actually a doublet in the recording and in the simulation in Fig.8.39a ($I = 200$ pA).

Stellate cells in the entorhinal cortex of adult animals can exhibit damped or sustained subthreshold oscillations in a frequency range from 5 to 15 Hz. The oscillations can be seen clearly when the cell is depolarized by injected DC current, as in Fig.8.39b. The stronger the current, the higher the amplitude and frequency of oscillations, which occasionally result in spikes or even bursts of spikes (Alonso and Klink 1993). The simple model also exhibits slow damped oscillations because its resting state is a stable focus. The focus loses stability via subcritical Andronov-Hopf bifurcation, and hence it coexists with a spiking limit cycle. To enable sustained oscillations and random spikes, we add channel noise to the $v$-equation (White et al. 2000).

In Fig.8.39c we explain the mechanism of random transitions between subthreshold oscillations and spikes, which is similar to the mechanism of stuttering in RS and FS neurons. When weak DC current is injected (left), the attraction domain of the resting state (shaded region) is separated from the rest of the phase space by the stable manifold to the saddle equilibrium (denoted separatrix). Noisy perturbations evoke small, sustained noisy oscillations around the resting state with an occasional spike when the separatrix is crossed. Increasing the level of injected DC current results in the series of bifurcations similar to those in Fig.8.15. As a result, there is a coexistence of a large amplitude (spiking) limit cycle attractor and a small unstable limit cycle, which encompasses the attraction domain of the resting state (right). Noisy perturbations can randomly switch the activity between these attractors, resulting in the random bursting activity in Fig.8.39b.

### 8.4.5   Mitral Neurons of the Olfactory Bulb

Mitral cells recorded in slices of rat main olfactory bulb exhibit intrinsic bistability of membrane potentials (Heyward et al. 2001). They spontaneously alternate between two membrane potentials separated by 10 mV: a relatively depolarized (up-state) and hyperpolarized (down-state). The membrane potential can be switched between the states by a brief depolarizing or hyperpolarizing pulse of current, as we show in Fig.7.36. In response to stimulation, the cells are more likely to fire in the up-state than in the down-state.

Current-voltage (I-V) relations of such mitral cells have three zeros in the subthreshold voltage range confirming that there are three equilibria: two stable ones corresponding to the up-state and the down-state, and one unstable, the saddle. There are no subthreshold oscillations in the down-state, hence it is a node, and the cell is an integrator. There are small-amplitude 40 Hz oscillations in the up-state; hence it is a focus, and the cell is a resonator.

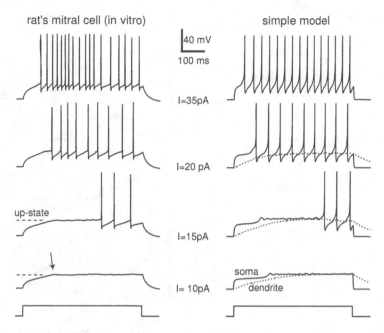

Figure 8.40: Comparison of in vitro recordings of mitral neurons of rat olfactory bulb with simulations of the simple two-compartment model. Soma: $40\dot{v} = (v+55)(v+50) + 0.5(v_d-v)-u+I$, $\dot{u} = 0.4\{(U(v)-u\}$ with $U(v) = 0$ when $v < v_b$ and $U(v) = 20(v-v_b)$ when $v \geq v_b = -48$ mV. If $v \geq 35$, then $v \leftarrow -50$. Passive dendrite (dotted curve): $\dot{v}_d = 0.0125(v - v_d)$. Weak noise was added to simulations to unmask subthreshold oscillations in the up-state. The membrane potential of the neuron is held at $-75$ mV by injecting a strong negative current, and then stimulated with steps of positive current. (Data provided by Philip Heyward.)

To model the bistability, we use the simple model with a piecewise linear slow nullcline that approximates nonlinear activation functions $n_\infty(v)$ near the "threshold" of the current and a passive dendritic compartment. In many respects, the model is similar to the one for late spiking (LS) cortical interneurons. In Fig.8.40 we fine-tune the model to simulate responses of a rat mitral cell to pulses of current of various amplitudes. To prevent noise-induced spontaneous transitions between the up-state and the down-state, the cell in the figure was held at $-75$ mV by injection of a large negative current. Its responses to weak positive pulses of current show a fast-rising phase followed by an abrupt step (arrow in the figure) to a constant value corresponding to the up-state. Increasing the magnitude of stimulation elicits trains of spikes with a considerable latency whose cause has yet to be determined experimentally. The latency could be the result of slow activation of an inward current, slow inactivation of an outward current (e.g., the K$^+$ A-current), or just slow charging of the dendritic compartment. All three cases correspond to additional slow variable in the simple model, which we interpret as a membrane potential of a passive dendritic compartment.

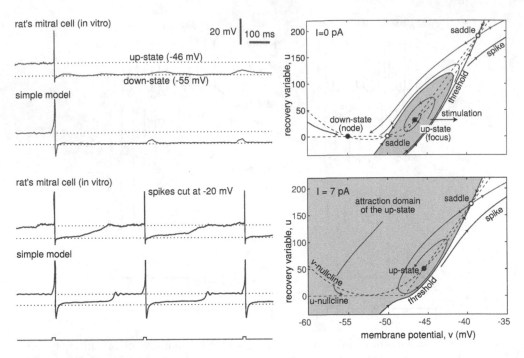

Figure 8.41: Voltage responses of a rat mitral cell and a simple model from Fig.8.40 at two different values of the holding current. *Right:* Phase portraits of somatic compartments show coexistence of stable node (down-state) and stable focus (up-state) equilibria. Spikes are emitted only from the up-state.

To understand the dynamics of the simple model, and hopefully of the mitral cell, we simulate its responses in Fig.8.41 to the activation of the olfactory nerve (ON). At the top of Fig.8.41, the cell is held at $I = 0$ pA. Its phase portrait clearly shows the coexistence of a stable node and focus equilibria separated by a saddle. The shaded region corresponds to the attraction domain of the focus equilibrium. To fire a spike from the up-state, noise or external stimulation must push the state of the system from the shaded region over the threshold to the right. The cell returns to the down-state immediately after the spike. Much stronger stimulation is needed to fire the cell from the down-state. Typically, the cell is switched to the up-state first, spends some time oscillating at 40 Hz, and then fires a spike (Heyward et al. 2001).

At the bottom of Fig.8.41, the cell is held at a slightly depolarizing current $I = 7$ pA. The node equilibrium disappears via saddle-node bifurcation, so there is no down-state, but only its ghost. Stimulation at the up-state results in a spike, after-hyperpolarization, and slow transition through the ghost of the down-state back to the up-state. Further increasing the holding current results in the stable manifold to the upper saddle (marked "threshold" in the figure) making a loop, then becoming a homoclinic trajectory to the saddle, giving birth to an unstable limit cycle which shrinks to the focus and makes it lose stability via subcritical Andronov-Hopf bifurcation. Note that this phase portrait and the bifurcation scenario are different from the one in Fig.7.36. However, in both cases, the neuron is an integrator in the down-state and a resonator in the up-state! The same property is exhibited by cerebellar Purkinje cells (see Fig.7.37), and possibly by other neurons kept in the up-state (intrinsically or extrinsically).

---

## Review of Important Concepts

- An integrate-and-fire neuron is a linear model having a stable *node* equilibrium, an artificial threshold, and a reset.

- A resonate-and-fire neuron is a linear model having a stable *focus* equilibrium, an artificial threshold, and a rest.

- Though technically not spiking neurons, these models are useful for analytical studies, that is, to prove theorems.

- The quadratic integrate-and-fire model captures the nonlinearity of the spike generation mechanism of real neurons having Class 1 excitability (saddle-node on invariant circle bifurcation).

- Its simple extension, model (8.5, 8.6), quantitatively reproduces subthreshold, spiking, and bursting activity of all known types of cortical and thalamic neurons in response to pulses of DC current.

- The simple model makes testable hypotheses on the dynamic mechanisms of excitability in these neurons.

- The model is especially suitable for simulations of large-scale models of the brain.

---

## Bibliographical Notes

Many people have used the integrate-and-fire neuron, treating it as a folklore model. It was Tuckwell's *Introduction to Theoretical Neurobiology* (1988) that gave appropriate credit to its inventor, Lapicque (1907). Although better models, such as the quadratic integrate-and-fire model, are available now, many scientists continue to favor the leaky integrate-and-fire neuron mostly because of its simplicity. Such an attitude is understandable when one wants to derive analytical results. However, purely computational papers can suffer from using the model because of its weird properties, such as the logarithmic F-I curve and fixed threshold.

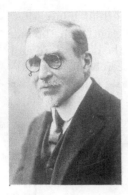

Figure 8.42: Louis Lapicque, the discoverer of the integrate-and-fire neuron.

The resonate-and-fire model was introduced by Izhikevich (2001a), and then by Richardson, Brunel, and Hakim (2003) and Brunel, Hakim, and Richardson (2003). These authors initially called the model "resonate-and-fire", but then changed its name to "generalized integrate-and-fire" (GIF), possibly to avoid confusion.

A better choice is the quadratic integrate-and-fire neuron in the normal form (8.2) or in the $\vartheta$-form (8.8); see exercise 7. The $\vartheta$-form was first suggested in the context of circle/circle (parabolic) bursting by Ermentrout and Kopell (1986a,b). Later, Ermentrout (1996) used this model to generalize numerical results of Hansel et al. (1995) on synchronization of Class 1 excitable systems, discussed in chapter 10. Hoppensteadt and Izhikevich (1997) introduced the canonical model approach, provided many examples of canonical models, and proved that the quadratic integrate-and-fire model is canonical in the sense that all Class 1 excitable systems can be transformed into this model by a piecewise continuous change of variables. They also suggested calling the model the "Ermentrout-Kopell canonical model" to honor its inventors, but most scientists follow Ermentrout and call it the "theta-neuron".

The model presented in section 8.1.4 was first suggested by Izhikevich (2000a; equations (4) and (5), with voltage reset discussed in Sect. 2.3.1) in the $\vartheta$-form. The form presented here first appeared in Izhikevich (2003). The representation of the function $I + v^2$ in the form $(v - v_r)(v - v_t)$ was suggested by Latham et al. (2000).

We stress that the simple model is useful only when one wants to simulate large-scale networks of spiking neurons. He or she still needs to use the Hodgkin-Huxley-type conductance-based models to study the behavior of one neuron or a small network of neurons. The parameter values that match firing patterns of biological neurons presented in this chapter are only educated guesses (the same is true for conductance-based models). More experiments are needed to reveal the true spike generation mechanism of any particular neuron. An additional insight into the question, "which model is more realistic?" is in Fig.1.8.

Looking at the simple model, one gets an impression that the spike generation mechanism of RS neurons is the simplest in the neocortex. This is probably true; however, the complexity of the RS neurons, most of which are pyramidal cells, is hidden in their extensive dendritic trees having voltage- and $Ca^{2+}$-gated currents. Dendritic dynamics is a subject for a 500-page book by itself, and we purposely omitted it. An interested reader is recommended to study *Dendrites* by Stuart et al. (1999), recent reviews by Hausser and Mel (2003) and Williams and Stuart (2003), and the seminal paper by Arshavsky et al. (1971; Russian language edition, 1969).

# Exercises

1. (Integrate-and-fire network) The simplest implementation of a pulse-coupled integrate-and-fire neural network has the form

$$\dot{v}_i = b_i - v_i + \sum_{j \neq i} c_{ij}\delta(t - t_j) \, ,$$

   where $t_j$ is the moment of firing of the $j$th neuron, that is, the moment $v_j(t_j) = 1$. Thus, whenever the $j$th neuron fires, the membrane potentials of the other neurons are instantaneously adjusted by $c_{ij}, \ i \neq j$. Show that the same initial conditions may result in different solutions, depending on the implementation details.

2. (Latham et al. 2000) Determine the relationship between the normal form for saddle-node bifurcation (6.2) and the equation

$$\dot{V} = a(V - V_{\text{rest}})(V - V_{\text{thresh}}) \, .$$

3. Show that the period of oscillations in the quadratic integrate-and-fire model (8.2) is

$$T = \frac{1}{\sqrt{b}} \left( \text{atan} \frac{v_{\text{peak}}}{\sqrt{b}} - \text{atan} \frac{v_{\text{reset}}}{\sqrt{b}} \right)$$

   when $b > 0$.

4. Show that the period of oscillations in the quadratic integrate-and-fire model (8.2) with $v_{\text{peak}} = 1$ is

$$T = \frac{1}{2\sqrt{|b|}} \left( \ln \frac{1 - \sqrt{|b|}}{1 + \sqrt{|b|}} - \ln \frac{v_{\text{reset}} - \sqrt{|b|}}{v_{\text{reset}} + \sqrt{|b|}} \right)$$

   when $b < 0$ and $v_{\text{reset}} > \sqrt{|b|}$.

5. Justify the bifurcation diagram in Fig.8.3.

6. Brizzi et al. (2004) have shown that shunting inhibition of cat motoneurons raises the firing threshold, and the rheobase current, and shifts the F-I curve to the right without changing the shape of the curve. Use the quadratic integrate-and-fire model to explain the effect. (Hint: Consider $\dot{v} = b - gv + v^2$ with $g \geq 0$, $v_{\text{reset}} = -\infty$, and $v_{\text{peak}} = +\infty$.)

7. (Theta neuron) Determine when the quadratic integrate-and-fire neuron (8.2) is equivalent to the theta neuron

$$\dot{\vartheta} = (1 - \cos \vartheta) + (1 + \cos \vartheta)r \,, \tag{8.8}$$

where $r$ is the bifurcation parameter and $\vartheta \in [-\pi, \pi]$ is a phase variable on the unit circle.

8. (Another theta neuron) Show that the quadratic integrate-and-fire neuron (8.2) is equivalent to

$$\dot{\vartheta} = \vartheta^2 + (1 - |\vartheta|)^2 r \,.$$

where $\vartheta \in [-1, 1]$ and $r$ have the same meaning as in exercise 7. Are there any other "theta-neurons"?

9. When is the linear version of (8.3, 8.4),

$$
\begin{aligned}
\dot{v} &= I - v - u & \text{if } v = 1, \text{ then} \\
\dot{u} &= a(bv - u) & v \leftarrow 0, \ u \leftarrow u + d,
\end{aligned}
$$

equivalent to the integrate-and-fire or resonate-and-fire model?

10. Show that the simple model (8.3, 8.4) with $b < 0$ is equivalent to the quadratic integrate-and-fire neuron with a passive dendritic compartment.

11. All membrane potential responses in Fig.8.8 were obtained using model (8.3, 8.4) with appropriate values of the parameters. Use MATLAB to experiment with the model and reproduce the figure.

12. Simulate the FS spiking neuron in Fig.8.27, using the simple model (8.5, 8.6) with linear equation for $u$. What can you say about its possible bifurcation structure?

13. Fit the recordings of the RS neuron in Fig.8.12, using the model

$$
\begin{aligned}
C\dot{v} &= I - g(v - v_{\mathrm{r}}) + p(v - v_{\mathrm{t}})_+^2 - u & \text{if } v = v_{\mathrm{peak}}, \text{ then} \\
\dot{u} &= a(b(v - v_{\mathrm{r}}) - u) & v \leftarrow c, \ u \leftarrow u + d,
\end{aligned}
$$

where $x_+ = x$ when $x > 0$ and $x_+ = 0$ when otherwise. This model better fits the upstroke of the action potential.

14. Explore numerically the model (8.3, 8.4) with a nonlinear after-spike reset $v \leftarrow f(u), u \leftarrow g(u)$, where $f$ and $g$ are some functions.

15. [M.S.] Analyze the generalization of the system (8.3, 8.4)

$$
\begin{aligned}
\dot{v} &= I + v^2 + evu - u & \text{if } v = 1, \text{ then} \\
\dot{u} &= a(bv - u) & v \leftarrow c, \ u \leftarrow u + d
\end{aligned}
$$

where $e$ is another parameter.

16. [**M.S.**] Analyze the generalization of the following system, related to the exponential integrate-and-fire model

$$\dot{v} = I - v + ke^v - u \qquad \text{if } v = 1, \text{ then}$$
$$\dot{u} = a(bv - u) \qquad\qquad v \leftarrow c,\, u \leftarrow u + d$$

where $k$ is another parameter.

17. [**M.S.**] Analyze the system

$$\dot{v} = I - v + kv_+^2 - u \qquad \text{if } v = 1, \text{ then}$$
$$\dot{u} = a(bv - u) \qquad\qquad v \leftarrow c,\, u \leftarrow u + d$$

where $v_+ = v$ when $v > 0$ and $v_+ = 0$ otherwise.

18. [**M.S.**] Find an analytical solution to the system (8.3, 8.4) with time-dependent input $I = I(t)$.

19. [**M.S.**] Determine the complete bifurcation diagram of the system (8.3, 8.4).

# Chapter 9

# Bursting

A burst is two or more spikes followed by a period of quiescence. Neurons can fire single spikes or stereotypical bursts of spikes, depending on the nature of stimulation and the intrinsic neuronal properties. Typically, bursting occurs due to the interplay of fast currents responsible for spiking activity and slow currents that modulate the activity. In this chapter we study this interplay in detail.

To understand the geometry of bursting, it is customary to assume that the fast and slow currents have drastically different time scales. In this case we can dissect a burster, that is, freeze its slow currents and use them as parameters that control the fast spiking subsystem. During bursting, the slow parameters drive the fast subsystem through bifurcations of equilibria and limit cycles. We provide a topological classification of bursters based on these bifurcations, and show that different topological types have different neurocomputational properties.

## 9.1   Electrophysiology

Many spiking neurons can exhibit bursting activity if manipulated, for instance, pharmacologically. In Fig.9.1 we depict a few well-known examples of neurons that burst under natural conditions without any manipulation. Some require an injected DC current to bias the membrane potential, while others do not. One can only be amazed by the diversity of bursting patterns and time scales. In this chapter we consider electrophysiological and bifurcation mechanisms responsible for the generation of these patterns.

Is a zebra a black animal with white stripes or a white animal with black stripes? This seemingly silly question is pertinent to every bursting pattern: Does bursting activity correspond to an infinite period of quiescence interrupted by groups of spikes, or does it correspond to an infinite spike train interrupted by short periods of quiescence? Biologists are mostly concerned with the question of what makes the neuron fire the first spike in a burst and what keeps it in the spiking regime afterward. The question of why the spiking stops is often forgotten. It turns out that to fully understand the ionic mechanism of bursting, we need to concentrate on the second question, that is, we

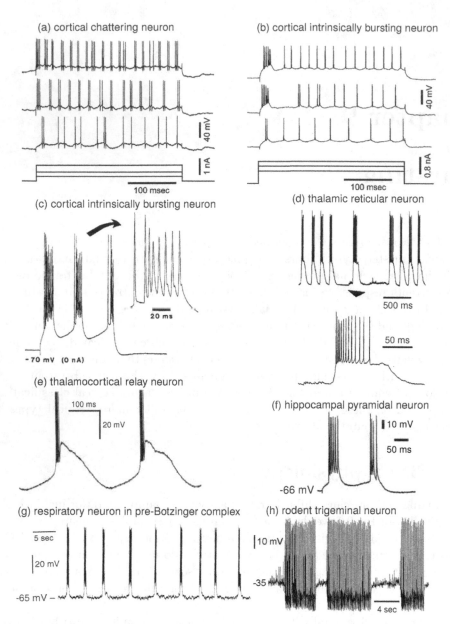

Figure 9.1: Examples of intrinsic bursters. (a) and (b) cat primary visual cortical neurons (modified from Nowak et al. 2003). (c) cortical neuron in anesthetized cat (modified from Timofeev et al. 2000). (d) thalamic reticular (RE) neuron (modified from Steriade 2003). (e) Cat thalamocortical relay neuron (modified from McCormick and Pape 1990). (f) CA1 pyramidal neuron exhibiting grade II low-threshold bursting pattern (modified from Su et al. 2001). (g) respiratory neuron in the pre-Botzinger complex (modified from Butera et al. 1999). (h) Trigeminal interneuron from rat brainstem (modified from Del Negro et al. 1998).

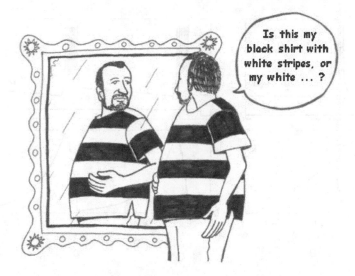

Figure 9.2: Is bursting a spiking state interrupted by periods of quiescence, or is it a quiescent state interrupted by groups of spikes?

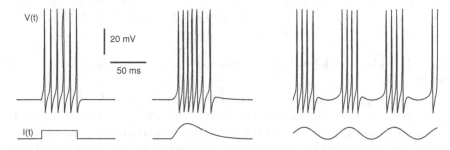

Figure 9.3: Forced bursting in the $I_{\mathrm{Na,p}}+I_{\mathrm{K}}$-model with parameters as in Fig.4.1a and time-dependent injected current $I(t)$.

need to treat bursting as an infinite spike train that is chopped into short bursts by a slow (resonant) current that builds up during the spiking phase and recovers during the quiescent phase. Before proceeding to a general case, let us consider a simple example.

### 9.1.1   Example: The $I_{\mathrm{Na,p}}+I_{\mathrm{K}}+I_{\mathrm{K(M)}}$-Model

Any model neuron capable of spiking can also burst, as, for instance, the $I_{\mathrm{Na,p}}+I_{\mathrm{K}}$-model in Fig.9.3. However, this example is not interesting because the neuron is forced to burst by the time-dependent input $I(t)$.

In contrast, a modification of the $I_{\mathrm{Na,p}}+I_{\mathrm{K}}$-model in Fig.9.4 fires a burst of spikes in response to a brief pulse of current. The first spike in the burst is caused by the stimulation, whereas the subsequent spikes are generated autonomously due to the intrinsic properties of the neuron, and they outlast the stimulation. Such a burst is

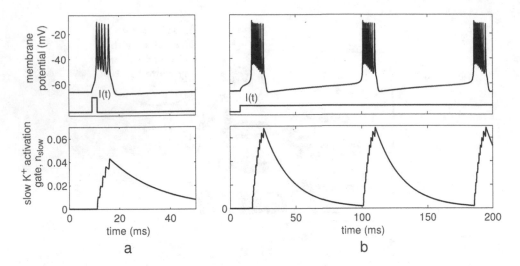

Figure 9.4: Intrinsic bursting in the $I_{\text{Na,p}}+I_K+I_{K(M)}$-model (7.1), consisting of the $I_{\text{Na,p}}+I_K$-model with parameters as in Fig.4.1a, and a fast $K^+$ current ($g_K = 9, \tau(V) = 0.152$) and a slow $K^+$ current with $g_{\text{slow}} = 5$, $V_{1/2} = -20$ mV, $k = 5$ mV, and $\tau_{\text{slow}}(V) = 20$ ms. (a) Burst excitability when $I = 0$. (b) Periodic bursting when $I = 5$.

stereotypical and fairly independent of the amplitude or the duration of the pulse that triggered it.

To make the $I_{\text{Na,p}}+I_K$-model burst, we took parameters as in Fig.6.7a, so that there is a coexistence of the resting and spiking states. The brief pulse of current excites the neuron, that is, moves its state into the attraction domain of the spiking limit cycle and initiates periodic activity. Without any other modification, the model will produce an infinite spike train. To stop the train, we added a slower high-threshold persistent $K^+$ current similar to $I_{K(M)}$ that provides a negative feedback. This M-current is not activated at rest. However, during the active (spiking) phase, the current slowly activates, as indicated by the slow buildup of its gating variable $n_{\text{slow}}$ in the figure. The neuron becomes less and less excitable, and eventually cannot sustain spiking activity. If, instead of a pulse of current, a constant current is applied, the neuron can burst periodically, as in Fig.9.4b.

This model presents only one of many possible examples of bursters, which we study in this chapter. However, it illustrates a number of important issues common to all bursters. For instance, in contrast to the forced bursting in Fig.9.3, this bursting is *intrinsic* or *autonomous*. This stereotypical bursting pattern results from the intrinsic voltage-sensitive currents, and not from a time-dependent input. The behavior in Fig.9.4a is called *burst excitability* to emphasize that the model is an excitable system, with the exception that superthreshold stimulation elicits a burst of spikes instead of a single spike. Hippocampal pyramidal neurons that are "grade III bursters", depicted in Fig.8.34Eb, exhibit burst excitability.

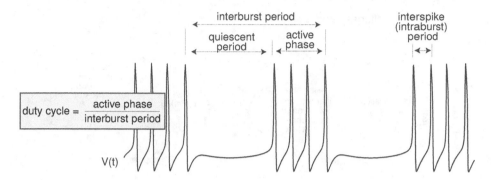

Figure 9.5: Basic characteristics of bursting dynamics.

Biologists sometimes refer to the bursting in Fig.9.4b as *conditional*, because repetitive bursting occurs when a certain condition is satisfied, for instance, positive $I$ is injected. From a mathematical point of view, every burster is conditional, since it exists for some values of the parameters but not for others.

## 9.1.2 Fast-Slow Dynamics

In general, every bursting pattern consists of oscillations with two time scales: a fast spiking oscillation within a single burst (*intra*burst oscillation, or spiking), and one modulated by a slow oscillation between the bursts (*inter*burst oscillation); see Fig.9.5. Typically, though not necessarily (see exercises at the end of this chapter), two time scales result from two interacting processes involving fast and slow currents. For example, the spiking in Fig.9.4 is generated by the fast $I_{Na,p}+I_K$-subsystem and modulated by the slow $I_{K(M)}$-subsystem.

There are two questions associated with each bursting pattern:

- What *initiates* sustained spiking during the burst?

- What *terminates* sustained spiking (temporarily) and ends the burst?

The answer to the first question is relatively simple. Repetitive spiking is initiated and sustained by the positive injected current $I$ or some other source of persistent inward current that causes the neuron to fire (most biologists are interested in identifying this source, and they would not consider this question trivial). Surprisingly, the second question is the more important for building a model of bursting. While the neuron fires, relatively slow processes somehow make it non-excitable and eventually terminate the firing. Such slow processes result in a slow buildup of an outward current or in a slow decrease of an inward current needed to sustain the spiking. During the quiescent phase, the neuron slowly recovers and regains the ability to generate action potentials.

Let us discuss possible ionic mechanisms responsible for the termination of spiking within a burst. Suppose we are given a neuronal model that is capable of sustained

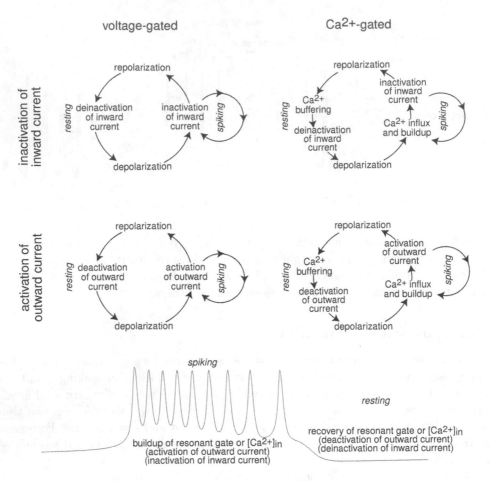

Figure 9.6: Four major classes of bursting models are defined by the slow resonant gating variables that modulate spiking activity.

spiking activity, at least when a positive $I$ is injected. To transform an infinite spike train into a finite burst of spikes, it suffices to add a slow *resonant* current or gating variable (see section 5.1.1) that modulates the spiking via a slow negative feedback. The resonant gating variable can describe inactivation of an inward current or activation of an outward current, either voltage- or $Ca^{2+}$-dependent (see Fig.5.17). Hence, there are four major classes of bursting models, summarized in Fig.9.6:

- *Voltage-gated inactivation of an inward current*, e.g., slow inactivation of a persistent $Na^+$ current or inactivation of a $Ca^{2+}$ transient T-current, or inactivation of the h-current (most biologists refer to this as activation of the h-current by hyperpolarization). Repetitive spiking slowly inactivates (turns off) the inward current, and makes the neuron less excitable and unable to sustain spiking activity. After a while, the spiking stops and the membrane potential repolarizes. The inward current slowly de-inactivates (turns on) and depolarizes the membrane potential, possibly resulting in a new burst.

- *Voltage-gated activation of an outward current*, e.g., slow activation of a persistent $K^+$ current, such as the M-current. Repetitive spiking slowly activates the outward current, which eventually terminates the spiking activity. While at rest, the outward current slowly deactivates (turns off) and unmasks inward currents that can depolarize the membrane potential, possibly initiating another burst.

- $Ca^{2+}$-*gated inactivation of an inward current*, e.g., slow inactivation of high-threshold $Ca^{2+}$-currents $I_{Ca(L)}$ or $I_{Ca(N)}$. Entry of calcium during repetitive spiking leads to its intracellular accumulation and slow inactivation of $Ca^{2+}$-channels that provide an inward current needed for repetitive spiking. As a result, the neuron cannot sustain spiking activity, and becomes quiescent. During this period, intracellular $Ca^{2+}$ ions are removed, $Ca^{2+}$ channels are de-inactivated, and the neuron is primed to start a new burst.

- $Ca^{2+}$-*gated activation of an outward current*, e.g., slow activation of the $Ca^{2+}$-dependent $K^+$-current $I_{AHP}$. Calcium entry and buildup during repetitive spiking slowly activate the outward current and make the neuron less and less excitable. When the spiking stops, intracellular $Ca^{2+}$ ions are removed, the $Ca^{2+}$-gated outward current deactivates (turns off), and the neuron is no longer hyperpolarized and is ready to fire a new burst of spikes.

In addition, the slow process may include $Na^+$-, $K^+$-, or $Cl^-$-gated currents, such as the "slack and slick" family of $Na^+$-gated $K^+$ currents, or slow change of ionic concentrations in the vicinity of the cell membrane (the Hodgkin-Frankenhaeuser layer), which leads to slow change of the Nernst potential for ionic species. We do not elaborate these cases in this book.

Note that in some cases, the slow process modulates fast currents responsible for spiking, while in other cases it produces an independent slow current that impedes spiking. In any case, the slow process is directly responsible for the termination of continuous spiking, and indirectly responsible for its initiation and maintenance.

The four mechanisms in Fig.9.6 and their combinations are ubiquitous in neurons, as we summarize in Fig.9.7. However, there could be other, less obvious bursting mechanisms. In exercises 8–10 we provide examples of bursters having slowly activating persistent inward current, such as $I_{Na,p}$. These surprising examples show that buildup of the inward current (or any other amplifying gate) can also be responsible for the termination of the active phase and for the repolarization of the membrane potential. To understand these mechanisms, one needs to study the geometry of bursting.

| neuron | slow dynamics | | | | references |
|---|---|---|---|---|---|
| | voltage-gated | | Ca$^{2+}$-gated | | |
| | activation of outward | inactivation of inward | activation of outward | inactivation of inward | |
| neocortical chattering neurons | $I_{K(M)}$ $I_{Kslow}$ | | | | Wang (1999) |
| pre-Botzinger complex (respiratory rhythm) | $I_{Kslow}$ | $I_{Naslow}$ | | | Butera et al. (1999) |
| thalamic relay neurons | | $I_{Ca(T)}$ $I_h$ | | | Huguenard and McCormick (1992) |
| thalamic reticular neurons | | $I_{Ca(T)}$ | | | Destexhe et al. (1994) |
| hippocampal CA3 neurons | | | $I_{AHP}$ | | Traub et al. (1991) |
| subiculum bursting neurons | | | $I_{AHP}$ | | Stanford et al. (1998) |
| midbrain dopaminergic neurons | | | $I_{K(Ca)}$ | $I_{Ca(L)}$ | Amini et al. (1999) |
| anterior bursting (AB) neuron in lobster stomatogastric ganglion | | | $I_{K(Ca)}$ | $I_{Ca(L)}$ | Harris-Warrick and Flamm (1987) |
| Aplysia abdominal ganglion R15 neuron | | | | $I_{Ca(L)}$ | Canavier et al. (1991) |

Figure 9.7: Slow dynamics in bursting neurons.

## 9.1.3 Minimal Models

Let us follow the ideas presented in section 5.1 and determine minimal models for bursting. That is, we are interested in classification of all fast-slow electrophysiological models that can exhibit sustained bursting activity, as in Fig.9.4b, at least for some values of parameters. A bursting model is *minimal* if removal of any current or gating variable eliminates the ability to burst.

One way to build a fast-slow minimal model for bursting is to take a minimal model for spiking, which consists of an amplifying gate and a resonant gate (see Fig.5.17) and add another slow resonant gate. Since there are many minimal spiking models in Fig.5.17 and four choices of slow resonant gates in Fig.9.6, there are quite a few combinations, which fill the squares in Fig.9.8. We present only a few reasonable models in the figure; the reader is asked to fill in the blanks. Completing the table is an excellent test of one's knowledge and understanding of how different currents interact to produce nontrivial firing patterns.

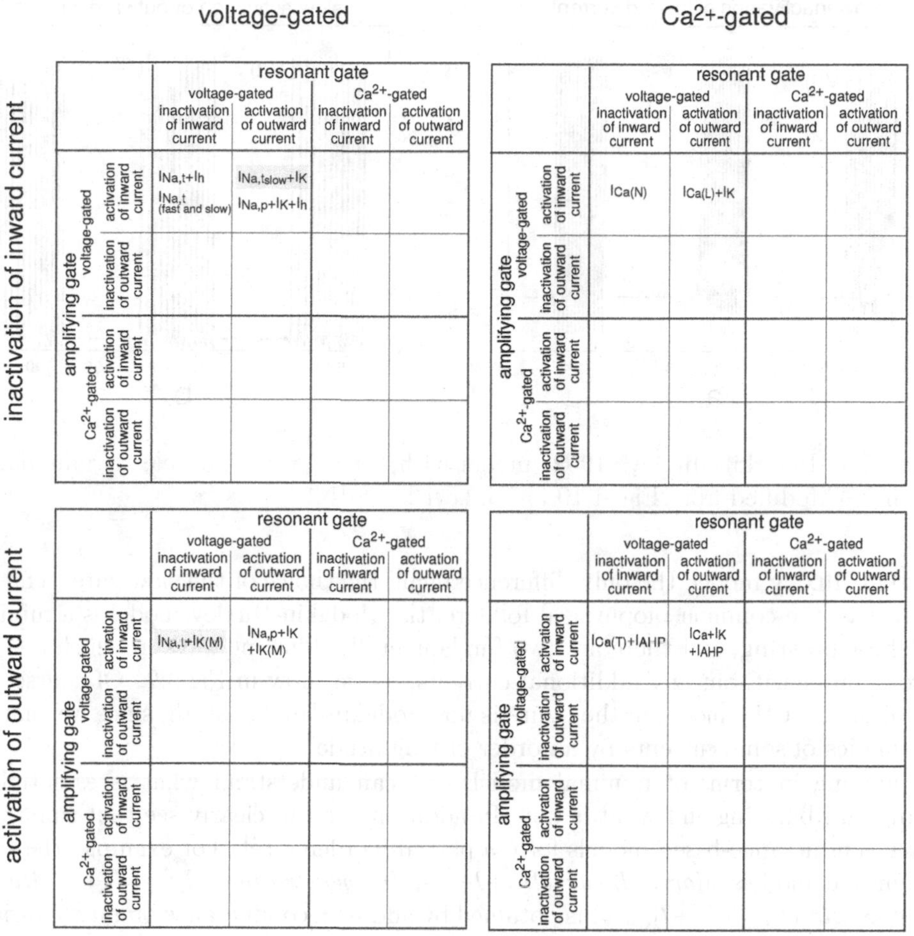

voltage-gated        Ca$^{2+}$-gated

**inactivation of inward current**

*Top-left panel (voltage-gated column):*

| | resonant gate | | | |
| | voltage-gated | | Ca$^{2+}$-gated | |
| | inactivation of inward current | activation of outward current | inactivation of inward current | activation of outward current |
|---|---|---|---|---|
| **amplifying gate** — voltage-gated — activation of inward current | $I_{Na,t}+I_h$; $I_{Na,t}$ (fast and slow) | $I_{Na,tslow}+I_K$; $I_{Na,p}+I_K+I_h$ | | |
| voltage-gated — inactivation of outward current | | | | |
| Ca$^{2+}$-gated — activation of inward current | | | | |
| Ca$^{2+}$-gated — inactivation of outward current | | | | |

*Top-right panel (Ca$^{2+}$-gated column):*

| | resonant gate | | | |
| | voltage-gated | | Ca$^{2+}$-gated | |
| | inactivation of inward current | activation of outward current | inactivation of inward current | activation of outward current |
|---|---|---|---|---|
| **amplifying gate** — voltage-gated — activation of inward current | $I_{Ca(N)}$ | $I_{Ca(L)}+I_K$ | | |
| voltage-gated — inactivation of outward current | | | | |
| Ca$^{2+}$-gated — activation of inward current | | | | |
| Ca$^{2+}$-gated — inactivation of outward current | | | | |

**activation of outward current**

*Bottom-left panel (voltage-gated column):*

| | resonant gate | | | |
| | voltage-gated | | Ca$^{2+}$-gated | |
| | inactivation of inward current | activation of outward current | inactivation of inward current | activation of outward current |
|---|---|---|---|---|
| **amplifying gate** — voltage-gated — activation of inward current | $I_{Na,t}+I_{K(M)}$ | $I_{Na,p}+I_K+I_{K(M)}$ | | |
| voltage-gated — inactivation of outward current | | | | |
| Ca$^{2+}$-gated — activation of inward current | | | | |
| Ca$^{2+}$-gated — inactivation of outward current | | | | |

*Bottom-right panel (Ca$^{2+}$-gated column):*

| | resonant gate | | | |
| | voltage-gated | | Ca$^{2+}$-gated | |
| | inactivation of inward current | activation of outward current | inactivation of inward current | activation of outward current |
|---|---|---|---|---|
| **amplifying gate** — voltage-gated — activation of inward current | $I_{Ca(T)}+I_{AHP}$ | $I_{Ca}+I_K+I_{AHP}$ | | |
| voltage-gated — inactivation of outward current | | | | |
| Ca$^{2+}$-gated — activation of inward current | | | | |
| Ca$^{2+}$-gated — inactivation of outward current | | | | |

Figure 9.8: Some minimal models for bursting.

Some of the minimal models for bursting might seem too bizarre at first glance. Yet Fig.9.8, upon completion, might prove to be a valuable tool that could allow experimenters to formulate various ionic hypotheses. For example, if one uses pharmacological agents (e.g., TEA or Ba$^{2+}$) to block Ca$^{2+}$-gated K$^+$ channels and shows that bursting persists, then the possible electrophysiological mechanisms of bursting are confined to the left column in Fig.9.8. Minimal models in this column would provide testable hypotheses for the ionic basis of bursting, and they could guide novel experiments. If a block abolishes bursting, we cannot conclude that the blocked current drives the bursting – it may merely be necessary for providing background stimulation.

Note that the $I_{Na,t_{slow}} + I_K$-model and the $I_{Na,t} + I_{K(M)}$-model in the figure (see the shaded rectangles) consist of the same gating variables: Na$^+$ activation gate $m$, inactivation gate $h$, and K$^+$ activation gate $n$. Both models are equivalent to the

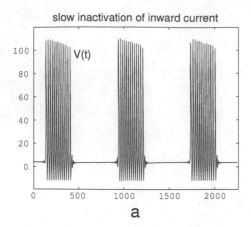
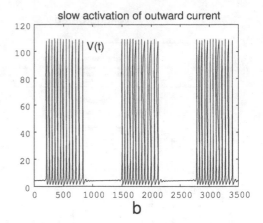

Figure 9.9: Hodgkin-Huxley (1952) model with three gating variables is minimal for bursting. (Modified from Fig. 1.10 in Izhikevich 2001b.)

Hodgkin-Huxley model, the only difference being the choice of the slow gate. Thus, in contrast to the common biophysical folklore, the Hodgkin-Huxley model is a minimal model for bursting, and there are two fundamentally different ways in which one can make it burst without any additional currents, as we show in Fig.9.9. Of course, one may argue that the model in the figure is not Hodgkin-Huxley at all, since we changed the kinetics of some currents by an order of magnitude.

Thinking in terms of minimal models, we can understand what is essential for spiking and bursting and what is not. In addition, we can clearly see that some well-known conductance-based models form a partially ordered set. For example, the chain of neuronal models *Morris-Lecar* ($I_{Ca}+I_K$) ≺ *Hodgkin-Huxley* ($I_{Na,t}+I_K$) ≺ *Butera-Rinzel-Smith* ($I_{Na,t}+I_K+I_{K,slow}$) is obtained by adding a conductance or gating variable to one model to get the next one. Here, $A \prec B$ means $A$ is a subsystem of $B$.

Understanding the ionic bases of bursting is an important step in analysis of bursting dynamics. However, such an understanding may not provide sufficient information on why the bursting pattern looks as it does, what the neurocomputational properties of the neuron are, and how they depend on the parameters of the system. Indeed, we showed in chapter 5 that spiking models based on quite different ionic mechanisms can have identical dynamics and vice versa. This is true for bursting models as well.

## 9.1.4   Central Pattern Generators and Half-Center Oscillators

Bursting can also appear in small circuits of coupled spiking neurons, such as the two mutually inhibitory oscillators in Fig.9.10, called half-center oscillators. While one cell fires, the other is inhibited; then they switch roles; and so on. Such small circuits, suggested by Brown (1911), are the building blocks of central pattern generators in the pyloric network of the lobster stomatogastric ganglion, the medicinal leech heartbeat,

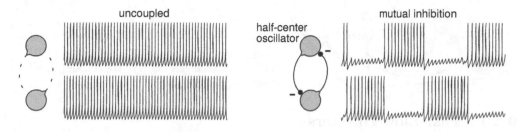

Figure 9.10: Central pattern generation by mutually inhibitory oscillators.

fictive motor patterns, and the swimming patterns of many vertebrates and inverte-brates (Marder and Bucher 2001). We show later that this bursting is of cycle-cycle type.

What makes the oscillators in Fig.9.10 alternate? Wang and Rinzel (1992) suggested two mechanisms, *release* and *escape*, which were later refined to *intrinsic* and *synaptic* by Skinner et al. (1994):

- *Intrinsic release*: The active cell stops spiking, terminates inhibition, and allows the inhibited cell to fire.

- *Intrinsic escape*: The inhibited cell recovers, starts to fire, and shuts off the active cell.

- *Synaptic release*: The inhibition weakens (e.g., due to spike frequency adaptation or short-term synaptic depression) and allows the inhibited cell to fire.

- *Synaptic escape*: The inhibited cell depolarizes above a certain threshold and starts to inhibit the active cell.

All four mechanisms assume that in addition to fast variables responsible for spiking, there are slow adaptation variables responsible for slowing or termination of spiking, recovery, or synaptic depression. Thus, similar to the minimal models above, the circuit has at least two time scales, that is, it is a fast-slow system.

## 9.2 Geometry

To understand the neurocomputational properties of bursters, we need to study the geometry of their phase portraits. In general, it is quite a difficult task. However, it can be accomplished in the special case of fast-slow dynamics.

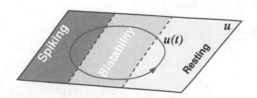

Figure 9.11: Parameter $u$ can control spiking behavior of the fast subsystem in (9.1). When $u$ changes slowly, the model exhibits bursting behavior.

### 9.2.1   Fast-Slow Bursters

We say that a neuron is a *fast-slow burster* if its behavior can be described by a fast-slow system of the form

$$
\begin{aligned}
\dot{x} &= f(x, u) & \text{(fast spiking)}, \\
\dot{u} &= \mu g(x, u) & \text{(slow modulation)}.
\end{aligned} \tag{9.1}
$$

The vector $x \in \mathbb{R}^m$ describes fast variables responsible for spiking. It includes the membrane potential $V$, activation and inactivation gating variables for fast currents, and so on. The vector $u \in \mathbb{R}^k$ describes relatively slow variables that modulate fast spiking (e.g., gating variable of a slow K$^+$ current, an intracellular concentration of Ca$^{2+}$ ions, etc.). The small parameter $\mu$ represents the ratio of time scales between spiking and modulation. When we analyze models, we assume that $\mu \ll 1$; that is, it can be as small as we wish. The results obtained via such an analysis may not have any sense when $\mu$ is of the order 0.1 or greater.

To analyze bursters, we first assume that $\mu = 0$, so that we can consider the fast and slow systems separately. This constitutes the method of *dissection* of neural bursting pioneered by Rinzel (1985). In fact, we have done this many times in the previous chapters when we substituted $m = m_\infty(V)$ into the voltage equation. The fast subsystem can be resting (but excitable), bistable, or spiking, depending on the value of $u$; see Fig.9.11. Bursting occurs when $u$ visits the spiking and quiescent areas periodically. Many important aspects of bursting behavior can be understood via phase portrait analysis of the fast subsystem

$$
\dot{x} = f(x, u), \qquad x \in \mathbb{R}^m,
$$

treating $u \in \mathbb{R}^k$ as a vector of slowly changing bifurcation parameters.

We say that the burster is of the "$m+k$" type when the fast subsystem is $m$-dimensional and the slow subsystem is $k$-dimensional. There are some "1+1" and "2+0" bursters (see exercises 1–4), though they do not correspond to any known neuron. Most of the bursting models in this chapter are of the "2+1" or "2+2" type.

### 9.2.2   Phase Portraits

Since most bursting models are at least of the "2+1" type, their phase space is at least three-dimensional. Analyzing and depicting multidimensional phase portraits is challenging. Even understanding the geometry of the single bursting trajectory depicted in Fig.9.12 is difficult unless one uses a stereoscope.

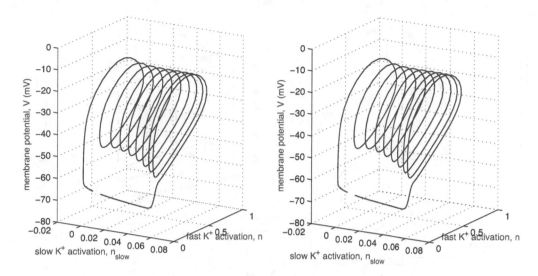

Figure 9.12: Stereoscopic image of a bursting trajectory of the $I_{\text{Na,p}}+I_{\text{K}}+I_{\text{K(M)}}$-model in the three-dimensional phase space $(V, n, n_{\text{slow}})$ (for cross-eye viewing).

In Fig.9.13 we geometrically investigate the $I_{\text{Na,p}}+I_{\text{K}}+I_{\text{K(M)}}$-model, which is a fast-slow burster of the "2+1" type. The naked bursting trajectory is shown in the lower left corner. We set $\mu = 0$ (i.e., $\tau_{\text{slow}}(V) = +\infty$) and slice the three-dimensional space by planes $n_{\text{slow}}$ =const, shown in the top right corner. Phase portraits of the two-dimensional fast subsystem with fixed $n_{\text{slow}}$ are shown in the middle of the figure. Note how the limit cycle attractors and the equilibria of the fast subsystem depend on the value of $n_{\text{slow}}$. Gluing the phase portraits together, we see that there is a manifold of limit cycle attractors (shaded cylinder) that starts when $n_{\text{slow}} < 0$ and ends in a saddle homoclinic orbit bifurcation when $n_{\text{slow}} = 0.066$. There is also a locus of stable and unstable equilibria that appears via a saddle-node bifurcation when $n_{\text{slow}} = 0.0033$.

Once we understand the transitions from one phase portrait to another as the slow variable changes, we can understand the geometry of the burster. Suppose $\mu > 0$ (i.e., $\tau_{\text{slow}}(V) = 20$ ms), so that $n_{\text{slow}}$ can evolve according to its gating equation.

Let us start with the membrane potential at the stable equilibrium corresponding to the resting state. The parameters of the $I_{\text{Na,p}}+I_{\text{K}}+I_{\text{K(M)}}$-model (see caption of Fig.9.4) are such that the slow K$^+$ M-current deactivates at rest, that is, $n_{\text{slow}}$ slowly decreases, and the bursting trajectory slides along the bold half-parabola corresponding to the locus of stable equilibria. After a while, the K$^+$ current becomes so small that it cannot hold the membrane potential at rest. This happens when $n_{\text{slow}}$ passes the value 0.0033, the stable equilibrium coalesces with an unstable equilibrium (saddle), and they annihilate each other via saddle-node bifurcation. Since the resting state no longer exists (see the phase portrait at the top left of Fig.9.13), the trajectory jumps up to the stable limit cycle corresponding to repetitive spiking. This jumping corresponds to the transition from resting to spiking behavior.

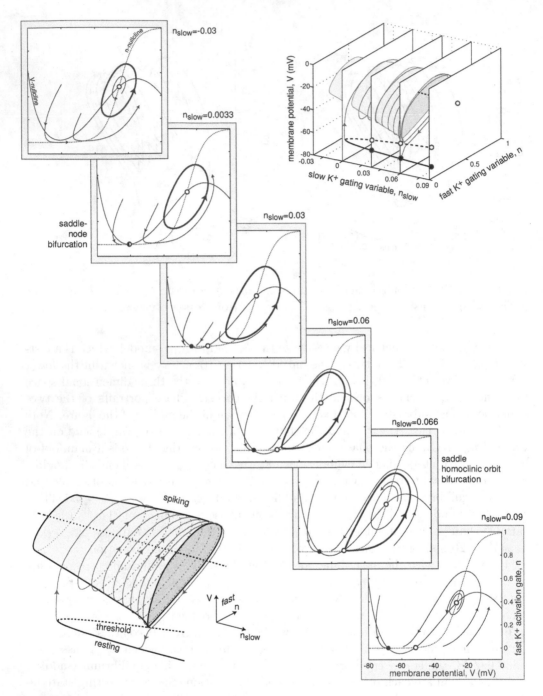

Figure 9.13: Bursting trajectory of the $I_{\mathrm{Na,p}}+I_{\mathrm{K}}+I_{\mathrm{K(M)}}$-model in three-dimensional phase space and its slices $n_{\mathrm{slow}} = \mathrm{const}$.

While the fast subsystem fires spikes, the K$^+$ M-current slowly activates, that is, $n_{\text{slow}}$ slowly increases. The bursting trajectory winds up around the cylinder corresponding to the manifold of limit cycles. Each rotation corresponds to firing a spike. After the ninth spike in the figure, the K$^+$ current becomes so large that repetitive spiking cannot be sustained. This happens when $n_{\text{slow}}$ passes the value 0.066, the limit cycle becomes a homoclinic orbit to a saddle, and then disappears. The bursting trajectory jumps down to the stable equilibrium corresponding to the resting state. This jumping corresponds to the termination of the active phase of bursting and transition to resting. While at rest, the K$^+$ current deactivates, $n_{\text{slow}}$ decreases, and so on.

Figure 9.13 presents the inner structure of the geometrical mechanism of bursting of the $I_{\text{Na,p}}+I_{\text{K}}+I_{\text{K(M)}}$-model with parameters as in Fig.9.4. Other values of the parameters can result in different geometrical mechanisms, summarized in section 9.3. In all cases, our approach is the same: freeze the slow subsystem by setting $\mu = 0$; analyze phase portraits of the fast subsystem, treating the slow variable as a bifurcation parameter; glue the phase portraits; let $\mu \neq 0$ but small; and see how the evolution of the slow subsystem switches the fast subsystem between spiking and resting states. The method usually breaks down if $\mu$ is not small enough, because evolution of the "slow" variable starts to interfere with that of the fast variable. How small is *small* depends on the particulars of the equations describing bursting activity. One should worry when $\mu$ is greater than 0.1.

### 9.2.3   Averaging

What governs the evolution of the slow variable $u$? To study this question, we describe a well-known and widely used method that reduces the fast-slow system (9.1) to its slow component. In fact, we have already used this method in chapters 3 and 4 to reduce the dimension of neuronal models via the substitution $m = m_\infty(V)$. Using essentially the same ideas, we take advantage of the two time scales in (9.1) and get rid of the fast subsystem by means of the substitution $x = x(u)$.

When the neuron is resting, its membrane potential is at an equilibrium and all fast gating variables are at their steady-state values, so that $x = x_{\text{rest}}(u)$. Using this function in the slow equation in (9.1), we obtain

$$\dot{u} = \mu g(x_{\text{rest}}(u), u) \qquad \text{(reduced slow subsystem)}, \qquad (9.2)$$

which easily can be studied using the geometrical methods presented in Chapters 3 and 4.

Let us illustrate all the steps involved using the $I_{\text{Na,p}}+I_{\text{K}}+I_{\text{K(M)}}$-model, with $n_{\text{slow}}$ being the gating variable of the slow K$^+$ M-current. First, we freeze the slow subsystem, that is, set $\tau_{\text{slow}}(V) = \infty$ so that $\mu = 1/\tau_{\text{slow}} = 0$, and numerically determine the resting potential $V_{\text{rest}}$ as a function of the slow variable $n_{\text{slow}}$. The function $V = V_{\text{rest}}(n_{\text{slow}})$ is depicted in Fig.9.14 (top) and it coincides with the solid half-parabola in Fig.9.13. Then, we use this function in the gating equation for the M-current to obtain (9.2)

$$\dot{n}_{\text{slow}} = (n_{\infty,\text{slow}}(V_{\text{rest}}(n_{\text{slow}})) - n_{\text{slow}})/\tau_{\text{slow}}(V_{\text{rest}}(n_{\text{slow}})) = \bar{g}(n_{\text{slow}}),$$

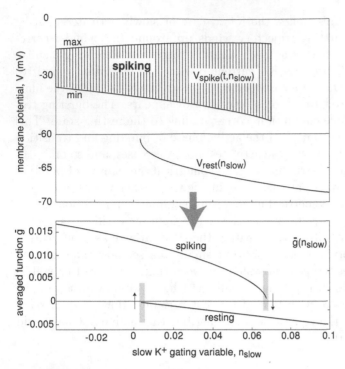

Figure 9.14: Spiking solutions $V(t) = V_{\text{spike}}(t, u_{\text{slow}})$, resting membrane potential $V = V_{\text{rest}}(n_{\text{slow}})$, and the reduced slow subsystem $\dot{n}_{\text{slow}} = \bar{g}(n_{\text{slow}})$ of the $I_{\text{Na,p}} + I_{\text{K}} + I_{\text{K(M)}}$-model. The reduction is not valid in the shaded regions.

depicted in Fig.9.14 (bottom). Note that $\bar{g} < 0$, meaning that $n_{\text{slow}}$ decreases while the fast subsystem rests. The rate of decrease is fairly small when $n_{\text{slow}} \approx 0$.

A similar method of reduction, with an extra step, can be used when the fast subsystem fires spikes. Let $x(t) = x_{\text{spike}}(t, u)$ be a periodic function corresponding to an infinite spike train of the fast subsystem when $u$ is frozen. Slices of this function are shown in Fig.9.14 (top). Let $T(u)$ be the period of spiking oscillation. The periodically forced slow subsystem

$$\dot{u} = \mu g(x_{\text{spike}}(t, u), u) \qquad \text{(slow subsystem)} \tag{9.3}$$

can be averaged and reduced to a simpler model,

$$\dot{w} = \mu \bar{g}(w) \qquad \text{(averaged slow subsystem)}, \tag{9.4}$$

by a near-identity change of variables $w = u + o(\mu)$, where $o(\mu)$ denotes small terms of order $\mu$ or less. Here,

$$\bar{g}(w) = \frac{1}{T(w)} \int_0^{T(w)} g(x_{\text{spike}}(t, w), w)\, dt$$

is the average of $g$, shown in Fig.9.14 (bottom), for the $I_{\text{Na,p}} + I_{\text{K}} + I_{\text{K(M)}}$-model. (The reader should check that $\bar{g}(w) = g(x_{\text{rest}}(w), w)$ when the fast subsystem is resting.)

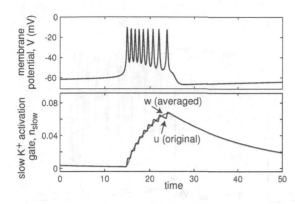

Figure 9.15: The $I_{\mathrm{Na,p}}+I_{\mathrm{K}}+I_{\mathrm{K(M)}}$-model burster with original and averaged slow variable.

Limit cycles of the averaged slow subsystem correspond to bursting dynamics, whereas equilibria correspond to either resting or periodic spiking states of the full system (9.1) – the result is known as the Pontryagin–Rodygin (1960) theorem. Interesting regimes correspond to the coexistence of limit cycles and equilibria of the slow averaged system.

The main purpose of averaging consists in replacing the wiggle trajectory of $u(t)$ with a smooth trajectory of $w(t)$, as we illustrate in Fig.9.15. We purposely used a different letter, $w$, for the new slow variable to stress that (9.4) is not equivalent to (9.3). Their solutions are $o(\mu)$-close to each other only when certain conditions are satisfied; see Guckenheimer and Holmes (1983) or Hoppensteadt and Izhikevich (1997). In particular, this straightforward averaging breaks down when $u$ slowly passes the bifurcation values. For example, the period, $T(u)$, of $x_{\mathrm{spike}}(t, u)$ may go to infinity, as happens near saddle-node on invariant circle and saddle homoclinic orbit bifurcations, or transients may take as long as $1/\mu$, or the averaged system (9.4) is not smooth. All these cases are encountered in bursting models. Thus, one can use the reduced slow subsystem only when the fast subsystem is sufficiently far from a bifurcation, that is, away from the shaded regions in Fig.9.14.

### 9.2.4 Equivalent Voltage

Let us consider a "2+1" burster with a slow subsystem depending only on the slow variable and the membrane potential $V$, as in the $I_{\mathrm{Na,p}}+I_{\mathrm{K}}+I_{\mathrm{K(M)}}$-model. The nonlinear equation

$$g(V, u) = \bar{g}(u) \tag{9.5}$$

can be solved for $V$. The solution, $V = V_{\mathrm{equiv}}(u)$, is referred to as the *equivalent voltage* (Kepler et al. 1992; Bertram et al. 1995) because it replaces the periodic function $x_{\mathrm{spike}}(t, u)$ in (9.3) with an "equivalent" value of the membrane potential, so that the reduced slow subsystem (9.3) has the same form,

$$\dot{u} = \mu g(V_{\mathrm{equiv}}(u), u) \qquad \text{(slow subsystem)}, \tag{9.6}$$

as in (9.1). (The reader should check that $V_{\mathrm{equiv}}(u) = V_{\mathrm{rest}}(u)$ when the fast subsystem is resting.) An interesting mathematical possibility occurs when $V_{\mathrm{equiv}}$ during spiking

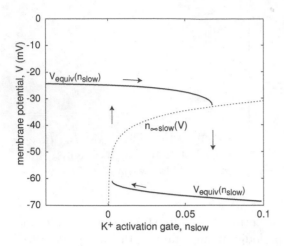
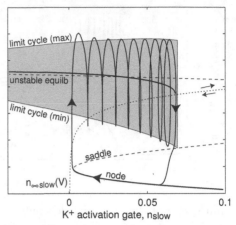

Figure 9.16: Projection of bursting trajectory of the $I_{\text{Na,p}}+I_{\text{K}}+I_{\text{K(M)}}$-model onto the $(n_{\text{slow}}, V)$ plane.

is below $V_{\text{rest}}$, leading to bizarre bursters having amplifying slow currents, such as the one in exercise 10.

We depict the equivalent voltage of the $I_{\text{Na,p}}+I_{\text{K}}+I_{\text{K(M)}}$-model in Fig. 9.16 (left) (variable $u$ corresponds to $n_{\text{slow}}$). In the same figure we depict the steady-state activation function $n = n_{\infty,\text{slow}}(V)$ (notice the flipped coordinate system). We interpret the two curves as fast and slow nullclines of the reduced $(V, n_{\text{slow}})$ system. During the active (spiking) phase of bursting, the reduced system slides along the upper branch of $V_{\text{equiv}}(n_{\text{slow}})$ to the right. When it reaches the end of the branch, it falls downward to the lower branch corresponding to resting, and slides along this branch to the left. When it reaches the left end of the lower branch, it jumps to the upper branch, and thereby closes the hysteresis loop. Figure 9.16 (right) summarizes all the information needed to understand the transitions between resting and spiking states in this model. It depicts the bursting trajectory, loci of equilibria of the fast subsystem, and the voltage range of the spiking limit cycle as a function of the slow gate $n_{\text{slow}}$. With some experience, one can read this complicated figure and visualize the three-dimensional geometry underlying bursting dynamics.

## 9.2.5 Hysteresis Loops and Slow Waves

Sustained bursting activity of the fast-slow system (9.1) corresponds to periodic (or chaotic) activity of the reduced slow subsystem (9.6). Depending on the dimension of $u$, that is, on the number of slow variables, there could be two fundamentally different ways the slow subsystem oscillates.

If the slow variable $u$ is one-dimensional, then there must be a bistability of resting and spiking states of the fast subsystem so that $u$ oscillates via a hysteresis loop. That is, the reduced equation (9.6) consists of two parts: one for $V_{\text{equiv}}(u)$, corresponding

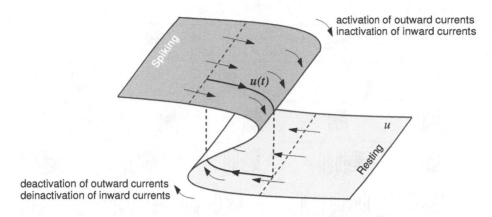

Figure 9.17: Hysteresis loop periodic bursting.

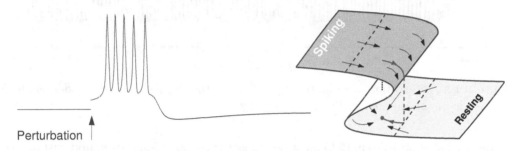

Figure 9.18: Burst excitability: a perturbation causes a burst of spikes.

to spiking, and one for $V_{\text{equiv}}(u)$, corresponding to resting of the fast subsystem, as in Fig.9.16 (left). Such a hysteresis loop bursting can also occur when $u$ is multidimensional, as we illustrate in Fig.9.17. The vector field on the top (spiking) leaf pushes $u$ outside the spiking area, whereas the vector field on the bottom (resting) leaf pushes $u$ outside the resting area. As a result, $u$ visits the spiking and resting areas periodically, and the model exhibits *hysteresis loop* bursting.

If resting $x$ does not push $u$ into the spiking area, but leaves it in the bistable area, then the neuron exhibits *burst excitability*. It has quiescent excitable dynamics, but its response to perturbations is not a single spike, rather, it is a burst of spikes, as we illustrate in Fig.9.18. Grade III bursters of the hippocampus (Fig.8.34Eb) produce such a response, often called a *complex spike* response, to brief stimuli. In general, many bistable models are bistable only because they neglect slow currents and other homeostatic processes present in real neurons. If the currents are taken into account, then the models become bistable on a short time scale and burst excitable on a longer time scale. This justifies why many researchers refer to bistable systems as excitable, implicitly assuming that the response to superthreshold perturbations is either a single spike or a long train of spikes.

If the fast subsystem does not have a coexistence of resting and spiking states, then

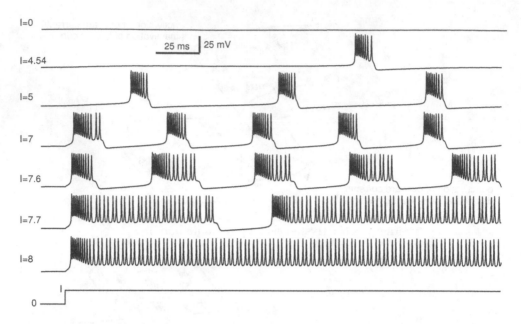

Figure 9.19: Bifurcations of bursting solutions in the $I_{Na,p}+I_K+I_{K(M)}$-model as the magnitude of the injected DC current $I$ changes.

the reduced slow subsystem (9.6) must be at least two-dimensional to exhibit sustained autonomous oscillation (however, see exercise 6). Such an oscillation produces a depolarization wave that drives the fast subsystem to spiking and back, as in Fig.9.3. We refer to such bursters as *slow-wave* bursters. Quite often, however, the slow subsystem of a slow-wave burster needs the feedback from the fast subsystem to oscillate. For example, in section 9.3.2 we consider slow-wave bursting in the $I_{Na,p}+I_K+I_{Na,slow} + I_{K(M)}$-model, whose slow subsystem consists of two uncoupled equations, and hence cannot oscillate by itself unless the fast subsystem is present.

## 9.2.6 Bifurcations "Resting ↔ Bursting ↔ Tonic Spiking"

Switching between spiking and resting states during bursting occurs because the slow variable drives the fast subsystem through bifurcations of equilibria and limit cycle attractors. These bifurcations play an important role in the classification of bursters and in understanding their neurocomputational properties. We discuss them in detail in section 9.3.

Since the fast subsystem goes through bifurcations, *does this mean that the entire system (9.1) undergoes bifurcations during bursting?* The answer is NO. As long as parameters of (9.1) are fixed, the system as a whole does not undergo any bifurcations, no matter how small $\mu$ is. The system can exhibit periodic, quasi-periodic, or even chaotic bursting activity, but its $(m + k)$-dimensional phase portrait does not change.

The only way to make system (9.1) undergo a bifurcation is to change its parameters. For example, in Fig.9.19 we change the magnitude of the injected DC current $I$ in the $I_{Na,p}+I_K+I_{K(M)}$-model. Apparently, no bursting exists when $I = 0$. Then, repetitive bursting appears with a large interburst period that decreases as $I$ increases. The value $I = 5$ was used to obtain bursting solutions in Fig.9.12 and Fig.9.13. Increasing $I$ further increases the duration of each burst, until it becomes infinite, that is, bursting turns into tonic spiking. When $I > 8$, the slow $K^+$ current is not enough to stop spiking.

In Fig.9.20 we depict the geometry of bursting in the $I_{Na,p}+I_K+I_{K(M)}$-model when $I = 3$ (just before periodic bursting appears) and when $I = 10$ (just after bursting turns into tonic spiking).

When $I = 3$, the nullcline of the slow subsystem $n_{slow} = n_{\infty,slow}(V)$ intersects the locus of stable equilibria of the fast subsystem. The intersection point is a globally stable equilibrium of the full system (9.1). Small perturbations, whether in the $V$ direction, the $n$ direction, or the $n_{slow}$ direction, subside, whereas a large perturbation (e.g., in the $V$ direction) that moves the membrane potential to the open square in the figure initiates a transient (phasic) burst of seven spikes. Increasing the magnitude of the injected current $I$ shifts the saddle-node parabola to the right. When $I \approx 4.54$, the nullcline of the slow subsystem does not intersect the locus of stable equilibria, and the resting state no longer exists, as in Fig.9.16 (right). There is still a global steady state, but it is not stable.

Further increase of the magnitude of the injected current $I$ results in the intersection of the nullcline of the slow subsystem with the equivalent voltage function $V_{equiv}(n_{slow})$. The intersection, marked by the black circle in Fig.9.20 (right), corresponds to a globally stable (spiking) limit cycle of the full system (9.1). A sufficiently strong perturbation can push the state of the fast subsystem into the attraction domain of the stable (resting) equilibrium. While the fast subsystem is resting, the slow variable decreases (i.e., the $K^+$ current deactivates), the resting equilibrium disappears, and repetitive spiking resumes.

Figures 9.19 and 9.20 illustrate possible transitions between bursting and resting, and bursting and tonic spiking. There could be other routes of emergence of bursting solutions from resting or spiking; some of them are in Fig.9.21. Each such route corresponds to a bifurcation in the full system (9.1) with some $\mu > 0$. For example, the case $a \to 0$ corresponds to supercritical Andronov-Hopf bifurcation; the case $c \to \infty$ corresponds to a saddle-node on invariant circle or saddle homoclinic orbit bifurcation; the case $d \to \infty$ corresponds to a periodic orbit with a homoclinic structure, e.g., blue-sky catastrophe, fold limit cycle on homoclinic torus bifurcation, or something more complicated. The transitions bursting $\leftrightarrow$ spiking often exhibit chaotic (irregular) activity, so Fig.9.21 is probably a great oversimplification. Understanding and classifying all possible bifurcations leading to bursting dynamics is an important but open problem; see exercise 27.

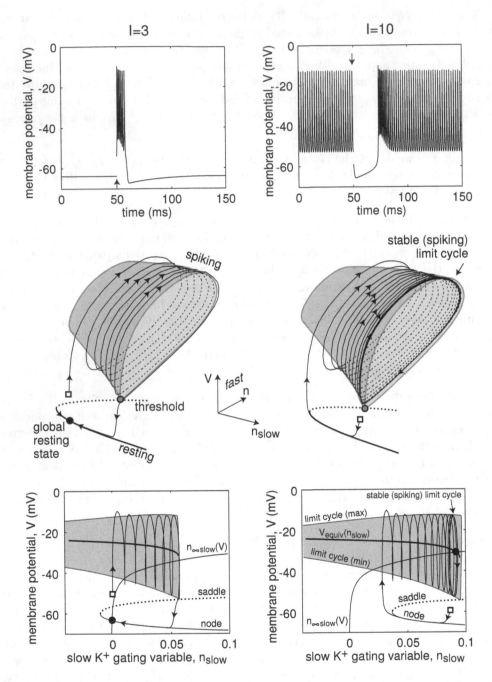

Figure 9.20: Burst excitability ($I = 3$, left) and periodic spiking ($I = 10$, right) in the $I_{Na,p}+I_K+I_{K(M)}$-model.

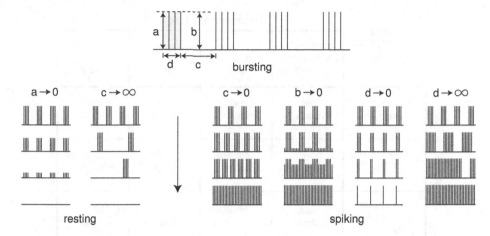

Figure 9.21: Possible transitions between repetitive bursting and resting, and repetitive bursting and repetitive spiking.

## 9.3 Classification

In Fig.9.22 we identify two important bifurcations of the fast subsystem that are associated with bursting activity in the fast-slow burster (9.1):

- *(resting → spiking)*. Bifurcation of an equilibrium attractor that results in transition from resting to repetitive spiking.

- *(spiking → resting)*. Bifurcation of the limit cycle attractor that results in transition from spiking to resting.

The ionic basis of bursting, that is, the fine electrophysiological details, determines the kinds of bifurcations in Fig.9.22. The bifurcations, in turn, determine the neurocomputational properties of fast-slow bursters, discussed in section 9.4.

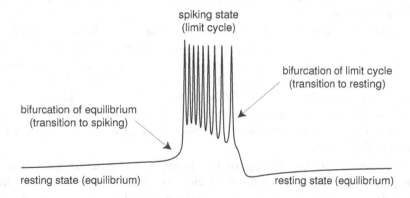

Figure 9.22: Two important bifurcations associated with fast-slow bursting.

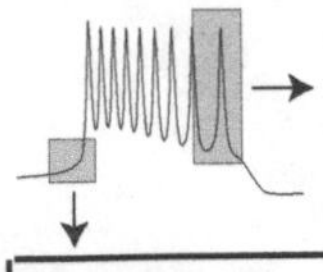

bifurcations of limit cycles

| | saddle-node on invariant **circle** | saddle **homoclinic** orbit | supercritical Andronov-**Hopf** | **fold** limit **cycle** |
|---|---|---|---|---|
| saddle-node **(fold)** | fold/ circle | fold/ homoclinic | fold/ Hopf | fold/ fold cycle |
| saddle-node on invariant **circle** | circle/ circle | circle/ homoclinic | circle/ Hopf | circle/ fold cycle |
| supercritical Andronov-**Hopf** | Hopf/ circle | Hopf/ homoclinic | Hopf/ Hopf | Hopf/ fold cycle |
| **sub**critical Andronov-**Hopf** | subHopf/ circle | subHopf/ homoclinic | subHopf/ Hopf | subHopf/ fold cycle |

bifurcations of equilibria

Figure 9.23: Classification of planar point-cycle fast-slow bursters based on the codimension-1 bifurcations of the resting and spiking states of the fast subsystem.

A complete topological classification of bursters based on these two bifurcations is provided by Izhikevich (2000a), who identified 120 different topological types. Here, we consider only 16 planar point-cycle codimension-1 fast-slow bursters. We say that a fast-slow burster is *planar* when its fast subsystem is two-dimensional. We emphasize planar bursters because they have a greater chance of being encountered in computer simulations (but not necessarily in nature). We say that a burster is of the *point-cycle* type when its resting state is a stable equilibrium point and its spiking state is a stable limit cycle. All bursters considered so far, including those in Fig.9.1, are of the point-cycle type. Other, less common types, such as cycle-cycle and point-point, are considered as exercises.

We consider here only bifurcations of codimension 1, that is, those that need only one parameter and hence are more likely to be encountered in nature. Having a two-dimensional fast subsystem imposes severe restrictions on possible codimension-1 bifurcations of the resting and spiking states. In particular, there are only four bifurcations of equilibria and four bifurcations of limit cycles, which we considered in chapter 6 and summarized in figures 6.46 and 6.47. Any combination of them results in a distinct topological type of fast-slow bursting; hence there are $4 \times 4 = 16$ such bursters, summarized in Fig.9.23.

We name the bursters according to the types of the bifurcations of the resting and spiking states. To keep the names short, we refer to saddle-node on invariant circle bifurcation as a "circle" bifurcation because it is the only codimension-1 bifurcation on a circle manifold $\mathbb{S}^1$. We refer to supercritical Andronov-Hopf bifurcation

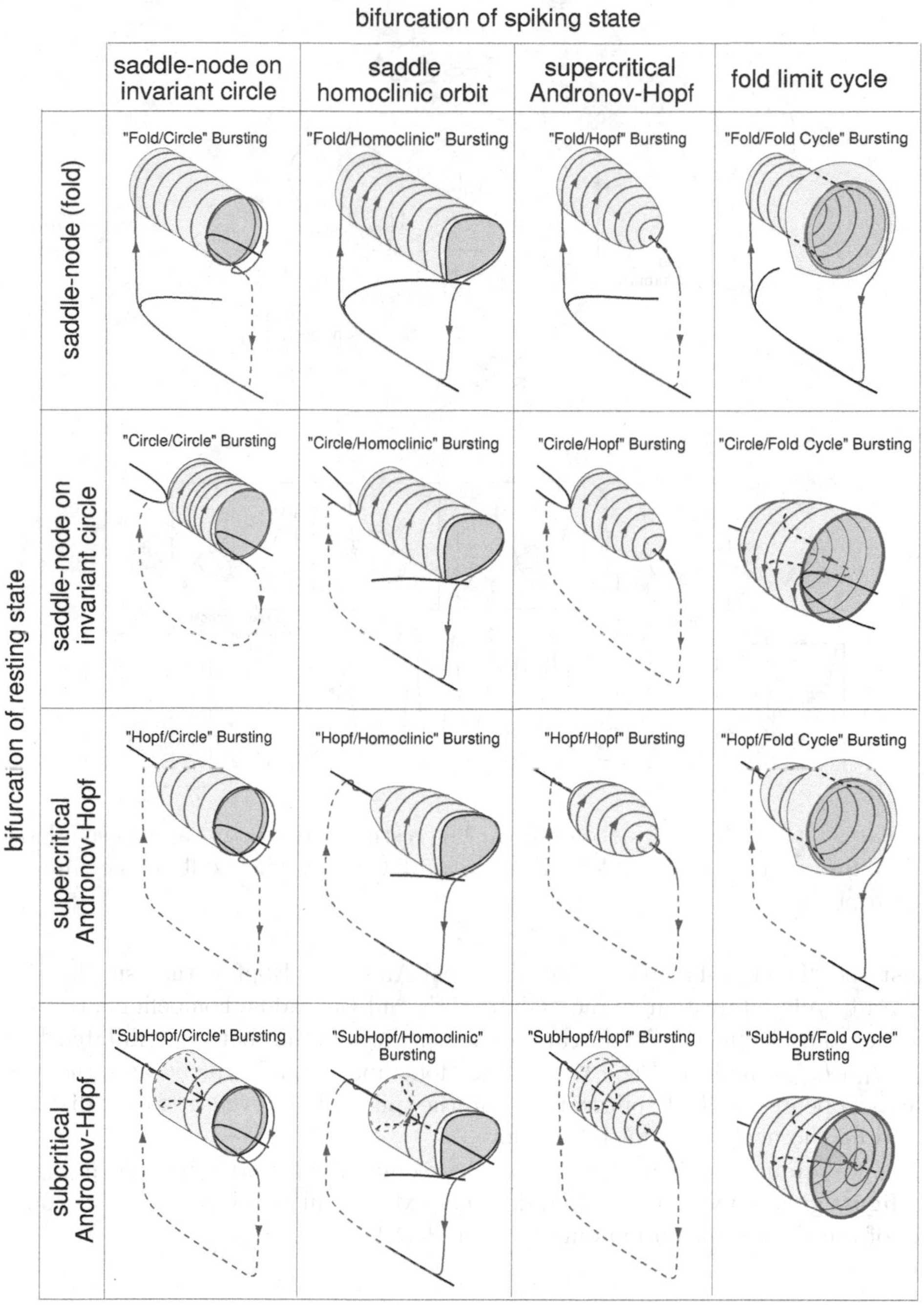

bifurcation of spiking state

Figure 9.24: Examples of "2+1" point-cycle fast-slow codimension-1 bursters of hysteresis-loop type (modified from Izhikevich 2000a). Dashed chains of arrows show transitions that might involve bifurcations not relevant to the bursting type.

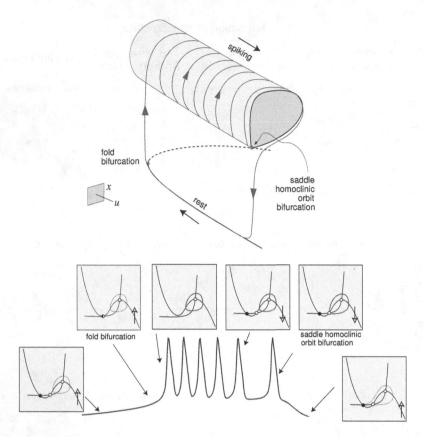

Figure 9.25: "Fold/homoclinic" bursting. The resting state disappears via saddle-node (fold) bifurcation, and the spiking limit cycle disappears via saddle homoclinic orbit bifurcation.

as just the "Hopf" bifurcation, the subcritical Andronov-Hopf as the "subHopf", the fold limit cycle bifurcation as the "fold cycle", and the saddle homoclinic orbit bifurcation as the "homoclinic" bifurcation. Thus, the bursting pattern exhibited by the $I_{\text{Na,p}}+I_{\text{K}}+I_{\text{K(M)}}$-model in Fig.9.13 is of the "fold/homoclinic" type because the resting state disappears via "fold" bifurcation, and the spiking limit cycle attractor disappears via saddle "homoclinic" orbit bifurcation.

In a way similar to Fig.9.13, we depict the geometry of the other bursters in Fig.9.24. This figure gives only examples, and does not exhaust all possibilities. Let us consider some of the most common bursting types in detail.

## 9.3.1   Fold/Homoclinic

When the resting state disappears via a saddle-node (fold) bifurcation and the spiking limit cycle disappears via a saddle homoclinic orbit bifurcation, the burster is said to

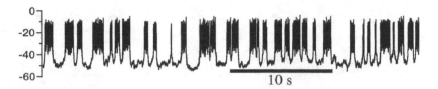

Figure 9.26: Putative "fold/homoclinic" bursting in a pancreatic $\beta$-cell. (Modified from Kinard et al. 1999.)

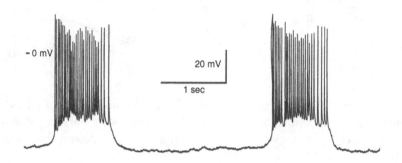

Figure 9.27: Putative "fold/homoclinic" bursting in a cell located in the pre-Botzinger complex of rat brain stem. (Data shared by Christopher A. Del Negro and Jack L. Feldman, Systems Neurobiology Laboratory, Department of Neurobiology, UCLA.)

be of the "fold/homoclinic" type depicted in Fig.9.25. Note the bistability of resting and spiking states, resulting in the hysteresis loop oscillation of the slow subsystem.

"Fold/homoclinic" bursting is quite common in neuronal models, such as in the $I_{Na,p}+I_K+I_{K(M)}$-model considered in this chapter; see Fig.9.13. It was first characterized in the context of the insulin-producing pancreatic $\beta$-cells in Fig.9.26, with intracellular concentration of $Ca^{2+}$ ions being the slow resonant variable (Chay and Keizer 1983). Neurons located in the pre-Botzinger complex, a region that is associated with generating the rhythm for breathing, also exhibit this kind of bursting (Butera et al. 1999), as shown in Fig.9.27. Intrinsic bursting (IB) and chattering (CH) behavior of the simple model in section 8.2 could be of the "fold/homoclinic" type too, provided the parameter $a$ is sufficiently small. Because of the distinct square-wave shape of oscillations of the membrane potential in figures 9.26 and Fig.9.27, this bursting was called "square-wave" bursting in earlier studies. Since many types of bursters resemble square waves, referring to a burster by its shape is misleading and should be avoided.

In Fig.9.25 (bottom) we depict a typical configuration of nullclines of the fast subsystem during "fold/homoclinic" bursting. The resting state of the membrane potential corresponds to the left stable equilibrium, which is the intersection of the left knee of the fast N-shaped nullcline with the slow nullcline. During resting, the N-shape null-

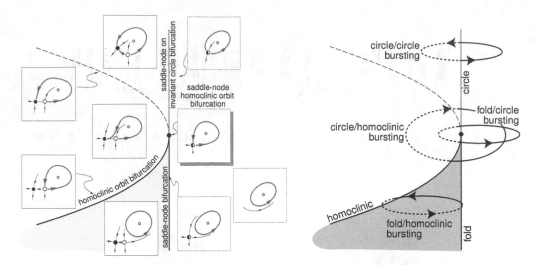

Figure 9.28: A neural system near codimension-2 saddle-node homoclinic orbit bifurcation (center dot) can exhibit four different types of fast-slow bursting, depending on
the trajectory of the slow variable $u \in \mathbb{R}^2$ in the two-dimensional parameter space.
Solid (dotted) lines correspond to spiking (resting) regimes.

cline slowly moves upward, until its knee touches the slow nullcline at a saddle-node
point. Right after this moment, the resting state disappears via saddle-node (fold)
bifurcation; hence the "fold" in the name of the burster. After the fold bifurcation,
the membrane potential jumps up to the stable limit cycle corresponding to repetitive
spiking. During the spiking state, the N-shaped nullcline slowly moves downward, and
the middle (saddle) equilibrium moves away from the resting state toward the limit
cycle. After a while, the limit cycle becomes a homoclinic trajectory to the saddle,
and then the cycle disappears via saddle homoclinic orbit bifurcation; hence the "homoclinic" in the name of the burster. After this bifurcation, the membrane potential
jumps down to the resting state and closes the hysteresis loop.

Suppose that the hysteresis loop oscillation of the slow variable $u$ has a small amplitude. That is, the saddle-node bifurcation and the saddle homoclinic orbit bifurcation
occur for nearby values of the parameter $u$. In this case, the fast subsystem of (9.1) is
near codimension-2 saddle-node homoclinic orbit bifurcation, depicted in Fig.9.28 and
studied in section 6.3.6. The figure shows a two-parameter unfolding of the bifurcation,
treating $u \in \mathbb{R}^2$ as the parameter. A stable equilibrium (resting state) exists in the left
half-plane, and a stable limit cycle (spiking state) exists in the right half-plane of the
figure and in the shaded (bistable) region. "Fold/homoclinic" bursting occurs when
the bifurcation parameter, being a slow variable, oscillates between the resting and
spiking states through the shaded region. Due to the bistability, the parameter could
be one-dimensional. Other trajectories of the slow parameter correspond to other types
of bursting.

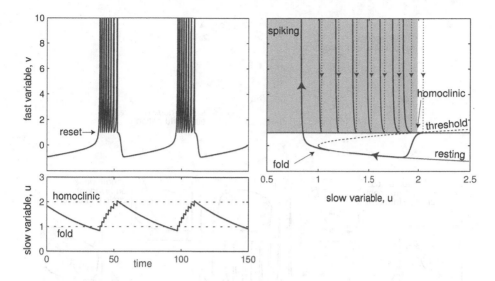

Figure 9.29: "Fold/homoclinic" bursting in the canonical model (9.7) with parameters $\mu = 0.02, I = 1$, and $d = 0.2$.

In exercise 16 we prove that there is a piecewise continuous change of variables that transforms any "fold/homoclinic" burster with a fast subsystem near such a bifurcation into the canonical model (see section 8.1.5)

$$
\begin{aligned}
\dot{v} &= I + v^2 - u \,, \\
\dot{u} &= -\mu u \,,
\end{aligned}
\tag{9.7}
$$

with an after-spike resetting

$$\text{if } v = +\infty, \quad \text{then} \quad v \leftarrow 1 \quad \text{and} \quad u \leftarrow u + d.$$

Here $v \in \mathbb{R}$ is the re-scaled membrane potential of the neuron; $u \in \mathbb{R}$ is the re-scaled net outward (resonant) current that provides a negative feedback to $v$; and $I, d$, and $\mu \ll 1$ are parameters. This model is related to the canonical model considered in section 8.1.4, and it is simplified further in exercise 15.

The fast subsystem $\dot{v} = (I - u) + v^2$ is the normal form for the saddle-node bifurcation, and with the resetting it is known as the quadratic integrate-and-fire neuron (section 3.3.8). When $u > I$, there is a stable equilibrium $v_{\text{rest}} = -\sqrt{u - I}$ corresponding to the resting state. While the parameter $u$ slowly decreases toward $u = 0$, the stable equilibrium and the saddle equilibrium $v_{\text{thresh}} = +\sqrt{u - I}$ approach and annihilate each other at $u = I$ via saddle-node (fold) bifurcation. When $u < I$, the membrane potential $v$ increases and escapes to infinity in a finite time, that is, it fires a spike. (Instead of infinity, any large value can be used in simulations.) The spike activates fast outward currents and resets $v$ to 1, as in Fig.9.29. It also activates slow currents and increments $u$ by $d$. If the reset value 1 is greater than the threshold potential $v_{\text{thresh}}$, the fast subsystem fires another spike, and so on, even when $u > I$; see

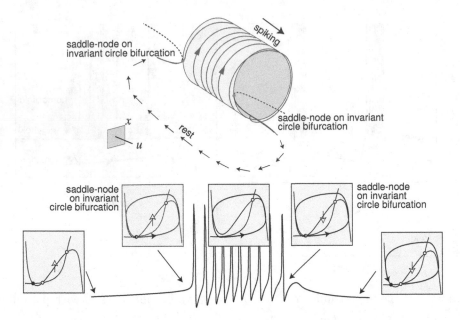

Figure 9.30: "Circle/circle" bursting. The resting state disappears via saddle-node on invariant circle bifurcation, and so does the spiking limit cycle.

Fig.9.29. Since each spike increases $u$, the repetitive spiking stops when $u = I + 1$ via saddle homoclinic orbit bifurcation. The membrane potential jumps downward to the resting state, the hysteresis loop is closed, and the variable $u$ decreases (recovers) to initiate another "fold/homoclinic" burst. One can vary $I$ in the canonical model (9.7) to study transitions from quiescence to bursting to tonic spiking, as in Fig.9.20.

## 9.3.2   Circle/Circle

When the equilibrium corresponding to the resting state disappears via a saddle-node on invariant *circle* bifurcation, and the limit cycle attractor corresponding to the spiking state disappears via another saddle-node on invariant *circle* bifurcation, the burster is said to be of the "circle/circle" type shown in Fig.9.30. Since the bifurcation does not produce a coexistence of attractors, there is usually no hysteresis loop, and the bursting is of the slow-wave type with at least two slow variables. (An unusual example of "circle/circle" hysteresis loop bursting in a "2+1" system is provided by Izhikevich (2000a)).

"Circle/circle" bursting is a prominent feature of the $R_{15}$ cells in the abdominal ganglion of the mollusk *Aplysia*, shown in Fig.9.31 (Plant 1981). It was called "parabolic" bursting in earlier studies because the interspike period depicted in Fig.9.32 was erroneously thought to be a parabola. In section 6.1.2 we showed that when a system undergoes a saddle-node on invariant circle bifurcation, its period scales as $1/\sqrt{\lambda}$, where $\lambda$ is the distance to the bifurcation. Two pieces of this function, put together

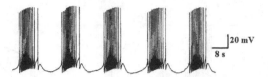

Figure 9.31: Putative "circle/circle" bursting pacemaker activity of neuron $R_{15}$ in the abdominal ganglion of the mollusk *Aplysia*. (Modified from Levitan and Levitan 1988.)

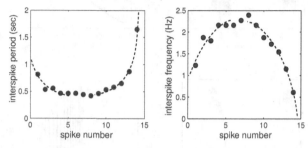

Figure 9.32: The interspike period in the "circle/circle" bursting in Fig.9.31 resembles a parabola, which led to the name "parabolic bursting" used in earlier studies.

as in Fig.9.32, do indeed resemble a parabola. But so does the interspike period of a "circle/homoclinic" burster.

To transform the $I_{Na,p}+I_K$-model to a "circle/circle" burster, take the parameters in Fig.4.1a so that there is a saddle-node on invariant circle bifurcation when $I = 4.51$ (see section 6.1.2). Its nullclines and phase portrait look similar to those in Fig.9.30. Then, add one amplifying and one resonant current with gating variables

$$\dot{m}_{slow} = (m_{\infty,slow}(V) - m_{slow})/\tau_{Na,slow}(V) \quad \text{(slow } I_{Na,slow}),$$
$$\dot{n}_{slow} = (n_{\infty,slow}(V) - n_{slow})/\tau_{K(M)}(V) \quad \text{(slow } I_{K(M)}),$$

having parameters as in Fig.9.33. Note that these equations are uncoupled and hence cannot oscillate by themselves without the feedback from variable $V$.

Let us describe the bursting mechanism in the full $I_{Na,p}+I_K+I_{Na,slow} + I_{K(M)}$-model with $I = 5$. Since $I > 4.51$, the resting state of the fast subsystem does not exist, and the model generates action potentials, depicted in Fig.9.33a. Each spike activates $I_{Na,slow}$, producing even more inward current and, hence, more spikes. This, however, activates a much slower $K^+$ current (see Fig.9.33b) and produces a net outward current that moves the fast nullcline downward and eventually terminates spiking. The transition from spiking to resting occurs via saddle-node on invariant circle bifurcation. While at rest, both currents deactivate and the fast nullcline slowly moves upward. The net inward current, consisting mostly of the injected DC current $I = 5$, drives the fast subsystem via the same saddle-node on invariant circle bifurcation and initiates another burst, as shown in Fig.9.33a.

Using the averaging technique described in section 9.2.3, one can reduce the four-dimensional $I_{Na,p} + I_K + I_{Na,slow} + I_{K(M)}$-model to a simpler, two-dimensional slow

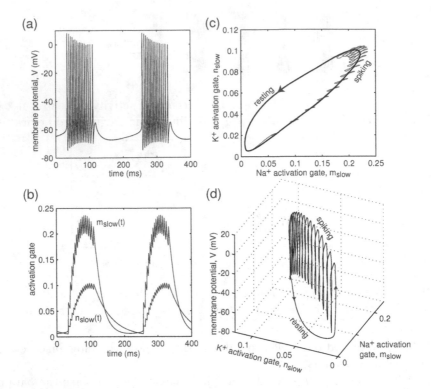

Figure 9.33: "Circle/circle" bursting in the $I_{Na,p}+I_K+I_{Na,slow}+I_{K(M)}$-model. Parameters of the fast $I_{Na,p}+I_K$-subsystem are the same as in Fig.4.1a with $I = 5$. Slow $Na^+$ current has $V_{1/2} = -40$ mV, $k = 5$ mV, $g_{Na,slow} = 3$, $\tau_{Na,slow}(V) = 20$ ms. Slow $K^+$ current has $V_{1/2} = -20$ mV, $k = 5$ mV, $g_{K(M)} = 20$, $\tau_{K(M)}(V) = 50$ ms.

$I_{Na,slow}+I_{K(M)}$-subsystem of the form (9.4). Bursting of the full model corresponds to a limit cycle attractor of the averaged slow subsystem depicted as a bold curve on the $(m_{slow}, n_{slow})$ plane in Fig.9.33c. Superimposed is the projection of the bursting solution of the full system (thin, wobbly curve). In Fig.9.33d we project a four-dimensional bursting trajectory onto the three-dimensional subspace $(V, m_{slow}, n_{slow})$.

The $I_{Na,p}+I_K+I_{Na,slow}+I_{K(M)}$-model in Fig.9.33 has a remarkable property: it generates slow-wave bursts even though its slow $I_{Na,slow} + I_{K(M)}$-subsystem consists of two uncoupled equations, and hence cannot oscillate by itself! Another example of this phenomenon is presented in exercise 12. Thus, the slow wave that drives the fast $I_{Na,p}+I_K$-subsystem through the two circle bifurcations is not autonomous: it needs feedback from $V$. In particular, the oscillation will disappear in a voltage-clamp experiment, that is, when the membrane potential is fixed.

Now consider a "circle/circle" burster with a slow subsystem performing small-amplitude oscillations so that the fast subsystem is always near the saddle-node on invariant circle bifurcation. If the slow subsystem has an autonomous limit cycle at-

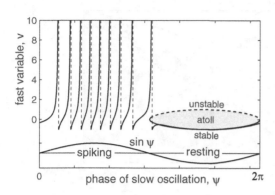

Figure 9.34: "Circle/circle" bursting in the Ermentrout-Kopell canonical model (9.8) with $r(\psi) = \sin\psi$ and $\omega = 0.1$. The fast variable fires spikes while $\sin\psi > 0$ and is quiescent while $\sin\psi < 0$. The shaded atoll is surrounded by the equilibria curves $\pm\sqrt{|\sin\psi|}$. The fast subsystem undergoes saddle-node on invariant circle bifurcation when $\sin\psi = 0$.

tractor that exists without feedback from $V$, then such a burster can be reduced to the Ermentrout-Kopell (1986) canonical model

$$
\begin{aligned}
\dot{v} &= v^2 + r(\psi), &\text{if } v = +\infty, \text{ then } v = -1, &\qquad (9.8)\\
\dot{\psi} &= \omega,
\end{aligned}
$$

which was originally written in the $\vartheta$-form; see exercise 13. Here, $\psi$ is the phase of autonomous oscillation of the slow subsystem, $\omega \approx 0$ is the frequency of the slow oscillation, and $r(\psi)$ is a periodic function that changes sign and slowly drives the fast quadratic integrate-and-fire neuron (9.8) back and forth through the bifurcation, as illustrated in Fig.9.34.

Alternatively, suppose that the slow subsystem cannot have sustained oscillations without the fast subsystem, that is, the slow subsystem has a stable equilibrium if $v$ is fixed. In exercise 17 we prove that there is a piecewise continuous change of variables that transforms any such "circle/circle" burster into one of the two canonical models below, depending on the type of equilibrium. If the equilibrium of the slow subsystem is a stable node, then the canonical model has the form

$$
\begin{aligned}
\dot{v} &= I + v^2 + u_1 - u_2,\\
\dot{u}_1 &= -\mu_1 u_1,\\
\dot{u}_2 &= -\mu_2 u_2.
\end{aligned}
\qquad (9.9)
$$

If the equilibrium of the slow subsystem is a stable focus, then the canonical model has the form

$$
\begin{aligned}
\dot{v} &= I + v^2 + u_1,\\
\dot{u}_1 &= -\mu_1 u_2,\\
\dot{u}_2 &= -\mu_2(u_2 - u_1),
\end{aligned}
\qquad (9.10)
$$

with $\mu_2 < 4\mu_1$. In both cases, there is an after-spike resetting:

$$
\text{if } v = +\infty, \quad \text{then} \quad v \leftarrow -1, \quad \text{and} \quad (u_1, u_2) \leftarrow (u_1, u_2) + (d_1, d_2).
$$

Similar to (9.7), the variable $v \in \mathbb{R}$ is the re-scaled membrane potential of the neuron. The positive feedback variable $u_1 \in \mathbb{R}$ describes activation of slow amplifying currents

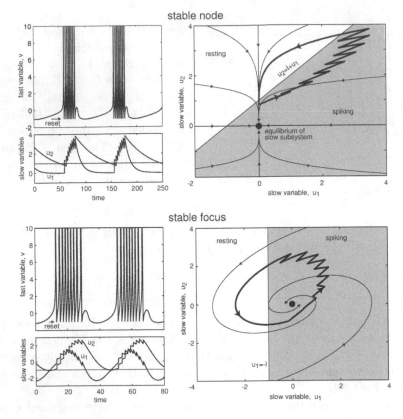

Figure 9.35: "Circle/circle" bursting in the canonical models (9.9) (top, parameters: $I = 1$, $\mu_1 = 0.1$, $\mu_2 = 0.02$, $d_1 = 1$, $d_2 = 0.5$) and (9.10) (bottom, parameters: $I = 1$, $\mu_1 = 0.2$, $\mu_2 = 0.1$, $d_1 = d_2 = 0.5$).

or potential at a dendritic compartment, whereas the negative feedback variable $u_2 \in \mathbb{R}$ describes activation of slow resonant currents. $I, d_1, d_2$, and $\mu_1, \mu_2 \ll 1$ are parameters.

When $\mu_2 > 4\mu_1$, the equilibrium of the slow subsystem in (9.10) is a stable node, so (9.10) can be transformed into (9.9) by a linear change of slow variables. If $d_1 = 0$, then $u_1 \to 0$ and (9.9) is equivalent to (9.7).

Both canonical models above exhibit "circle/circle" slow-wave bursting, as depicted in Fig.9.35. When $I > 0$, the equilibrium of the slow subsystem is in the shaded area corresponding to spiking dynamics of the fast subsystem. When the slow vector $(u_1, u_2)$ enters the shaded area, the fast subsystem fires spikes, prevents the vector from converging to the equilibrium, and eventually pushes it out of the area. While it is outside, the vector follows the curved trajectory of the linear slow subsystem and then reenters the shaded area. Such a slow wave oscillation corresponds to the thick limit cycle attractor in Fig.9.35, which looks remarkably similar to the one for the $I_{\text{Na,p}} + I_{\text{K}} + I_{\text{Na,slow}} + I_{\text{K(M)}}$-model in Fig.9.33.

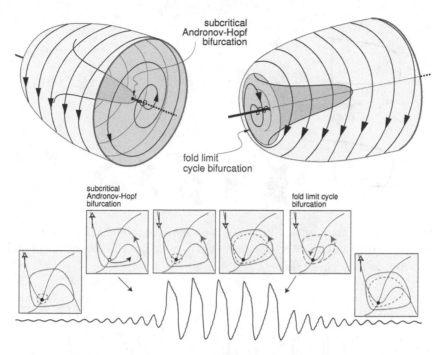

Figure 9.36: "SubHopf/fold cycle" burster: The middle equilibrium corresponding to the resting state loses stability via subcritical Andronov-Hopf bifurcation, and the outer limit cycle attractor corresponding to repetitive spiking disappears via fold limit cycle bifurcation. The two top images are different views of the same 3-D structure.

## 9.3.3   SubHopf/Fold Cycle

When the resting state loses stability via subcritical Andronov-Hopf bifurcation, and the spiking state disappears via fold limit cycle bifurcation, the burster is said to be of the "subHopf/fold cycle" type depicted in Fig.9.36. Because there is a coexistence of resting and spiking states, such bursting usually occurs via a hysteresis loop with only one slow variable.

This kind of bursting was one of the three basic types identified by Rinzel (1987). It was called "elliptic" in earlier studies because the profile of oscillation of the membrane potential resembles an ellipse, or at least a half-ellipse; see Fig.9.37. Rodent trigeminal interneurons in Fig.9.38, and dorsal root ganglia and mesV neurons in Fig.9.39 are "subHopf/fold cycle" bursters, yet the bursting profiles do not look like ellipses. Many models of "subHopf/fold cycle" bursters do not generate elliptic profiles either; hence, referring to this type of bursting by its shape is misleading and should be avoided.

It is quite easy to transform the $I_{\mathrm{Na,p}}+I_{\mathrm{K}}$-model into a "subHopf/fold cycle" burster. First, we chose the parameters of the model as in Fig.6.16, so that the phase portrait depicted in Fig.9.40 is the same as in Fig.9.36 (bottom). The coexistence of the stable equilibrium, an unstable limit cycle, and a stable limit cycle is essential for producing

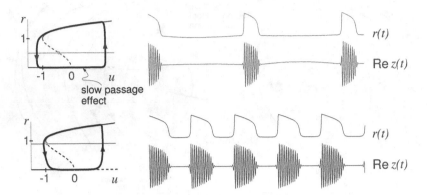

Figure 9.37: Phase portrait and solution of the canonical model (9.11) for $\mu = 0.1$, $\omega = 3$, and $a = 0.25$ (top) and $a = 0.8$ (bottom), where $r = |z|$ is the amplitude of oscillation (modified from Izhikevich 2000b).

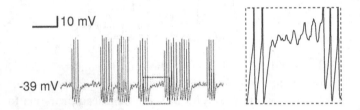

Figure 9.38: Putative "subHopf/fold cycle" bursting in rodent trigeminal neurons. (Modified from Del Negro et al. 1998.)

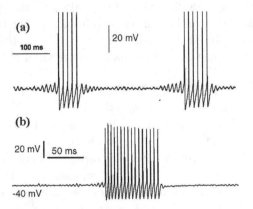

Figure 9.39: Putative "subHopf/fold cycle" bursting in (a) injured dorsal root ganglion (data modified from Jian et al. 2004) and in (b) rat mesencephalic layer 5 neurons.

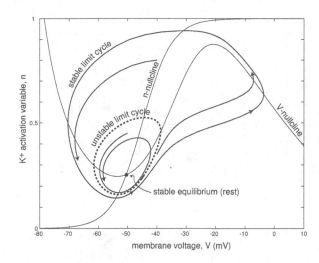

Figure 9.40: Phase portrait of the $I_{\mathrm{Na,p}}+I_{\mathrm{K}}$-model with parameters corresponding to subcritical Andronov-Hopf bifurcation and fold limit cycle bifurcation.

the hysteresis loop oscillation. Then, we add a slow $K^+$ M-current that activates while the fast subsystem fires spikes, and deactivates while it is resting. Such a resonant current provides a negative feedback to the fast subsystem, and the full $I_{\mathrm{Na,p}}+I_{\mathrm{K}}+I_{\mathrm{K(M)}}$-model exhibits "subHopf/fold cycle" bursting, shown in Fig.9.41.

As in the previous examples, the burster in this figure is conditional: it needs an injection of a DC current $I$, so that the equilibrium corresponding to the resting state of the fast subsystem is unstable. If the subsystem is near such an equilibrium, it slowly diverges from the equilibrium and jumps to the large-amplitude limit cycle attractor corresponding to spiking behavior, as one can see in Fig.9.41a. Each spike activates a slow $K^+$ M-current, see Fig.9.41b, and results in the buildup of a net outward current that makes the fast subsystem less and less excitable. Geometrically, the large-amplitude limit cycle attractor is approached by a smaller-amplitude unstable limit cycle; they coalesce, and annihilate each other via fold limit cycle bifurcation at $n_{\mathrm{slow}} \approx 0.14$; see Fig.9.41c. The trajectory jumps to the stable equilibrium corresponding to the resting state. At this moment, the slow $K^+$ current starts to deactivate, and the net outward current decreases. Since the activation gate $n_{\mathrm{slow}}$ moves in the opposite direction, the fold limit cycle bifurcation gives birth to large-amplitude stable and unstable limit cycles, but the trajectory remains on the steady-state branch. The unstable limit cycle slowly shrinks, and makes the resting equilibrium lose stability via subcritical Andronov-Hopf bifurcation. Once the resting state becomes unstable, the trajectory diverges from it and jumps back to the large-amplitude limit cycle, thereby closing the hysteresis loop.

A prominent feature of "subHopf/fold cycle" bursting, as well as any other type of fast-slow bursting involving Andronov-Hopf bifurcation ("subHopf/*" or "Hopf/*", where the wild card "*" means any bifurcation) is that the transition from resting to spiking does not occur at the moment the resting state becomes unstable. The fast subsystem remains at the unstable equilibrium for quite some time before it jumps rather abruptly to a spiking state, as we can clearly see in Fig.9.41. This delayed

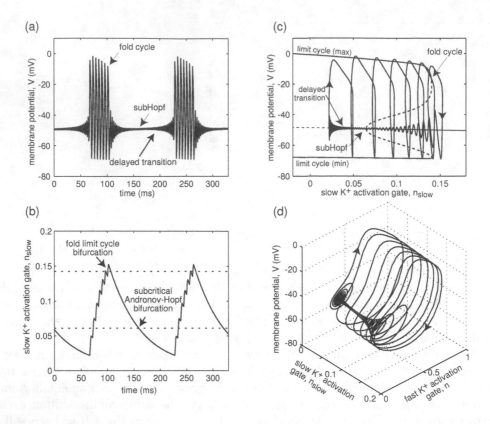

Figure 9.41: "SubHopf/fold cycle" bursting in the $I_{\text{Na,p}}+I_{\text{K}}+I_{\text{K(M)}}$-model. Parameters of the fast $I_{\text{Na,p}}+I_{\text{K}}$-subsystem are the same as in Fig.6.16 with $I = 55$. Slow K$^+$ M-current has $V_{1/2} = -20$ mV, $k = 5$ mV, $\tau(V) = 60$ ms, and $g_{\text{K(M)}} = 1.5$.

transition is due to the slow passage through Andronov-Hopf bifurcation, discussed in section 6.1.4. Delayed transitions through Andronov-Hopf bifurcation are ubiquitous in neuronal models, but they have never been seen in real neurons. Conductance noise, always present at physiological temperatures, constantly kicks the membrane potential away from the stable equilibrium, as one can see in the inset in Fig.9.38, so transition to spiking in real neurons is never delayed. Instead, it can occur even before the equilibrium becomes unstable, as we show in section 6.1.4.

Suppose that the hysteresis loop oscillation of the slow variable has a small amplitude. That is, the subcritical Andronov-Hopf bifurcation and the fold limit cycle bifurcation of the fast subsystem in (9.1) occur for nearby values of the parameter $u$. In this case, the fast subsystem is near a codimension-2 Bautin bifurcation, which was studied in section 6.3.5. Its two-parameter unfolding is depicted in Fig.9.42 (left). "SubHopf/fold cycle" bursting occurs when the bifurcation parameter, being a slow variable, oscillates between the resting and spiking regions through the shaded area.

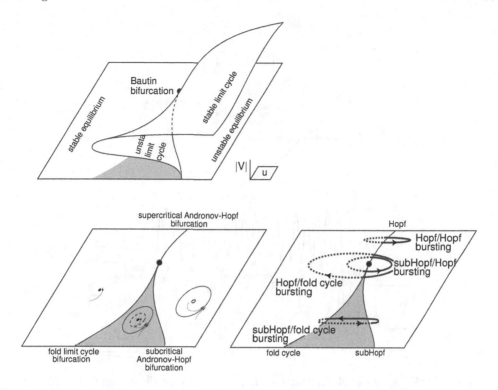

Figure 9.42: A neural system near codimension-2 Bautin bifurcation (central dot) can exhibit four different types of fast-slow bursting, depending on the trajectory of the slow variable $u \in \mathbb{R}^2$ in the parameter space. The "subHopf/fold cycle" bursting occurs via a hysteresis loop and requires only one slow variable. Solid (dotted) lines correspond to spiking (resting) regimes. (Modified from Izhikevich 2000a.)

Due to the bistability, the parameter could be one-dimensional. Other trajectories of the slow parameter correspond to other types of bursting shown in Fig.9.42 (right).

If the slow variable has an equilibrium near the Bautin bifurcation point, then the fast-slow burster (9.1) can be transformed into the following canonical "2+1" model by a continuous change of variables

$$\begin{aligned}
\dot{z} &= (u + i\omega)z + 2z|z|^2 - z|z|^4, \\
\dot{u} &= \mu(a - |z|^2),
\end{aligned} \qquad (9.11)$$

where $z \in \mathbb{C}$ and $u \in \mathbb{R}$ are the canonical fast and slow variables, respectively, and $a, \omega$, and $\mu \ll 1$ are parameters. In exercise 14 we show that the model exhibits the hysteresis loop periodic point-cycle bursting behavior depicted in Fig.9.37 when $0 < a < 1$.

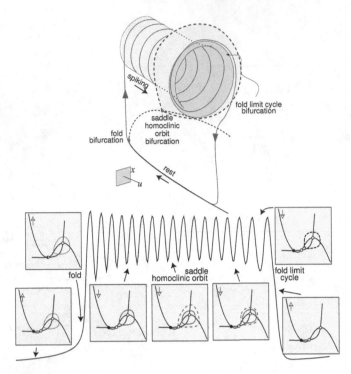

Figure 9.43: "Fold/fold cycle" bursting. The resting state disappears via saddle-node (fold) bifurcation, and the spiking limit cycle disappears via fold limit cycle bifurcation. (Modified from Izhikevich 2000a.)

### 9.3.4   Fold/Fold Cycle

When the stable equilibrium corresponding to the resting state disappears via saddle-node (fold) bifurcation and the limit cycle attractor corresponding to the spiking state disappears via fold limit cycle bifurcation, the burster is said to be of the "fold/fold cycle" type, as in Fig.9.43. This type was first discovered in the Chay-Cook (1988) model of a pancreatic $\beta$-cell by Bertram et al. (1995), who referred to it as being Type IV bursting (the three bursters we have considered so far are referred to as being Types I, II, and III). Since both bifurcations result in a coexistence of resting and spiking states, the "fold/fold cycle" bursting can occur via a hysteresis loop in a "2+1" system.

An interesting geometrical feature of the "fold/fold cycle" bursting is that an unstable limit cycle appears in the middle of a burst and participates in the "fold cycle" bifurcation to terminate the burst. The cycle appears via saddle homoclinic orbit bifurcation in Fig.9.43, but other scenarios are possible. It is a good exercise of one's geometrical intuition and understanding of the fast-slow bursting mechanisms to develop alternative scenarios of the "fold/fold cycle" bursting. For example, consider the case of the unstable limit cycle being inside the stable one.

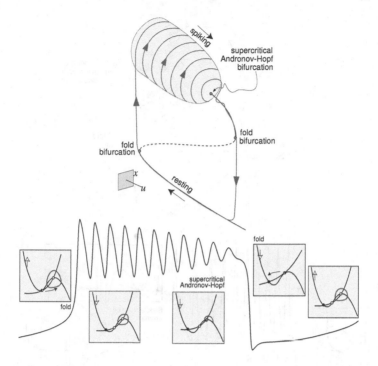

Figure 9.44: "Fold/Hopf" bursting: The resting state disappears via saddle-node (fold) bifurcation, and the spiking limit cycle shrinks to a point via supercritical Andronov-Hopf bifurcation. (Modified from Izhikevich 2000a.)

## 9.3.5 Fold/Hopf

When the stable equilibrium corresponding to the resting state disappears via saddle-node (fold) bifurcation and the limit cycle attractor corresponding to the spiking state shrinks to a point via supercritical Andronov-Hopf bifurcation, the burster is said to be of the "fold/Hopf" type (see Fig.9.44). This type of bursting, called "tapered" in some earlier studies, was found in models of insulin-producing pancreatic $\beta$-cells (Smolen et al. 1993; Pernarowski 1994) and in models of certain enzymatic systems (Holden and Erneux 1993a, 1993b).

As one can see in the figure, the fast subsystem undergoes two bifurcations while in the excited state: One corresponds to the termination of repetitive spiking via supercritical Andronov-Hopf bifurcation, and the other corresponds to the transition from the excited equilibrium to resting equilibrium via saddle-node (fold) bifurcation. The first bifurcation (i.e., bifurcation of a spiking limit cycle attractor) determines the topological type of bursting. The second bifurcation is essential for the "fold/fold" hysteresis loop, and it determines only the subtype of the "fold/Hopf" bursting. Using ideas described in exercise 19, one can come up with another subtype of "fold/Hopf" burster having a "fold/subHopf" hysteresis loop.

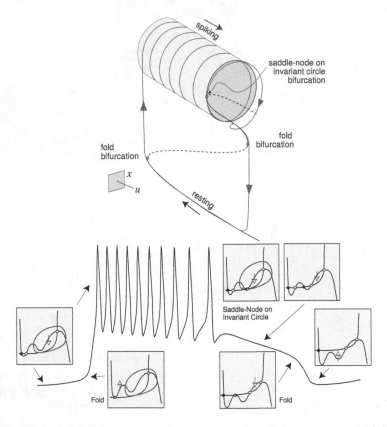

Figure 9.45: "Fold/circle" bursting: The resting state disappears via fold bifurcation and the spiking state disappears via saddle-node on invariant circle bifurcation. (Modified from Izhikevich 2000a.)

## 9.3.6   Fold/Circle

When the stable equilibrium corresponding to the resting state disappears via saddle-node (fold) bifurcation and the limit cycle attractor corresponding to the spiking state disappears via saddle-node on invariant circle bifurcation, the burster is said to be of the "fold/circle" type (see Fig.9.45). This type was first discovered in the model of the thalamocortical relay neuron by Rush and Rinzel (1994), and it was called "triangular" in earlier studies (Wang and Rinzel 1995) because of the shape of the voltage envelope.

As one can see in the figure, the fast subsystem can have five equilibria, two of which are stable nodes. This is a consequence of the quintic shape of the $V$-nullcline of the fast subsystem. While the trajectory is at the lower equilibrium, the $V$-nullcline moves upward, the equilibrium disappears via fold bifurcation, and the fast subsystem starts to fire spikes. During this active period, the $V$-nullcline slowly moves downward, and the spiking limit cycle disappears via saddle-node on invariant circle bifurcation. The fast subsystem, however, is at the second stable equilibrium corresponding to a depolarized state. The slow $V$-nullcline continues to move downward, and this equilibrium disappears via another fold bifurcation, thereby closing the "fold/fold" hysteresis loop. Alternatively, "fold/circle" bursting can be of the slow-wave type, depicted in Fig.9.28 having only three equilibria. The slow subsystem needs to be at least two-dimensional in this case, however.

# 9.4 Neurocomputational Properties

There is more to the topological classification of bursters than just a mathematical exercise. Indeed, in chapter 7 we showed that the neurocomputational properties of an excitable system depend on the type of bifurcation of the resting state. The same is valid for a burster: its neurocomputational properties depend on the kinds of bifurcations of the resting and spiking states, that is, on the burster's type. Knowing the topological type of a given bursting neuron, we know what the neuron can do - and, more importantly, what it cannot do – regardless of the model that describes its dynamics.

## 9.4.1 How to Distinguish?

First, we stress that the topological classification of bursters provided in the previous section is defined for mathematical models, and not for real neurons. Moreover, the types are defined for models of the fast-slow form (9.1) assuming that the ratio of time scales, $\mu$, is sufficiently small. Not all neurons can be described adequately by such models, so extending the classification to those neurons may be worthless. A typical example of classification failure is the model of bursting of the sensory processing neuron in weakly electric fish, known as the "ghostburster" (Doiron et al. 2002), in which $\mu > 0.1$.

If a bursting neuron can be described accurately by a model having a fast-slow form (9.1), then there is no problem in determining its topological type – just freeze the slow subsystem, that is, set $\mu = 0$, and find bifurcations of the fast subsystem treating $u$ as a parameter. Software packages such as XPPAUT, AUTO, and MATLAB-based MATCONT, are helpful in bifurcation analyses of such systems.

What if a neuron has an apparent fast-slow dynamics but its model is not known at present? To determine the types of bifurcations of the fast subsystem, we first use noninvasive observations: presence or absence of fast subthreshold oscillations, changes in intraburst (interspike) frequency, changes in spike amplitudes, and so on. Each piece of information excludes some bifurcations and narrows the set of possible types of bursting. Then, we can use invasive methods, e.g., small perturbations, to test the coexistence of resting and spiking states, and narrow the choice of bifurcations further. With some luck, we can exclude enough bifurcations and determine exactly the type of bursting without knowing the details of the mathematical model that describes it.

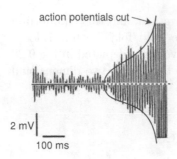

Figure 9.46: The conductance noise destabilizes the focus equilibrium in a mesencephalic V neuron before subcritical Andronov-Hopf bifurcation takes place, thereby giving an impression of a supercritical Andronov-Hopf bifurcation. (Data modified from Wu et al. 2001.)

### 9.4.2   Integrators vs. Resonators

A conspicuous feature of neuronal systems near Andronov-Hopf bifurcation, whether subcritical or supercritical, is the existence of fast subthreshold oscillations of the membrane potential. Quite often, these oscillations are visible in recordings of the membrane potential. If they are not, then they can be evoked by a brief, small pulse of current. Apparently, a bursting neuron exhibiting such oscillations in the quiescent state is either of the "Hopf/*" type or of the "subHopf/*" type, where the wild card "*" denotes any appropriate bifurcation of the spiking state. All such bursters are in the lower half of Fig.9.23.

To discern whether the bifurcation is supercritical or subcritical, one needs to study the amplitude of emerging oscillations, which can be tricky. In models, slow passage through supercritical Andronov-Hopf bifurcations often results in a delayed transition to oscillations with an intermediate or large amplitude; hence such a bifurcation may look like a subcritical one. In recordings like the ones in Fig.9.39a and Fig.9.46, noise destabilizes the focus equilibrium before the subcritical Andronov-Hopf bifurcation takes place and gives the impression that the amplitude increases gradually, that is, as if the bifurcation were supercritical.

The existence of fast subthreshold oscillations indicates that the bursting neuron acts as a resonator, at least right before the onset of a burst. In section 7.2.2 we showed that such neurons prefer a certain resonant frequency of stimulation that matches the frequency of subthreshold oscillations. A resonant input may excite the neuron and initiate a burst, or it may delay the transition to the burst, depending on its phase relative to the phase of subthreshold oscillations.

In contrast, all bursters in the upper half of the table in Fig.9.23 (i.e., "fold/*" and "circle/*" types) do not have fast subthreshold oscillations, at least before the onset of each burst (see exercise 5). The fast subsystem of such bursters acts as an integrator: it prefers high-frequency inputs; the higher the frequency, the sooner the transition to the spiking state. The phase of the input does not play any role here.

### 9.4.3   Bistability

Suppose the transition from resting to spiking state occurs via saddle-node bifurcation (off an invariant circle) or subcritical Andronov-Hopf bifurcation of the fast subsystem,

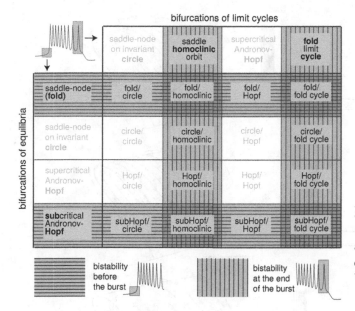

Figure 9.47: Bistability (i.e., coexistence of resting and spiking states) depends on the topological type of bursting.

as in Fig.6.46. In these cases, the trajectory jumps to a preexisting limit cycle attractor corresponding to the spiking state (not shown in the figure). In contrast, saddle-node on invariant circle bifurcation or supercritical Andronov-Hopf bifurcation creates such a limit cycle attractor. Thus, there must be a coexistence of stable resting and stable spiking states in the former case, but not necessarily in the latter case. This simple observation has far-reaching consequences described below. In particular, it implies that all "fold/*" and "subHopf/*" bursters exhibit bistability, at least before the onset of a burst, while "circle/*" and "Hopf/*" bursters may not (see Fig.9.47).

Similarly, if the transition from spiking to resting state of the fast subsystem occurs via saddle homoclinic orbit bifurcation or fold limit cycle bifurcation, then there is a preexisting stable equilibrium, and hence a coexistence of attractors. Thus, "*/homo-clinic" and "*/fold cycle" bursters also exhibit bistability, at least at the end of a burst, while "*/circle" and "*/Hopf" bursters may not, as we summarize in Fig.9.47.

An obvious consequence of bistability is that an appropriate stimulus can switch the system from resting to spiking and back. We illustrate this phenomenon in Fig.9.48, using the $I_{Na,p}+I_K+I_{K(M)}$-model, which exhibits a hysteresis loop "fold/homoclinic" bursting when $I = 5$. All three simulations in the figure start with the same initial conditions. In Fig.9.48b we apply a brief pulse of current while the fast subsystem is at the resting state. This stimulation pushes the membrane potential over the threshold state into the attraction domain of the spiking limit cycle of the fast subsystem, thereby evoking a burst.

Note that the evoked burst is one spike shorter than the control burst in Fig.9.48a. This is expected, since the $K^+$ M-current did not have enough time to recover from the previous burst (not shown in the figure); therefore, there is a residual outward

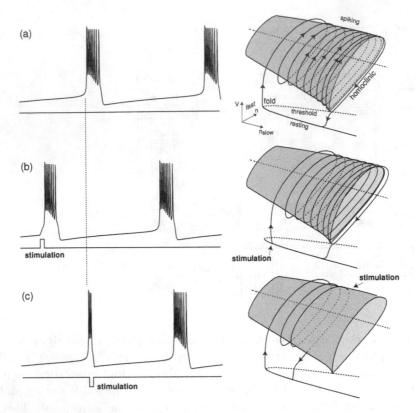

Figure 9.48: Bistability of resting and spiking states in a "fold/homoclinic" burster. A brief stimulus can initiate a premature transition to the spiking state (b) or to quiescent state (c). Shown are simulations of the $I_{Na,p}+I_K+I_{K(M)}$-model with parameters as in Fig.9.4b.

current that shortens the active phase. From the geometrical point of view, this occurs because the transition to the spiking manifold in Fig.9.48b (right) occurs before the slow variable reaches the fold knee; hence the distance to the homoclinic bifurcation is shorter. An interesting observation is that the first spike in the evoked burst actually corresponds to the second spike in the control burst in Fig.9.48a. The earlier the stimulation acts, the sooner the trajectory jumps to the spiking manifold and the fewer spikes the evoked burst has.

In Fig.9.48c we applied a brief pulse of current in the middle of a burst to switch the system to the resting state. Note that the quiescent period, that is, the time to the second burst, is shorter than the control period in Fig.9.48a or 9.48b. This is also to be expected, since the $K^+$ M- current was not fully activated during the interrupted burst and therefore does not need much time to deactivate during the resting period. Geometrically, the short duration of the resting phase is a consequence of the distance the slow variable needs to travel to get to the fold knee being small.

## 9.4.4  Bursts as a Unit of Neuronal Information

There are many hypotheses on the importance of bursting activity in neural computation (Izhikevich 2006).

- *Bursts are more reliable than single spikes* in evoking responses in postsynaptic cells. Indeed, excitatory post-synaptic potentials (EPSP) from each spike in a burst add up and may result in a superthreshold EPSP.

- *Bursts overcome synaptic transmission failure.* Indeed, postsynaptic responses to a single presynaptic spike may fail (release does not occur), however in response to a bombardment of spikes, i.e., a burst, synaptic release is more likely (Lisman 1997).

- *Bursts facilitate transmitter release whereas single spikes do not* (Lisman 1997). Indeed, a synapse with strong short-term facilitation would be insensitive to single spikes or even short bursts, but not to longer bursts. Each spike in the longer burst facilitates the synapse so the effect of the last few spikes may be quite strong.

- *Bursts evoke long-term potentiation* and hence affect synaptic plasticity much greater, or differently than single spikes (Lisman 1997).

- *Bursts have higher signal-to-noise ratio than single spikes* (Sherman 2001). Indeed, burst threshold is higher than spike threshold, i.e., generation of bursts requires stronger inputs.

- *Bursts can be used for selective communication* if the postsynaptic cells have subthreshold oscillations of membrane potential. Such cells are sensitive to the frequency content of the input. Some bursts resonate with oscillations and elicit a response, others do not, depending on the interburst frequency (Izhikevich et al. 2003).

- *Bursts can resonate with short-term synaptic plasticity* making a synapse a band-pass filter (Izhikevich et al. 2003). A synapse having short-term facilitation and depression is most sensitive to a burst having certain resonant interspike frequency. Such a burst evokes just enough facilitation, but not too much depression, so its effect on the postsynaptic target is maximal.

- *Bursts encode different features* of sensory input than single spikes (Gabbiani et al. 1996, Oswald et al. 2004). For example, neurons in the electrosensory lateral-line lobe (ELL) of weakly electric fish fire network induced-bursts in response to communication signals and single spikes in response to prey signals (Doiron et al. 2003). In the thalamus of the visual system bursts from pyramidal neurons encode stimuli that inhibit the neuron for a period of time and then rapidly excite the neuron (Lesica and Stanely, 2004). Natural scenes are often composed of such events.

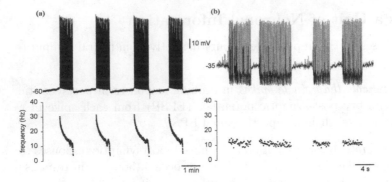

Figure 9.49: The instantaneous spike frequency of a trigeminal motor neuron (a) and a trigeminal interneuron (b) of a rodent. (Modified from Del Negro et al. 1998.)

- *Bursts have more informational content* than single spikes when analyzed as unitary events (Reinagel et al. 1999). This information may be encoded into the burst duration or in the fine temporal structure of interspike intervals within a burst.

In summary, burst input is more likely to have a stronger impact on the postsynaptic cell than single spike input, so some believe that bursts are all-or-none events, whereas single spikes may be noise.

### 9.4.5   Chirps

An important information may be carried in the intraburst frequency. Consider the effect of a burst on a postsynaptic resonator neuron, that is, a neuron with a resting state near an Andronov-Hopf bifurcation. Such a neuron is sensitive to the frequency content of the burst (i.e., whether it is resonant or not, as discussed in section 7.2.2). Some types of bursters have relatively constant intraburst (instantaneous interspike) frequencies, as in Fig.9.49b, which may be resonant for some postsynaptic neurons but not for others. In contrast, other topological types of bursters have widely varying instantaneous interspike frequencies, as in Fig.9.49a, that scan or sweep a broad frequency range going all the way to zero.

When the bifurcation from resting to spiking state is of the saddle-node on invariant circle type (i.e., the system is Class 1 excitable), the frequency of emerging spiking is first small, and then increases. Therefore, all "circle/*" bursters generate chirps with instantaneous interspike frequencies increasing from zero to a relatively large value, at least at the beginning of the burst. Similarly, when the bifurcation of the spiking state is of the saddle-node on invariant circle or saddle homoclinic orbit type, the frequency of spiking at the end of the burst decreases to zero, so all "*/circle" and "*/homoclinic" bursters also generate chirps, as in Fig.9.49a. In summary, all shaded bursters in Fig.9.50 have sweeping interspike frequencies, so that one part of the burst is resonant for one neuron and another part of the same burst is resonant for another neuron.

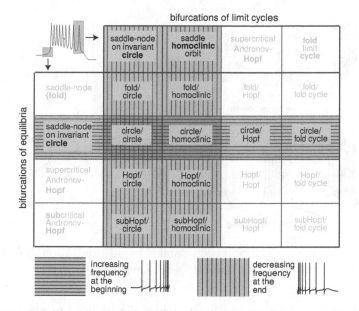

Figure 9.50: Topological types of bursters in the shaded regions can produce chirp-bursts that sweep a frequency range.

## 9.4.6 Synchronization

Consider two coupled bursting neurons of the fast-slow type. Since each burster has two time scales, one for rhythmic spiking and one for repetitive bursting, there are two synchronization regimes:

- Spike synchronization, as in Fig.9.51 (left).
- Burst synchronization, as in Fig.9.51 (right).

One of them does not imply the other. Of course, there is an additional regime in which spikes and bursts are synchronized. We will study synchronization phenomena

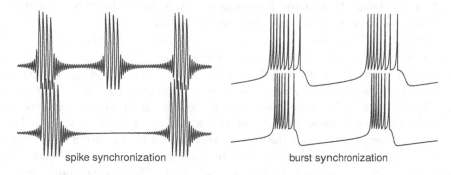

Figure 9.51: Various regimes of synchronization of bursters.

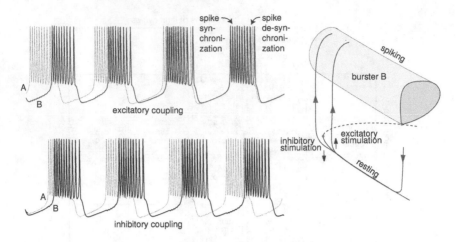

Figure 9.52: Burst synchronization and desynchronization of two coupled "fold/homoclinic" bursters. (Modified from Izhikevich 2000a.)

in detail in chapter 10; here we just mention how they depend on the topological type of bursting.

Let us consider spike synchronization first. Since we are interested in the fast time scale, we neglect the slow variable dynamics for now and treat two bursters as coupled oscillators. A necessary condition for synchronization of two weakly coupled oscillators is that they have nearly equal frequencies. How near is "near" depends on the strength of the coupling. Thus, spike synchronization depends crucially on the instantaneous interspike frequency, which may vary substantially during a burst. Indeed, a small perturbation of the slow variable may result in large perturbations of the interspike frequency in any shaded burster in Fig.9.50; hence such a burster would be unlikely to exhibit spike synchronization unless the coupling is strong.

Studying burst synchronization of weakly coupled neurons involves the same mathematical methods as studying synchronization of strongly coupled relaxation oscillators, which we consider in detail in chapter 10. The mechanisms of synchronization depend on whether the bursting is of the hysteresis loop type or of the slow wave type, and whether the resting state is an integrator or a resonator.

In Fig.9.52 we illustrate the geometry of burst synchronization of two coupled "fold/homoclinic" bursters of the hysteresis loop type. Burster A is slightly ahead of burster B, so that A starts the spiking phase while B is still resting. If the synaptic connections between the bursters are excitatory, firing of A causes B to jump to the spiking state prematurely, thereby shortening the time difference between the bursts. In addition, the evoked burst of B is shorter, which also speeds up the synchronization process. In contrast, when the connections are inhibitory, firing of A delays the transition of B to the spiking state, thereby increasing the time difference between the bursts and desynchronizing the bursters. Thus, the "fold/homoclinic" burster behaves according to the principle *excitation means synchronization, inhibition means desynchronization.* Since the instantaneous interspike frequency of "fold/homoclinic" bursting decays to zero, small deviations of the slow variable result in large deviations of the period of oscillation. Typically, the periods of fast oscillations of the two bursters can diverge slowly from each other. As a result, spikes may start synchronized and then desynchronize during the burst, as we indicate in the figure.

If the bursting neuron is a resonator, that is, it is of the "Hopf/*" or "subHopf/*" type, then both excitation and inhibition may evoke premature spiking, as we have shown in chapter 7, and lead to burst synchronization. An important feature here is that the interspike frequency of one burster must be resonant to the subthreshold oscillations of the other one. We study these and other issues related to synchronization in chapter 10.

---

## Review of Important Concepts

- A burst of spikes is a train of action potentials followed by a period of quiescence.

- Bursting activity typically involves two time scales: fast spiking and slow modulation via a resonant current.

- Many mathematical models of bursters have the fast-slow form

$$\begin{aligned} \dot{x} &= f(x, u) && \text{(fast spiking)}, \\ \dot{u} &= \mu g(x, u) && \text{(slow modulation)}. \end{aligned}$$

- To dissect a burster, one freezes its slow subsystem (i.e., sets $\mu = 0$) and uses the slow variable $u$ as a bifurcation parameter to study the fast subsystem.

- The fast subsystem undergoes two important bifurcations during a burst: (1) bifurcation of an equilibrium resulting in transition to the spiking state and (2) bifurcation of a limit cycle attractor resulting in transition to the resting state.

- Different types of bifurcations result in different topological types of bursting.

- There are 16 basic types of bursting, summarized in Fig.9.23.

- Different topological types of bursters have different neurocomputational properties.

| *Bifurcations* | *Saddle-Node on Invariant* **Circle** | *Saddle* **Homoclinic** *Orbit* | *Supercritical Andronov-* **Hopf** | **Fold** *Limit* **Cycle** |
|---|---|---|---|---|
| **Fold** | triangular | square-wave Type I | tapered Type V | Type IV |
| *Saddle-Node on Invariant* **Circle** | parabolic Type II | | | |
| *Supercritical Andronov-* **Hopf** | | | | |
| **Sub**critical Andronov- **Hopf** | | | | elliptic Type III |

Figure 9.53: Bifurcation mechanisms and classical nomenclature of the six bursters known in the twentieth century. Compare with Fig.9.23 and Fig.9.24.

# Bibliographical Notes

The history of formal classification of bursting starts with the seminal paper by Rinzel (1987), who contrasted the bifurcation mechanisms of the "square-wave", "parabolic", and "elliptic" bursters. Bertram et al. (1995) followed Rinzel's suggestion and referred to the bursters using Roman numerals, adding a new burster, Type IV. Another, "tapered" type of bursting was studied simultaneously and independently by Holden and Erneux (1993a, 1993b), Smolen et al. (1993), and Pernarowski (1994). Later, de Vries (1998) suggested referring to it as a Type V burster. A "triangular" type of bursting was studied by Rush and Rinzel (1994), making the total of identified bursters six. To honor these pioneers, we described these six *classical* bursters in the order of the numbering of Bertram et al. (1995). Their bifurcation mechanisms are summarized in Fig.9.53.

The complete classification of bursters, provided by Izhikevich (2000a), was motivated by Guckenheimer et al. (1997). There is a drastic difference between Izhikevich's approach and that of the scientists mentioned above. The latter used a *bottom-up* approach; that is, they considered biophysically plausible conductance-based models describing experimentally observable cellular behavior, then determined the types of bursting these models exhibited. In contrast, Izhikevich (2000a) used the *top-down*

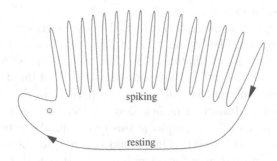

Figure 9.54: A hedgehog-like limit cycle attractor results in bursting dynamics even in two-dimensional systems; see exercise 1. (Modified from Hoppensteadt and Izhikevich 1997.)

approach and considered all possible pairs of codimension-1 bifurcations of rest and spiking states, which resulted in different types of bursting. (It was an easy task to provide a conductance-based model exhibiting each bursting type.) Thus, many of the bursters are "theoretical" in the sense that they have yet to be seen in experiments.

A challenging problem was to suggest a naming scheme for the bursters. The names should be self-explanatory, and easy to remember and understand. Thus, the numbering scheme suggested by Bertram et al. (1995) could lead to bursters of Type XXVII, Type LXIII, Type CLXVI, and so on. We cannot use descriptions such as "elliptic", "parabolic", "hyperbolic", "triangular", "rectangular", and such because they are misleading. In this book we follow Izhikevich (2000a) and name the bursters according to the two bifurcations involved, as in Fig.9.23.

Not all bursters can be represented in the fast-slow form with a clear separation of the time scales. Those that cannot, are referred to as hedgehog bursters (Izhikevich 2000a), since they have a limit cycle (or a more complicated attractor) with some spiky parts corresponding to repetitive spiking and some smooth parts corresponding to quiescence, as in Fig.9.54. An interesting example of the hedgehog burster is the model of the sensory processing neuron of weakly electric fish (Doiron et al. 2002). The authors refer to the model as "ghostburster" because repetitive spiking corresponds to a slow transition of the full system through the ghost of a fold limit cycle attractor. As a dynamical system, the ghostburster is near a codimension-2 bifurcation of limit cycle attractor, and it exhibits chaotic dynamics.

Betram et al. (1995) noticed that bursting often occurs when the fast subsystem is near a codimension-2 bifurcation. Izhikevich (2000a) suggested that many simple models of bursters could be obtained by considering unfoldings of various degenerate bifurcations of high codimension (organizing centers) and treating the unfolding parameters as slow variables rotating around the bifurcation point, as in Fig.9.28 or Fig.9.42. Considering the Bautin bifurcation, Izhikevich (2001) obtained the canonical model for the "subHopf/fold cycle" ("elliptic") burster (9.11). Golubitsky et al. (2001) applied this idea to other local bifurcations (spiking with infinitesimal amplitude). Global bifurcations are considered in exercise 26.

Izhikevich and Hoppensteadt (2004) extend the classification of bursters to one- and two-dimensional mappings, identifying 3 and 20 different classes, respectively. A recent book *Bursting: The Genesis of Rhythm in the Nervous System* edited by Coombes and Bressloff (2005), presents recent developments in the field of bursting dynamics.

Studying bursting dynamics is still one of the hardest problems in applied mathematics. The method of dissection of fast-slow bursters of the form (9.1), pioneered by Rinzel (1987), is part of the asymptotic theory of singularly perturbed dynamical systems (Mishchenko et al. 1994). One would expect the theory to suggest other, quantitative methods of analyzing fast-slow bursters. However, the basic assumption of the theory is that the fast subsystem has only equilibria, e.g., up- and down-states, as in the point-point hysteresis loops in exercise 19. This assumption is violated when the neuron fires a burst of spikes, since repetitive spikes correspond to limit cycles. Thus, the theory is of no help in studying fast-slow point-cycle bursters. An exception is Pontryagin's problem, which is related to "fold cycle/fold cycle" bursting; see exercise 21 and section 7 in Mishchenko et al. (1994). Pontryagin and Rodygin (1960) pioneered the method of averaging of the fast subsystem, which was used in the context of bursters by Rinzel and Lee (1986), Pernarowski et al. (1992), Smolen et al. (1993), and Baer et al. (1995). Shilnikov et al. (2005) introduced an average nullcline of the slow subsystem, and showed how the averaging method can be used to study coexistence of spiking and bursting states in a model neuron, and bifurcations in bursters in general. Some of the transitions "resting ↔ bursting ↔ tonic spiking" were considered by Ermentrout and Kopell (1986a), Terman (1991), Destexhe and Gaspard (1993), Shilnikov and Cymbalyuk (2004, 2005), and Medvedev (2005).

The averaging method, like many other classical methods of analysis of dynamical systems, breaks down when the fast subsystem slowly passes a bifurcation point. The development of early dynamical system theory was largely motivated by studies of periodic oscillators. It is reasonable to expect that the next major developments of this theory will come from studies of bursters.

## Exercises

1. (Planar burster) Invent a planar system of ODEs having a hedgehog limit cycle attractor (as in Fig.9.54) and capable of exhibiting periodic bursting activity.

2. (Noise-induced bursting) Explain why the $I_{Na,p}+I_K$-model with a phase portrait as in Fig.9.55 bursts even though it has only two dimensions.

3. (Noise-induced bursting) Explore numerically the $I_{Na,p}+I_K$-model with phase portrait as in Fig.6.7 (top) and make it burst as in Fig.9.56, without adding any new current or gating variable.

4. (Rebound bursting) Explain the mechanism of rebound bursting in the two-dimensional FitzHugh-Nagumo oscillator (4.11, 4.12), shown in Fig.9.57.

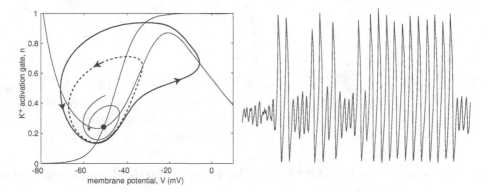

Figure 9.55: Bursting in two-dimensional $I_{\mathrm{Na,p}}+I_{\mathrm{K}}$-model with parameters as in Fig.6.16 and $I = 43$.

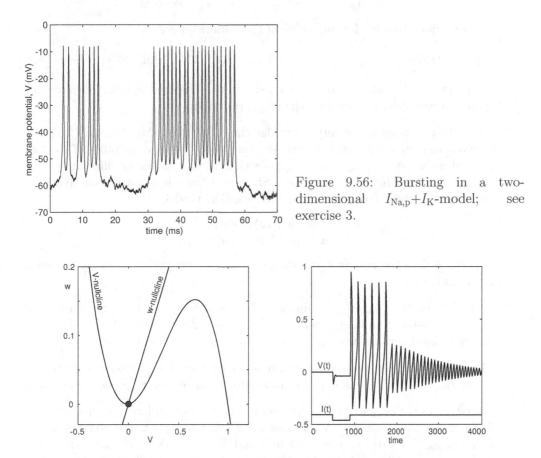

Figure 9.56: Bursting in a two-dimensional $I_{\mathrm{Na,p}}+I_{\mathrm{K}}$-model; see exercise 3.

Figure 9.57: Rebound bursting in the FitzHugh-Nagumo oscillator; see exercise 4.

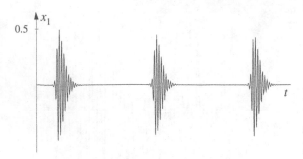

Figure 9.58: Hopf/Hopf bursting without coexistence of attractors; see exercise 6. (Modified from Hoppensteadt and Izhikevich 1997.)

5. Can "circle/*" and "fold/*" bursters have fast subthreshold oscillations of membrane potential? Explain.

6. (Hopf/Hopf bursting) The system

$$\dot{x} = (y + \mathrm{i})x - x|x|^2, \qquad x = x_1 + \mathrm{i}x_2 \in \mathbb{C},$$

has a unique attractor for any value of the parameter $y \in \mathbb{R}$. If

$$\dot{y} = \mu\left(2aS\left(\frac{y}{a} - a\right) - |x|\right), \quad \mu = 0.05, \quad a = \sqrt{\mu/20}, \quad \text{and} \quad S(u) = \frac{1}{1 + e^{-u}},$$

then the "2+1" system above can burst, as we show in Fig.9.58. Explore the system numerically and explain the origin of bursting.

7. (Hopf/Hopf canonical model) Consider the "2+1" fast-slow burster (9.1) and suppose that $x_0$ is the supercritical Andronov-Hopf bifurcation point of the fast subsystem when $u = u_0$. Also suppose that $u_0$ is a stable equilibrium of the slow subsystem when $x = x_0$ is fixed. Show that there is a continuous change of variables that transforms (9.1) into the canonical model

$$z' = (u + \mathrm{i}\omega)z - z|z|^2,$$
$$u' = \mu(\pm 1 \pm u - a|z|^2),$$

where $z \in \mathbb{C}$ is the new fast variable, $u \in \mathbb{R}$ is a slow variable, and $\omega, a$, and $\mu$ are parameters.

8. (Bursting in the $I_{\mathrm{Na,t}} + I_{\mathrm{Na,slow}}$-model) Take advantage of the phenomenon of inhibition-induced spiking described in section 7.2.8 to show that a slow persistent inward current, say $I_{\mathrm{Na,slow}}$, can stop spiking and create bursts.

9. Modify the example above to obtain repetitive bursting in a model consisting of a fast $I_{\mathrm{Na,t}}$ current, a leak current, and a slow passive dendritic compartment.

10. (Bursting in the $I_{\mathrm{Na,p}} + I_{\mathrm{K}} + I_{\mathrm{Na,slow}}$-model) Numerically explore this model with a fast subsystem as in Fig.6.16 and a slow Na$^+$ current with parameters $g_{\mathrm{Na,slow}} = 0.5$, $m_{\infty,\mathrm{slow}}(V)$ with $V_{1/2} = -50$ mV and $k = 10$ mV, and $\tau_{\mathrm{slow}}(V) = 5 + 100\exp(-(V + 20)^2/25^2)$. Explain the origin of bursting oscillations when $I = 27$ in Fig.9.59.

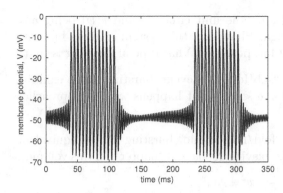

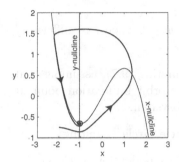

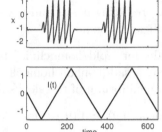

Figure 9.59: Bursting in the $I_{\mathrm{Na,p}}+I_{\mathrm{K}}+I_{\mathrm{Na,slow}}$-model; see exercise 10.

Figure 9.60: The phase portrait of the system in exercise 11 shows that there is only one stable equilibrium for any value of $I$. Nevertheless, the system bursts when $I$ is periodically modulated.

11. The Bonhoeffer–van der Pol oscillator

$$\dot{x} = I + x - x^3/3 - y \,,$$
$$\dot{y} = 0.2(1.05 + x) \,,$$

with nullclines as in Fig.9.60, is Class 3 excitable. It has a unique stable equilibrium for any value of $I$. Periodic modulations of $I$ shift the $x$-nullcline upward and downward but do not change the stability of the equilibrium. Why does the system burst in Fig.9.60? Explore the phenomenon numerically and explain the existence of repetitive spikes without a limit cycle.

12. Prove (without simulations) that the fast-slow "2+2" system

$$\dot{z} = (1 + u + i\omega)z - z|z|^2 \,, \qquad z \in \mathbb{C} \,,$$
$$\dot{u} = \mu(u - u^3 - w) \,,$$
$$\dot{w} = \mu(|z|^2 - 1) \,,$$

is a slow-wave burster, even though the slow subsystem cannot oscillate for any fixed value of the fast subsystem $z$.

13. (Ermentrout and Kopell 1986) Consider the system

$$\dot{\vartheta} = 1 - \cos\vartheta + (1 + \cos\vartheta)r(\psi) \,,$$
$$\dot{\psi} = \omega \,,$$

with $\vartheta$ and $\psi$ being phase variables on the unit circle $\mathbb{S}^1$ and $r(\psi)$ being any continuous function that changes sign. Show that this system exhibits bursting activity when $\omega$ is sufficiently small but positive. What type of bursting is that?

14. Prove that the canonical model for "subHopf/fold cycle" bursting (9.11) exhibits sustained bursting activity when $0 < a < 1$. What happens when $a$ approaches 0 or 1?

15. Show that the canonical model for "fold/homoclinic" bursting (9.7) is equivalent to a simpler model (equation 27 in Izhikevich 2000a and chapter 8 in this volume),

$$\begin{aligned} \dot{v} &= v^2 + w, \\ \dot{w} &= \mu, \end{aligned}$$

with after-spike ($v = +\infty$) resetting $v \leftarrow 1$ and $w \leftarrow w - d$, when $I$ is sufficiently large and $\mu$ and $d$ are sufficiently small.

16. Derive the canonical model for "fold/homoclinic" bursting (9.7), assuming that the fast subsystem is near a saddle-node homoclinic orbit bifurcation point at some $u = u_0$, which is an equilibrium of the slow subsystem.

17. Derive the canonical models (9.9) and (9.10) for "circle/circle" bursting.

18. Show that the averaged slow subsystems of the canonical models for "circle/circle" bursters (9.9) and (9.10) have the form

$$\begin{aligned} \dot{u}_1 &= -\mu_1 u_1 + d_1 f(I + u_1 - u_2), \\ \dot{u}_2 &= -\mu_2 u_2 + d_2 f(I + u_1 - u_2), \end{aligned}$$

and

$$\begin{aligned} \dot{u}_1 &= -\mu_1 u_2 + d_1 f(I + u_1), \\ \dot{u}_2 &= -\mu_2 (u_2 - u_1) + d_2 f(I + u_1), \end{aligned}$$

respectively, where

$$f(u) = \frac{\sqrt{u}}{\pi/2 + \operatorname{arcot} \sqrt{u}}$$

is the frequency of spiking of the fast subsystem (in Hz).

19. (Point-point hysteresis loops) Consider (9.1) and suppose that the fast subsystem has only equilibria for any value of the one-dimensional slow variable $u$. If there is a coexistence of equilibrium points of the fast subsystem, then (9.1) can exhibit point-point hysteresis loop oscillation. Classify all codimension-1 point-point hysteresis loops.

20. (Point-point bursting) In Fig.9.61 we present two geometrical examples of point-point bursters that have no limit cycle attractors, yet are capable of exhibiting spike like dynamics in the active phase. Construct a model for each type of point-point burster in the figure. Use phase portrait snapshots at the bottom of the figure as hints. What makes such bursting possible?

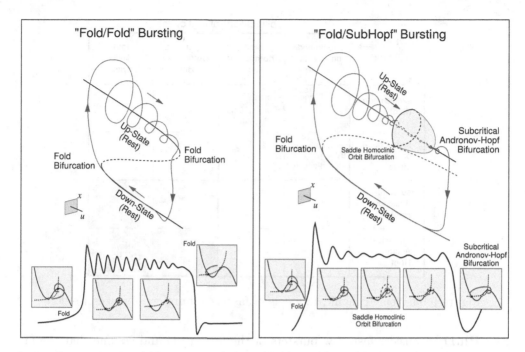

Figure 9.61: Two examples of point-point (not fast-slow) bursters. (Modified from Izhikevich 2000a.)

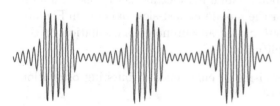

Figure 9.62: A cycle-cycle bursting: The resting state is not an equilibrium, but a small-amplitude limit cycle attractor.

21. (Cycle-cycle bursters) Consider a fast-slow burster (9.1) and suppose that the resting state is not an equilibrium, but a limit cycle attractor, as in Fig.9.62. Such a bursting is called cycle-cycle. Classify all codimension-1 planar cycle-cycle fast-slow bursters. Is bursting in Fig.9.10 of the cycle-cycle type?

22. (Minimal models for bursting) Fill in the blank squares in Fig.9.8.

23. Choose a minimal model from Fig.9.8 and simulate it. Change the parameters to get as many different bursting types as possible.

24. **[M.S.]** Determine the bifurcation diagram of the canonical model for "fold/homoclinic" bursting (9.7).

25. **[M.S.]** Determine the bifurcation diagrams of the canonical models for "circle/circle" bursters (9.9) and (9.10).

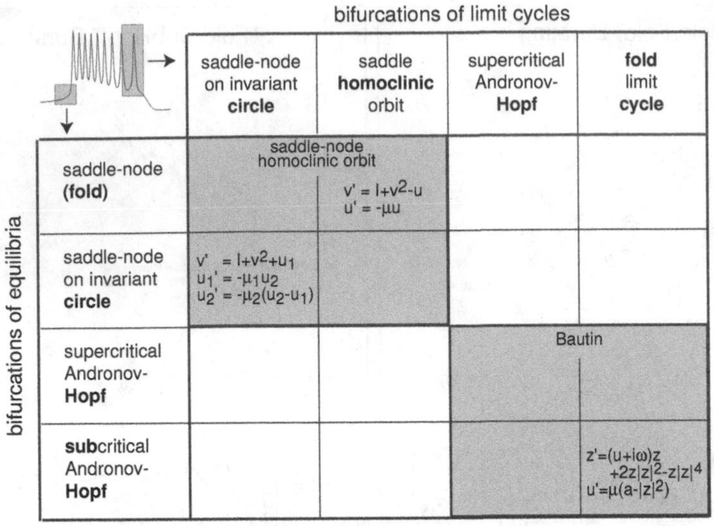

bifurcations of limit cycles

| | saddle-node on invariant **circle** | saddle **homoclinic** orbit | supercritical Andronov-**Hopf** | **fold** limit **cycle** |
|---|---|---|---|---|
| saddle-node **(fold)** | saddle-node homoclinic orbit | $v' = I+v^2-u$ $u' = -\mu u$ | | |
| saddle-node on invariant **circle** | $v' = I+v^2+u_1$ $u_1' = -\mu_1 u_2$ $u_2' = -\mu_2(u_2-u_1)$ | | | |
| supercritical Andronov-**Hopf** | | | Bautin | |
| **sub**critical Andronov-**Hopf** | | | | $z'=(u+i\omega)z$ $+2z\|z\|^2-z\|z\|^4$ $u'=\mu(a-\|z\|^2)$ |

Figure 9.63: Some canonical models of fast-slow bursters; see exercise 26.

26. [**Ph.D.**] Consider fast-slow bursters of the form (9.1) and assume that the fast subsystem is near a bifurcation of high codimension, as in Fig.9.28 or in Fig.9.42. Treating the bifurcation point as an organizing center for the fast subsystem (Bertram et al. 1995; Izhikevich 2000a; Golubitsky et al. 2001), use unfolding theory to derive canonical models for the remaining fast-slow bursters in Fig.9.63. Do not assume that the slow subsystem has an autonomous oscillation or that the fast oscillations have small amplitude.

27. [**Ph.D.**] Classify all possible mechanisms of emergence of bursting oscillations from resting or spiking, as in Fig.9.19.

28. [**Ph.D.**] Develop an asymptotic theory of singularly perturbed systems of the form
$$\dot{x} = f(x,u) \qquad \text{(fast subsystem)},$$
$$\dot{u} = \mu g(x,u) \qquad \text{(slow modulation)}$$
that can deal with transitions between equilibria and limit cycle attractors of the fast subsystem.

# Chapter 10

# Synchronization

This chapter, found on the author's Web page (www.izhikevich.com), considers networks of tonically spiking neurons. Like any other kind of physical, chemical, or biological oscillators, such neurons could synchronize and exhibit collective behavior that is not intrinsic to any individual neuron. For example, partial synchrony in cortical networks is believed to generate various brain oscillations, such as the alpha and gamma EEG rhythms. Increased synchrony may result in pathological types of activity, such as epilepsy. Coordinated synchrony is needed for locomotion and swim pattern generation in fish. There is an ongoing debate on the role of synchrony in neural computation (see, e.g., the special issue of *Neuron* [September 1999] devoted to the binding problem).

Depending on the circumstances, synchrony can be good or bad, and it is important to know what factors contribute to synchrony and how to control it. This is the subject of the present chapter, the most advanced chapter of the book. It provides a nice application of the theory developed earlier and hopefully gives some insight into why the previous chapters may be worth mastering. Unfortunately, it is too long to be included into the book, so reviewers recommended putting it on the Web.

The goal of this chapter is to understand how the behavior of coupled neurons depends on their intrinsic dynamics. First, we introduce the method of description of an oscillation by its phase. Then, we describe various methods of reduction of coupled oscillators to phase models. The reduction method and the exact form of the phase model depend on the type of coupling (i.e., whether it is pulsed, weak, or slow) and on the type of bifurcations of the limit cycle attractor generating tonic spiking. Finally, we show how to use phase models to understand the collective dynamics of many coupled oscillators.

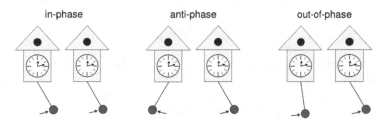

Figure 10.1: Different types of synchronization.

# Review of Important Concepts

- Oscillations are described by their phase variables $\vartheta$ rotating on a circle $\mathbb{S}^1$. We define $\vartheta$ as the time since the last spike.

- The phase response curve, PRC $(\vartheta)$, describes the magnitude of the phase shift of an oscillator caused by a strong pulsed input arriving at phase $\vartheta$.

- PRC depends on the bifurcations of the spiking limit cycle, and it defines synchronization properties of an oscillator.

- Two oscillators are synchronized in-phase, anti-phase, or out-of-phase when their phase difference, $\vartheta_2 - \vartheta_1$, equals 0, half-period, or some other value, respectively; see Fig.10.1.

- Synchronized states of pulse-coupled oscillators are fixed points of the corresponding Poincare phase map.

- Weakly coupled oscillators

$$\dot{x}_i = f(x_i) + \varepsilon \sum g_{ij}(x_j)$$

can be reduced to phase models

$$\dot{\vartheta}_i = 1 + \varepsilon \, Q(\vartheta_i) \sum g_{ij}(x_j(\vartheta_j)) \, ,$$

where $Q(\vartheta)$ is the infinitesimal PRC defined by Malkin's equation.

- Weak coupling induces a slow phase deviation of the natural oscillation, $\vartheta_i(t) = t + \varphi_i$, described by the averaged model

$$\dot{\varphi}_i = \varepsilon \left( \omega_i + \sum H_{ij}(\varphi_j - \varphi_i) \right) ,$$

where the $\omega_i$ denote the frequency deviations, and

$$H_{ij}(\varphi_j - \varphi_i) = \frac{1}{T} \int_0^T Q(t) \, g_{ij}(x_j(t + \varphi_j - \varphi_i)) \, dt$$

describe the interactions between the phases.

- Synchronization of two coupled oscillators correspond to equilibria of the one-dimensional system

$$\dot{\chi} = \varepsilon(\omega + G(\chi)) \, , \qquad \chi = \varphi_2 - \varphi_1 \, ,$$

where $G(\chi) = H_{21}(-\chi) - H_{12}(\chi)$ describes how the phase difference $\chi$ compensates for the frequency mismatch $\omega = \omega_2 - \omega_1$.

# Solutions to Exercises

## Solutions for chapter 2

1. $T = 20°C \approx 293°F$.

$$E_{\text{Ion}} = \frac{RT}{zF} \ln \frac{[\text{Ion}]_{\text{out}}}{[\text{Ion}]_{\text{in}}} = \frac{8315 \cdot 293 \cdot \ln 10}{z \cdot 96480} \log_{10} \frac{[\text{Ion}]_{\text{out}}}{[\text{Ion}]_{\text{in}}} = \pm 58 \log_{10} \frac{[\text{Ion}]_{\text{out}}}{[\text{Ion}]_{\text{in}}}$$

when $z = \pm 1$. Therefore,

$$
\begin{aligned}
E_{\text{K}} &= 58 \log(20/430) = -77 \text{ mV} \\
E_{\text{Na}} &= 58 \log(440/50) = 55 \text{ mV} \\
E_{\text{Cl}} &= -58 \log(560/65) = -54 \text{ mV}
\end{aligned}
$$

2.

$$
\begin{aligned}
I &= \bar{g}_{\text{Na}} \, p \, (V - E_{\text{Na}}) + \bar{g}_{\text{K}} \, p \, (V - E_{\text{K}}) = p\{(\bar{g}_{\text{Na}} + \bar{g}_{\text{K}}) \, V - \bar{g}_{\text{Na}} \, E_{\text{Na}} - \bar{g}_{\text{K}} \, E_{\text{K}}\} \\
&= \underbrace{(\bar{g}_{\text{Na}} + \bar{g}_{\text{K}}) \, p}_{\bar{g}} \left( V - \underbrace{\frac{\bar{g}_{\text{Na}} \, E_{\text{Na}} + \bar{g}_{\text{K}} \, E_{\text{K}}}{\bar{g}_{\text{Na}} + \bar{g}_{\text{K}}}}_{E} \right)
\end{aligned}
$$

3. The answer follows from the equation

$$I - g_{\text{L}}(V - E_{\text{L}}) = -g_{\text{L}}(V - \widehat{E}_{\text{L}}), \qquad \text{where} \qquad \widehat{E}_{\text{L}} = E_{\text{L}} + I/g_{\text{L}}.$$

4. See Fig.S.1.

| Function | $V_{1/2}$ | $k$ | Function | $V_{\max}$ | $\sigma$ | $C_{\text{amp}}$ | $C_{\text{base}}$ |
|----------|-----------|-----|----------|------------|----------|------------------|-------------------|
| $n_\infty(V)$ | 12 | 15 | $\tau_n(V)$ | $-14$ | 50 | 4.7 | 1.1 |
| $m_\infty(V)$ | 25 | 9 | $\tau_m(V)$ | 27 | 30 | 0.46 | 0.04 |
| $h_\infty(V)$ | 3 | $-7$ | $\tau_n(V)$ | $-2$ | 20 | 7.4 | 1.2 |

Hodgkin and Huxley shifted $V_{1/2}$ and $V_{\max}$ by 65 mV so that the resting potential is at $V = 0$ mV.

5. (Willms et al. 1999)

$$
\begin{aligned}
\tilde{V}_{1/2} &= V_{1/2} - k \ln(2^{1/p} - 1), \\
\tilde{k} &= \frac{k}{2p(1 - 2^{-1/p})}.
\end{aligned}
$$

The first equation is obtained from the condition $m_\infty^p(\tilde{V}_{1/2}) = 1/2$. The second equation is obtained from the condition that the two functions have the same slope at $V = \tilde{V}_{1/2}$.

6. See author's Web page, www.izhikevich.com.

7. See author's Web page, www.izhikevich.com.

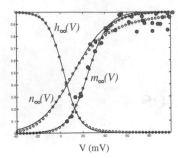
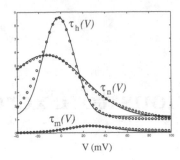

Figure S.1: *Open dots*: The steady-state (in)activation functions and voltage-sensitive time constants in the Hodgkin-Huxley model. *Filled dots*: steady-state Na$^+$ activation function $m_\infty(V)$ in the squid giant axon (experimental results by Hodgkin and Huxley 1952, figure 8). *Continuous curves*: Approximations by Boltzmann and Gaussian functions. See exercise 4.

# Solutions for chapter 3

1. Consider the limit case: (1) activation of the Na$^+$ current is instantaneous, and (2) conductance kinetics of the other currents are frozen. Then, the Na$^+$ current will result in the nonlinear term $g_{Na} m_\infty(V)(V - E_{Na})$ with the parameter $h_\infty(V_{rest})$ incorporated into $g_{Na}$, and all the other currents will result in the linear leak term.

   In Fig.3.15, the activation of the Na$^+$ current is not instantaneous; hence the sag right after the pulses. In addition, its inactivation, and the kinetics of the other currents are not slow enough; hence the membrane potential quickly reaches the excited state and then slowly repolarizes to the resting state.

2. See Fig.S.2. The eigenvalues are negative at each equilibrium marked as a filled circle (stable), and positive at each equilibrium marked as an open circle (unstable). The eigenvalue at the bifurcation point (left equilibrium in Fig.S.2b) is zero.

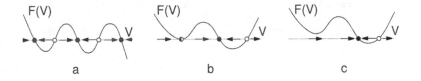

Figure S.2: Phase portraits of the system $\dot{V} = F(V)$ with given $F(V)$.

3. Phase portraits are shown in Fig.S.3.

   (a) The equation $0 = -1 + x^2$ has two solutions: $x = -1$ and $x = +1$; hence there are two equilibria in the system (a). The eigenvalues are the derivatives at each equilibrium, $\lambda = (-1 + x^2)' = 2x$, where $x = \pm 1$. Equilibrium $x = -1$ is stable because $\lambda = -2 < 0$. Equilibrium $x = +1$ is unstable because $\lambda = +2 > 0$. The same fact follows from the geometrical analysis in Fig.S.3.

(b) The equation $0 = x - x^3$ has three solutions: $x = \pm 1$ and $x = 0$; hence there are three equilibria in system (b). The eigenvalues are the derivatives at each equilibrium, $\lambda = (x - x^3)' = 1 - 3x^2$. The equilibria $x = \pm 1$ are stable because $\lambda = 1 - 3(\pm 1)^2 = -2 < 0$. The equilibrium $x = 0$ is unstable because $\lambda = 1 > 0$. The same conclusions follow from the geometrical analysis in Fig.S.3.

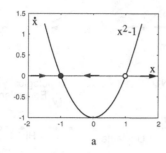
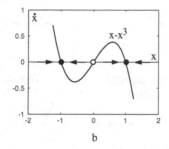

Figure S.3: Phase portraits of the systems (a) $\dot{x} = -1 + x^2$, and (b) $\dot{x} = x - x^3$.

4. The equilibrium $x = 0$ is stable in all three cases.

5. See Fig.S.4. Topologically equivalent systems are in (a), (b), and (c). In (d) there are different numbers of equilibria; no stretching or shrinking of the rubber phase line can produce new equilibria. In (e) the right equilibrium is unstable in $\dot{V} = F_1(V)$ but stable in $\dot{V} = F_2(V)$; no stretching or shrinking can change the stability of an equilibrium. In (f) the flow between the two equilibria is directed rightward in $\dot{V} = F_1(V)$ and leftward in $\dot{V} = F_2(V)$; no stretching or shrinking can change the direction of the flow.

6. (Saddle-node [fold] bifurcation in $\dot{x} = a + x^2$) The equation $0 = a + x^2$ has no real solutions when $a > 0$, and two solutions $x = \pm\sqrt{|a|}$ when $a \le 0$. Hence there are two branches of equilibria, depicted in Fig.S.5. The eigenvalues are

$$\lambda = (a + x^2)' = 2x = \pm 2\sqrt{|a|}.$$

The lower branch $-\sqrt{|a|}$ is stable ($\lambda < 0$), and the upper branch $+\sqrt{|a|}$ is unstable ($\lambda > 0$). They meet at the saddle-node (fold) bifurcation point $a = 0$.

7.

|   |   |   |
|---|---|---|
| (a) $x = -1$ at $a = 1$ | (b) $x = -1/2$ at $a = 1/4$ | (c) $x = 1/2$ at $a = 1/4$ |
| (d) $x = \pm 1/\sqrt{3}$ at $a = \pm 2/(3\sqrt{3})$ | (e) $x = \pm 1$ at $a = \mp 2$ | (f) $x = -1$ at $a = 1$ |

8. (Pitchfork bifurcation in $\dot{x} = bx - x^3$) The equation $0 = bx - x^3$ has one solution $x = 0$ when $b \le 0$, and three solutions $x = 0$, $x = \pm\sqrt{b}$ when $b > 0$. Hence there is only one branch of equilibria for $b < 0$ and three branches for $b > 0$ of the pitchfork curve depicted in Fig.S.6. The eigenvalues are

$$\lambda = (bx - x^3)' = b - 3x^2.$$

The branch $x = 0$ exists for any $b$, and its eigenvalue is $\lambda = b$. Thus, it is stable for $b < 0$ and unstable for $b > 0$. The two branches $x = \pm\sqrt{b}$ exist only for $b > 0$, but they are always stable because $\lambda = b - 3(\pm\sqrt{b})^2 = -2b < 0$. We see that the branch $x = 0$ loses stability when $b$ passes the pitchfork bifurcation value $b = 0$, at which point a pair of new stable branches bifurcates (hence the name *bifurcation*). In other words, the stable branch $x = 0$ divides (bifurcates) into two stable branches when $b$ passes 0.

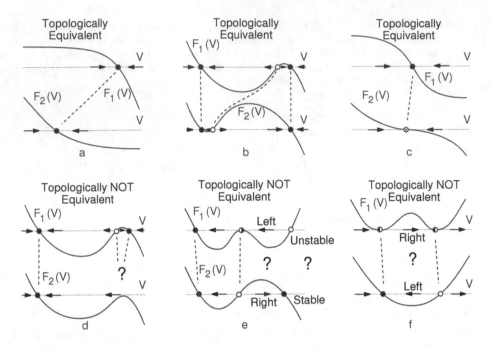

Figure S.4: Answer to chapter 3, exercise 5.

9. Recall that the current $I_{\text{Kir}}$ is turned off by depolarization and turned on by hyperpolarization. The dynamics of the $I_{\text{Kir}}$-model is similar to that of the $I_{\text{Na,p}}$-model in many respects. In particular, this system can also have coexistence of two stable equilibria separated by an unstable equilibrium, which follows from the N-shaped I-V relation. Indeed, when $V$ is hyperpolarized, the current $I_{\text{Kir}}$ is turned on (deinactivated), and it pulls $V$ toward $E_{\text{K}}$. In contrast, when $V$ is depolarized, the current is turned off (inactivated), and does not obstruct further depolarization of $V$.

Use (3.11) to find the curve

$$I = g_{\text{L}}(V - E_{\text{L}}) + g_{\text{Kir}} h_\infty(V)(V - E_{\text{K}}) ,$$

in Fig.S.8. (The curve may not be S-shaped if a different bifurcation parameter is used, as in exercise 12a below).

The bifurcation diagram of the $I_{\text{Kir}}$-model (3.11) in Fig.S.8 has three branches corresponding to the three equilibria. When the parameter $I$ is relatively small, the outward $I_{\text{Kir}}$ current dominates and the system has only one equilibrium in the low voltage range – the down-state. When the parameter $I$ is relatively large, the injected inward current $I$ dominates, and the system has one equilibrium in the intermediate voltage range – the up-state. When the parameter $I$ is in neighborhood of $I = 6$, the system exhibits bistability of the up-state and the down-state. The states appear and disappear via saddle-node bifurcations. The behavior of the $I_{\text{Kir}}$-model is conceptually (and qualitatively) similar to the behavior of the $I_{\text{Na,p}}$-model (3.5) even though the models have completely different ionic mechanisms for bistability.

10. The equilibrium satisfies the one-dimensional equation

$$0 = I - g_{\text{K}} n_\infty^4(V)(V - E_{\text{K}}) - g_{\text{Na}} m_\infty^3(V) h_\infty(V)(V - E_{\text{Na}}) - g_{\text{L}}(V - E_{\text{L}}) ,$$

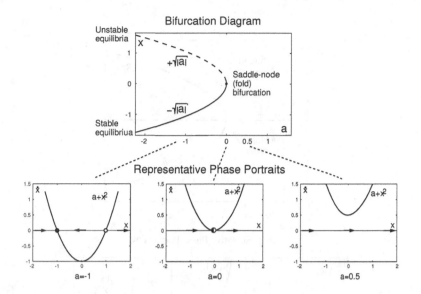

Figure S.5: Saddle-node (fold) bifurcation diagram and representative phase portraits of the system $\dot{x} = a + x^2$ (see chapter 3, exercise 6).

where all gating variables assume their asymptotic values. The solution

$$I = g_K n_\infty^4(V)(V - E_K) + g_{Na} m_\infty^3(V) h_\infty(V)(V - E_{Na}) + g_L(V - E_L)$$

is depicted in Fig.S.9. Since the curve in this figure does not have folds, there are no saddle-node bifurcations in the Hodgkin-Huxley model (with the original values of parameters).

11. The curves

$$\text{(a)} \qquad g_L(V) = -g_{Na} m_\infty(V)(V - E_{Na})/(V - E_L)$$

and

$$\text{(b)} \qquad E_L(V) = V + g_{Na} m_\infty(V)(V - E_{Na})(V - E_L)/g_L$$

are depicted in Fig.S.7.

12. The curves

$$\text{(a)} \qquad g_L(V) = \{I - g_{Kir} h_\infty(V)(V - E_K)\}/(V - E_L)$$

and

$$\text{(b)} \qquad g_{Kir}(V) = \{I - g_L(V - E_L)\}/\{h_\infty(V)(V - E_K)\}$$

are depicted in Fig.S.10. Note that the curve in Fig.S.10a does not have the S shape.

13.

$$F'(V) = -g_L - g_K m_\infty^4(V) - g_K 4 m_\infty^3(V) m'_\infty(V)(V - E_K) < 0$$

because $g_L > 0$, $m_\infty(V) > 0$, $m'_\infty(V) > 0$, and $V - E_K > 0$ for all $V > E_K$.

14.

$$F'(V) = -g_L - g_h h_\infty(V) - g_h h'_\infty(V)(V - E_h) < 0$$

because $g_L > 0$, $h_\infty(V) > 0$, but $h'_\infty(V) < 0$ and $V - E_h < 0$ for all $V < E_h$.

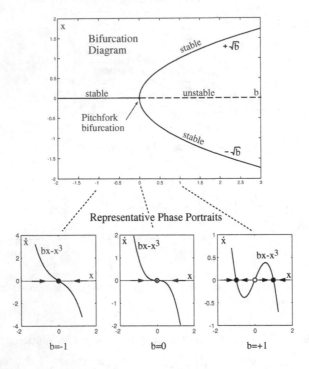

Figure S.6: Pitchfork bifurcation diagram and representative phase portraits of the system $\dot{x} = bx - x^3$ (see chapter 3, exercise 8).

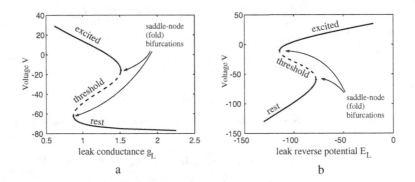

Figure S.7: Bifurcation diagrams of the $I_{\mathrm{Na,p}}$-model (3.5) with bifurcation parameters (a) $g_{\mathrm{L}}$ and (b) $E_{\mathrm{L}}$ (see chapter 3, exercise 11).

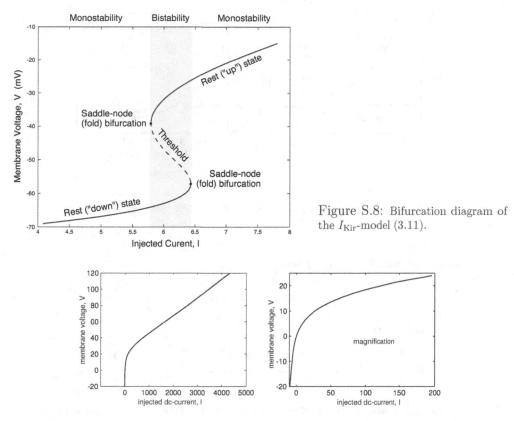

Figure S.8: Bifurcation diagram of the $I_{\mathrm{Kir}}$-model (3.11).

Figure S.9: Dependence of the position of equilibrium in the Hodgkin-Huxley model on the injected DC current; see exercise 10.

15. When $V$ is sufficiently large, $\dot{V} \approx V^2$. The solution of $\dot{V} = V^2$ is $V(t) = 1/(c - t)$ (check by differentiating), where $c = 1/V(0)$. Another way to show this is to solve (3.9) for $V$ and find the asymptote of the solution.

16. Each equilibrium of the system $\dot{x} = a + bx - x^3$ is a solution to the equation $0 = a + bx - x^3$. Treating $x$ and $b$ as free parameters, the set of all equilibria is given by $a = -bx + x^3$, and it looks like the cusp surface in Fig.6.34. Each point where the cusp surface folds, corresponds to a saddle-node (fold) bifurcation. The derivative with respect to $x$ at each such point is zero; alternatively, the vector tangent to the cusp surface at each such point is parallel to the $x$-axis. The set of all bifurcation points is projected to the $(a, b)$-plane at the bottom of the figure, and it looks like a curve having two branches. To find the equation for the bifurcation curves, one needs to remember that each bifurcation point satisfies two conditions:

   - It is an equilibrium; that is, $a + bx - x^3 = 0$.

   - The derivative of $a + bx - x^3$ with respect to $x$ is zero; that is, $b - 3x^2 = 0$.

Solving the second equation for $x$ and using the solution $x = \pm\sqrt{b/3}$ in the first equation yields $a = \mp 2(b/3)^{3/2}$. The point $a = b = 0$ is called a cusp bifurcation point.

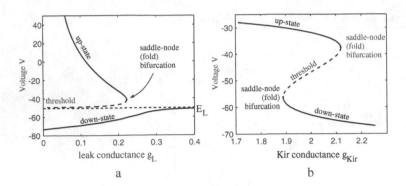

Figure S.10: Bifurcation diagrams of the $I_{Kir}$-model (3.11), $I = 6$, with bifurcation parameters (a) $g_L$ and (b) $g_{Kir}$ (see chapter 3, exercise 12).

17. (Gradient systems) For $\dot{V} = F(V)$ take

$$E(V) = -\int_c^V F(v)\, dv \, ,$$

where $c$ is any constant.

        a.  $E(V) = 1$         b.  $E(V) = -V$         c.  $E(V) = V^2/2$
        d.  $E(V) = V - V^3/3$   e.  $E(V) = -V^2/2 + V^4/4$   f.  $E(V) = -\cos V$

18. (c) implies (b) because $|x(t) - y| < \exp(-at)$ implies that $x(t) \to y$ as $t \to \infty$. (b) implies (a) according to the definition.

(a) does not imply (b) because $x(t)$ may not approach $y$. For example, $y = 0$ is an equilibrium in the system $\dot{x} = 0$ (any other point is also an equilibrium). It is stable, since $|x(t) - 0| < \varepsilon$ for all $|x_0 - 0| < \varepsilon$ and all $t \geq 0$. However, it is not asymptotically stable because $\lim_{t\to\infty} x(t) = x_0 \neq 0$ regardless of how close $x_0$ is to 0 (unless $x_0 = 0$).

(b) does not imply (c). For example, the equilibrium $y = 0$ in the system $\dot{x} = -x^3$ is asymptotically stable (check by differentiating that $x(t) = (2t + x_0^{-2})^{-1/2} \to 0$ is a solution with $x(0) = x_0$); however, $x(t)$ approaches 0 with a slower than exponential rate, $\exp(-at)$, for any constant $a > 0$.

# Solutions for chapter 4

1. See figures S.11–S.15.

2. See Fig.S.16.

3. See figures S.17–S.21.

4. The diagram follows from the form of the eigenvalues

$$\lambda = \frac{\tau \pm \sqrt{\tau^2 - 4\Delta}}{2} \, .$$

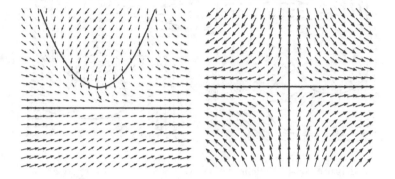

Figure S.11: Nullclines of the vector field; see also Fig.S.17.

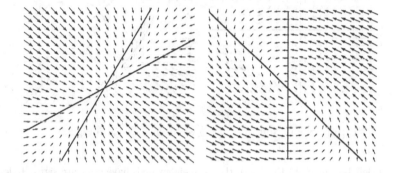

Figure S.12: Nullclines of the vector field; see also Fig.S.18.

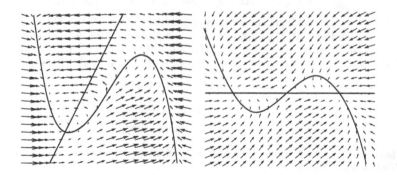

Figure S.13: Nullclines of the vector field; see also Fig.S.19.

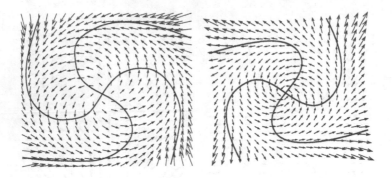

Figure S.14: Nullclines of the vector field; see also Fig.S.20.

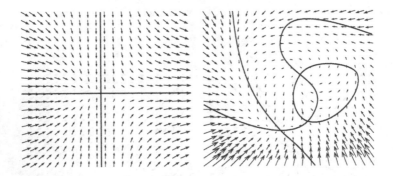

Figure S.15: Nullclines of the vector field; see also Fig.S.21.

If $\Delta < 0$ (left half-plane in Fig.4.15), then the eigenvalues have opposite signs. Indeed,

$$\sqrt{\tau^2 - 4\Delta} > \sqrt{\tau^2} = |\tau| \,,$$

whence

$$\tau + \sqrt{\tau^2 - 4\Delta} > 0 \qquad \text{and} \qquad \tau - \sqrt{\tau^2 - 4\Delta} < 0 \,.$$

The equilibrium is a saddle in this case. Now consider the case $\Delta > 0$. When $\tau^2 < 4\Delta$ (inside the parabola in Fig.4.15), the eigenvalues are complex-conjugate; hence the equilibrium is a focus. It is stable (unstable) when $\tau < 0$ ($\tau > 0$). When $\tau^2 > 4\Delta$ (outside the parabola in Fig.4.15), the eigenvalues are real. Both are negative (positive) when $\tau < 0$ ($\tau > 0$).

5. (van der Pol oscillator) The nullclines of the van der Pol oscillator,

$$y = x - x^3/3 \quad (x\text{-nullcline}) \,,$$
$$x = 0 \quad (y\text{-nullcline}) \,,$$

are depicted in Fig.S.22. There is a unique equilibrium $(0,0)$. The Jacobian matrix at the equilibrium has the form

$$L = \begin{pmatrix} 1 & -1 \\ b & 0 \end{pmatrix} \,.$$

Since $\operatorname{tr} L = 1 > 0$ and $\det L = b > 0$, the equilibrium is always an unstable focus.

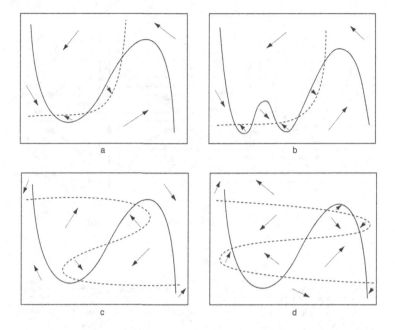

Figure S.16: Approximate directions of the vector in each region between the nullclines.

6. (Bonhoeffer–van der Pol oscillator) The nullclines of the Bonhoeffer–van der Pol oscillator with $c = 0$ have the form

$$y = x - x^3/3 \quad (x\text{-nullcline}) ,$$
$$x = a \quad (y\text{-nullcline}) ,$$

shown in Fig.S.23. They intersect at the point $x = a$, $y = a - a^3/3$. The Jacobian matrix at the equilibrium $(a, a - a^3/3)$ has the form

$$L = \begin{pmatrix} 1 - a^2 & -1 \\ b & 0 \end{pmatrix} .$$

Since $\operatorname{tr} L = 1 - a^2$ and $\det L = b > 0$, the equilibrium is a stable (unstable) focus when $|a| > 1$ ($|a| < 1$), as we illustrate in Fig.S.23.

7. (Hindmarsh-Rose spiking neuron) The Jacobian matrix at the equilibrium $(\bar{x}, \bar{y})$ is

$$L = \begin{pmatrix} f' & -1 \\ g' & -1 \end{pmatrix} ,$$

therefore

$$\operatorname{tr} L = f' - 1 \quad \text{and} \quad \det L = -f' + g' .$$

The equilibrium is a saddle ($\det L < 0$) when $g' < f'$, that is, in the region below the diagonal in Fig.S.24. When $g' > f'$, the equilibrium is stable ($\operatorname{tr} L < 0$) when $f' < 1$, which is the left half-plane in Fig.S.24. Using the classification in Fig.4.15, we conclude that it is a focus when $(f' - 1)^2 - 4(g' - f') < 0$, that is, when

$$g' > \frac{1}{4}(f' + 1)^2,$$

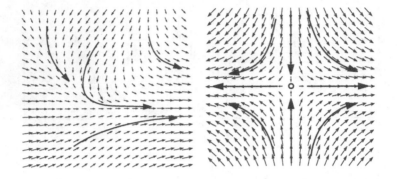

Figure S.17: *Left:* No equilibria. *Right:* Saddle equilibrium.

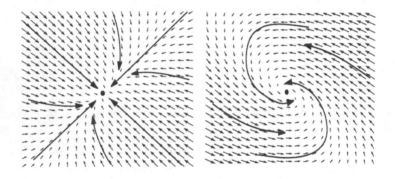

Figure S.18: *Left:* Stable node. *Right:* Stable focus.

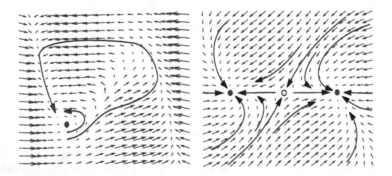

Figure S.19: *Left:* Excitable system having one stable equilibrium. *Right:* Two stable nodes separated by a saddle equilibrium.

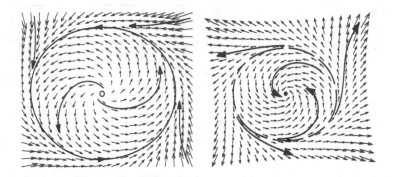

Figure S.20: *Left:* Unstable focus inside a stable limit cycle. *Right:* Stable focus inside an unstable limit cycle.

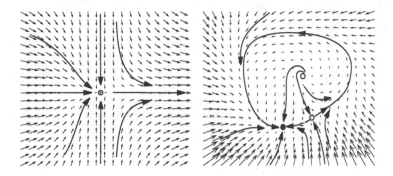

Figure S.21: *Left:* Saddle-node equilibrium. *Right:* Stable node and saddle equilibria connected by two heteroclinic trajectories, which form an invariant circle with an unstable focus inside.

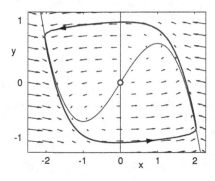

Figure S.22: Nullclines and phase portrait of the van der Pol oscillator ($b = 0.1$).

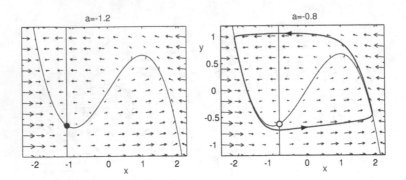

Figure S.23: Nullclines and phase portrait of the Bonhoeffer–van der Pol oscillator ($b = 0.05$ and $c = 0$).

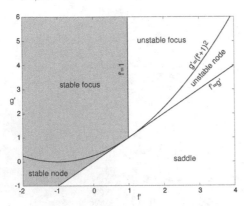

Figure S.24: Stability diagram of the Hindmarsh-Rose spiking neuron model; see exercise 7.

which is the upper part of the parabola in Fig.S.24.

8. ($I_K$-model) The steady-state I-V relation of the $I_K$-model is monotone; hence it has a unique equilibrium, which we denoted here as $(\bar{V}, \bar{m}) \in \mathbb{R}^2$, where $\bar{V} > E_K$ and $\bar{m} = m_\infty(\bar{V})$. The Jacobian at the equilibrium has the form

$$L = \begin{pmatrix} -(g_L + \bar{g}_K \bar{m}^4)/C & -4\bar{g}_K \bar{m}^3 (\bar{V} - E_K)/C \\ m'_\infty(\bar{V})/\tau(\bar{V}) & -1/\tau(\bar{V}) \end{pmatrix} ,$$

with the signs

$$L = \begin{pmatrix} - & - \\ + & - \end{pmatrix} .$$

Obviously, $\det L > 0$ and $\operatorname{tr} L < 0$; hence the equilibrium (focus or node) is always stable.

9. ($I_h$-model) The steady-state I-V relation of the $I_h$-model is monotone; hence it has a unique equilibrium denote here as $(\bar{V}, \bar{h}) \in \mathbb{R}^2$, where $\bar{V} < E_h$ and $\bar{h} = h_\infty(\bar{V})$. The Jacobian at the equilibrium has the form

$$L = \begin{pmatrix} -(g_L + \bar{g}_h \bar{h})/C & -\bar{g}_h (\bar{V} - E_h)/C \\ h'_\infty(\bar{V})/\tau(\bar{V}) & -1/\tau(\bar{V}) \end{pmatrix} ,$$

with the signs

$$L = \begin{pmatrix} - & + \\ - & - \end{pmatrix} .$$

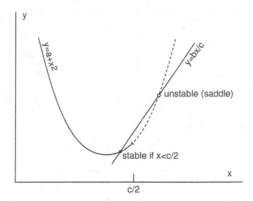

Figure S.25: The left equilibrium is stable when $x < c/2$; see exercise 11.

Obviously, $\det L > 0$ and $\operatorname{tr} L < 0$; hence the equilibrium is always stable.

10. (Bendixson's criterion) The divergence of the vector field of the $I_\text{K}$-model

$$\overbrace{(-g_\text{L} - \bar{g}_\text{K} m^4)/C}^{\partial f(x,y)/\partial x} + \overbrace{-1/\tau(V)}^{\partial g(x,y)/\partial y}$$

is always negative; hence the model cannot have a periodic orbit. Therefore, it cannot have sustained oscillations.

11. The $x$-nullcline is $y = a + x^2$ and the $y$-nullcline is $y = bx/c$, as in Fig.S.25. The equilibria (intersections of the nullclines) are

$$\bar{x} = \frac{b/c \pm \sqrt{(b/c)^2 - 4a}}{2}, \qquad \bar{y} = b\bar{x}/c,$$

provided that $a < \frac{1}{4}(b/c)^2$. The Jacobian matrix at $(\bar{x}, \bar{y})$ has the form

$$L = \begin{pmatrix} 2\bar{x} & -1 \\ b & -c \end{pmatrix}$$

with $\operatorname{tr} L = 2\bar{x} - c$ and

$$\det L = -2\bar{x}c + b = \mp\sqrt{b^2 - 4ac^2}.$$

Thus, the right equilibrium (i.e., $(b/c + \sqrt{(b/c)^2 - 4a})/2$) is always a saddle and the left equilibrium (i.e., $(b/c - \sqrt{(b/c)^2 - 4a})/2$) is always a focus or a node. It is always stable when it lies on the left branch of the parabola $y = a + x^2$ (i.e., when $\bar{x} < 0$), and also can be stable on the right branch if it is not too far from the parabola knee (i.e., if $\bar{x} < c/2$); see Fig.S.25.

# Solutions for chapter 5

1. The $I_\text{A}$-model with instantaneous activation has the form

$$C\dot{V} = I - \overbrace{g_\text{L}(V - E_\text{L})}^{\text{leak } I_\text{L}} - \overbrace{\bar{g}_\text{A} m_\infty(V) h(V - E_\text{K})}^{I_\text{A}}$$
$$\dot{h} = (h_\infty(V) - h)/\tau(V).$$

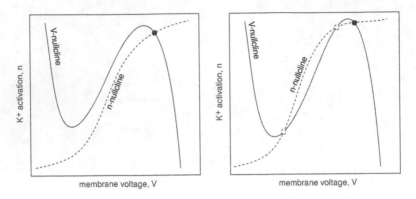

Figure S.26: Answer to exercise 2.

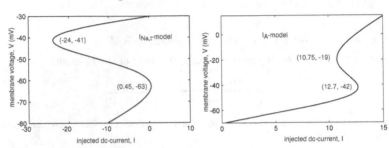

Figure S.27: The saddle-node bifurcation diagrams of the $I_{\mathrm{Na,t}}$- and $I_{\mathrm{A}}$-minimal models.

To apply the Bendixson criterion (chapter 4, exercise 10), we first determine the divergence of this vector field

$$\frac{\partial \dot{V}}{\partial V} + \frac{\partial \dot{h}}{\partial h} = -\{g_{\mathrm{L}} + \bar{g}_{\mathrm{A}} m'_{\infty}(V) h(V - E_{\mathrm{K}}) + \bar{g}_{\mathrm{A}} m_{\infty}(V) h\}/C - 1/\tau(V) < 0\,.$$

Since it is always negative, the $I_{\mathrm{A}}$-model cannot have limit cycle attractors (or any other closed loop orbit).

2. See Fig.S.26.

3. The curves

$$I = g_{\mathrm{L}}(V - E_{\mathrm{L}}) + \bar{g}_{\mathrm{Na}} m^3_{\infty}(V) h_{\infty}(V)(V - E_{\mathrm{Na}})$$

and

$$I = g_{\mathrm{L}}(V - E_{\mathrm{L}}) + \bar{g}_{\mathrm{A}} m_{\infty}(V) h_{\infty}(V)(V - E_{\mathrm{K}})$$

are depicted in Fig.S.27.

4. $g$ is not an absolute conductance, but is taken relative to the conductance at the resting state. Negative values occur because the initial holding voltage value in the voltage-clamp experiment described in Fig.5.22a corresponds to the resting potential, at which the $K^+$ conductance is partially activated. Indeed, in the $I_{\mathrm{Na,p}}+I_{\mathrm{K}}$-model the $K^+$ gating variable $n \approx 0.04$; hence the $K^+$ conductance is approximately 0.4 (because $\bar{g}_{\mathrm{K}} = 10$). According to the procedure, this value corresponds to $g = 0$. Any small decrease in conductance would result in negative values of $g$. If the initial holding voltage were very negative, say below $-100$ mV, then the slow conductance $g$ would have nonnegative values in the relevant voltage range (above $-100$ mV).

5. The curve $I_{\text{slow}}(V)$ defines slow changes of the membrane voltage. The curve $I - I_{\text{fast}}(V)$ defines fast changes. Its middle part, which has a positive slope, is unstable. If the I-V curves intersect in the middle part, the equilibrium is unstable, and the system exhibits periodic spiking: The voltage slowly slides down the left branch of the fast I-V curve toward the slow I-V curve until it reaches the left knee, and then jumps quickly to the right branch. After the jump, the voltage slowly slides up the right branch until it reaches the right knee, and then quickly jumps to the left branch along the straight line that connects the knee and the point $(E_{\text{K}}, 0)$ (see also previous exercise). Note that the direction of the jump is not horizontal, as in relaxation oscillators, but along a sloped line. On that line the slow conductance $g$ is constant, but the slow current $I_{\text{slow}}(V) = g(V - E_{\text{K}})$ changes quickly because the driving force $V - E_{\text{K}}$ changes quickly. When the I-V curves intersect at the stable point (negative slope of $I - I_{\text{fast}}(V)$), the voltage variable may produce a single action potential, then slide slowly toward the intersection, which is a stable equilibrium.

# Solutions for chapter 6

1. There are two equilibria: $x = 0$ and $x = b$. The stability is determined by the sign of the derivative

$$\lambda = (x(b - x))'_x = b - 2x$$

at the equilibrium. Since $\lambda = b$ when $x = 0$, this equilibrium is stable (unstable) when $b < 0$ ($b > 0$). Since $\lambda = -b$ when $x = b$, this equilibrium is unstable (stable) when $b < 0$ ($b > 0$).

2. (a) The system

$$\dot{x} = bx^2, \qquad b \neq 0$$

cannot exhibit saddle-node bifurcation: It has one equilibrium for any nonzero $b$, or an infinite number of equilibria when $b = 0$. The equilibrium $x = 0$ is non-hyperbolic, and the non-degeneracy condition is satisfied ($a = b \neq 0$). However, the transversality condition is not satisfied at the equilibrium $x = 0$. Another example is $\dot{x} = b^2 + x^2$.

(b) The system

$$\dot{x} = b - x^3$$

has a single stable equilibrium for any $b$. However, the point $x = 0$ is non-hyperbolic when $b = 0$ and the transversality condition is also satisfied. The non-degeneracy condition is violated, however.

3. It is easy to check (by differentiating) that

$$V(t) = \frac{\sqrt{c(b - b_{\text{sn}})}}{\sqrt{a}} \tan(\sqrt{ac(b - b_{\text{sn}})}\, t)$$

is a solution to the system. Since $\tan(-\pi/2) = -\infty$ and $\tan(+\pi/2) = +\infty$, it takes

$$T = \frac{\pi}{\sqrt{ac(b - b_{\text{sn}})}}$$

for the solution to go from $-\infty$ to $+\infty$.

4. The first system can be transformed into the second if we use complex coordinates $z = u + iv$. To obtain the third system, we use polar coordinates

$$re^{i\varphi} = z = u + iv \in \mathbb{C},$$

so that

$$\underbrace{\dot{z}}\qquad\qquad \overbrace{(c(b)+\mathrm{i}\omega(b))z+(a+\mathrm{i}d)z|z|^2}$$
$$\dot{r}e^{\mathrm{i}\varphi} + re^{\mathrm{i}\varphi}\mathrm{i}\dot{\varphi} = (c(b) + \mathrm{i}\omega(b))re^{\mathrm{i}\varphi} + (a + \mathrm{i}d)r^3 e^{\mathrm{i}\varphi} \ .$$

Next, we divide both sides of this equation by $e^{\mathrm{i}\varphi}$ and separate the real and imaginary parts to obtain

$$\{\dot{r} - c(b)r - ar^3\} + \mathrm{i}r\{\dot{\varphi} - \omega(b) - dr^2\} = 0 \ ,$$

which we can write in the polar coordinates form.

5.  (a) The equilibrium $r = 0$ of the system

$$\begin{aligned}\dot{r} &= br^3 \ , \\ \dot{\varphi} &= 1 \ , \end{aligned}$$

   has a pair of complex-conjugate eigenvalues $\pm \mathrm{i}$ for any $b$, and the non-degeneracy condition is satisfied for any $b \neq 0$. However, the transversality condition is violated, and the system does not exhibit Andronov-Hopf bifurcation (no limit cycle exists near the equilibrium).

   (b) The equilibrium $r = 0$ for $b = 0$

$$\begin{aligned}\dot{r} &= br \ , \\ \dot{\varphi} &= 1 \ , \end{aligned}$$

   has a pair of complex-conjugate eigenvalues $\pm \mathrm{i}$ and the transversality condition is satisfied. However, the bifurcation is not of the Andronov-Hopf type because no limit cycle exists near the equilibrium for any $b$.

6. The Jacobian matrix at the equilibrium $(u, v) = (0,0)$ has the form

$$L = \begin{pmatrix} b & -1 \\ 1 & b \end{pmatrix} \ .$$

It has eigenvalues $b\pm\mathrm{i}$. Therefore, the loss of stability occurs at $b = 0$, and the non-hyperbolicity and transversality conditions are satisfied. Since the model can be reduced to the polar-coordinate system (see exercise 4) and $a \neq 0$, the non-degeneracy condition is also satisfied, and the system undergoes an Andronov-Hopf bifurcation.

7. Since

$$(cr + ar^3)'_r = c + 3ar^2 = c + 3a|c/a| = \left\{ \begin{array}{ll} c + 3|c| & \text{when } a > 0, \\ c - 3|c| & \text{when } a < 0, \end{array} \right.$$

the limit cycle is stable when $a < 0$.

8. The sequence of bifurcations is similar to that of the RS neuron in Fig.8.15. The resting state is a globally asymptotically stable equilibrium for $I < 5.64$. At this value a stable (spiking) limit cycle appears via a big saddle homoclinic orbit bifurcation. At $I = 5.8$ a small-amplitude unstable limit cycle is born via another saddle homoclinic orbit bifurcation. This cycle shrinks to the equilibrium and makes it lose stability via subcritical Andronov-Hopf bifurcation at $I = 6.5$. This unstable focus becomes an unstable node when $I$ increases, and then it coalesces with the saddle (at $I = 7.3$) and disappears. Note that there is a saddle-node bifurcation according to the I-V relation, but it corresponds to the disappearance of an unstable equilibrium.

9. The Jacobian matrix of partial derivatives has the form

$$L = \begin{pmatrix} -I'_V(V,x) & -I'_x(V,x) \\ x'_\infty(V)/\tau(V) & -1/\tau(V) \end{pmatrix},$$

so that

$$\operatorname{tr} L = -\{I'_V(V,x) + 1/\tau(V)\}$$

and

$$\det L = \{I'_V(V,x) + I'_x(V,x)x'_\infty(V)\}/\tau(V) = I'_\infty(V)/\tau(V).$$

The characteristic equation

$$\lambda^2 - \lambda \operatorname{tr} L + \det L = 0$$

has two solutions

$$\overbrace{(\operatorname{tr} L)/2}^{c} \pm \overbrace{\sqrt{\{(\operatorname{tr} L)/2\}^2 - \det L}}^{\omega}$$

which might be complex-conjugate.

10. Let $z = re^{\varphi \mathbf{i}}$; then

$$\begin{aligned} r' &= ar + r^3 - r^5, \\ \varphi' &= \omega. \end{aligned}$$

Any limit cycle is an equilibrium of the amplitude equation, that is,

$$a + r^2 - r^4 = 0.$$

The system undergoes fold limit cycle bifurcation when the amplitude equation undergoes a saddle-node bifurcation, that is, when

$$a + 3r^2 - 5r^4 = 0$$

(check the non-degeneracy and transversality conditions). The two equations have the non-trivial solution $(a, r) = (-1/4, 1/\sqrt{2})$.

11. The projection onto the $v_1$-axis is described by the equation

$$\dot{x} = \lambda_1 x, \qquad x(0) = a.$$

The trajectory leaves the square when $x(t) = ae^{\lambda_1 t} = 1$; that is, when

$$t = -\frac{1}{\lambda_1} \ln a = -\frac{1}{\lambda_1} \ln \tau(I - I_b).$$

12. Equation (6.13) has two bifurcation parameters, $b$ and $v$, and the saddle-node homoclinic bifurcation occurs when $b = b_{sn}$ and $v = V_{sn}$. The saddle-node bifurcation curve is the straight line $b = b_{sn}$ (any $v$). This bifurcation is *on* an invariant circle when $v < V_{sn}$ and *off* otherwise. When $b > b_{sn}$, there are no equilibria and the normal form exhibits periodic spiking. When $b < b_{sn}$, the normal form has two equilibria,

$$\overbrace{V_{sn} - \sqrt{c|b - b_{sn}|/a}}^{\text{node}} \qquad \text{and} \qquad \overbrace{V_{sn} + \sqrt{c|b - b_{sn}|/a}}^{\text{saddle}}.$$

The saddle homoclinic orbit bifurcation occurs when the voltage is reset to the saddle, that is, when

$$v = V_{sn} + \sqrt{c|b - b_{sn}|/a}.$$

13. The Jacobian matrix at an equilibrium is

$$L = \begin{pmatrix} 2v & -1 \\ ab & -a \end{pmatrix}.$$

Saddle-node condition $\det L = -2va + ab = 0$ results in $v = b/2$. Since $v$ is an equilibrium, it satisfies $v^2 - bv + I = 0$; hence $b^2 = 4I$. The Andronov-Hopf condition $\operatorname{tr} L = 2v - a = 0$ results in $v = a/2$; hence $a^2/4 - ab/2 + I = 0$. The bifurcation occurs when $\det L > 0$, resulting in $a < b$. Combining the saddle-node and Andronov-Hopf conditions results in the Bogdanov-Takens conditions.

14. Change of variables (6.5), $v = x$ and $u = \sqrt{\mu}y$, transforms the relaxation oscillator into the form

$$\begin{aligned} \dot{x} &= f(x) - \sqrt{\mu}y \\ \dot{y} &= \sqrt{\mu}(x - b) \end{aligned} \quad \text{with the Jacobian} \quad L = \begin{pmatrix} f'(b) & -\sqrt{\mu} \\ \sqrt{\mu} & 0 \end{pmatrix}$$

at the equilibrium $v = x = b$, $u = \sqrt{\mu}y = f(b)$. The Andronov-Hopf bifurcation occurs when $\operatorname{tr} L = f'(b) = 0$ and $\det L = \mu > 0$. Using (6.7), we find that it is supercritical when $f'''(b) < 0$ and subcritical when $f'''(b) > 0$.

15. The Jacobian matrix at the equilibrium, which satisfies $F(v) - bv = 0$, is

$$L = \begin{pmatrix} F' & -1 \\ \mu b & -\mu \end{pmatrix}.$$

The Andronov-Hopf bifurcation occurs when $\operatorname{tr} L = F' - \mu = 0$ (hence $F' = \mu$) and $\det L = \omega^2 = \mu b - \mu^2 > 0$ (hence $b > \mu$). The change of variables (6.5), $v = x$ and $u = \mu x + \omega y$, transforms the system into the form

$$\begin{aligned} \dot{x} &= -\omega y + f(x) \\ \dot{y} &= \omega x + g(x), \end{aligned}$$

where $f(x) = F(x) - \mu x$ and $g(x) = \mu[bx - F(x)]/\omega$. The result follows from (6.7).

16. The change of variables (6.5) converts the system into the form

$$\begin{aligned} \dot{x} &= F(x) + \text{linear terms} \\ \dot{y} &= \mu(G(x) - F(x))/\omega + \text{linear terms}. \end{aligned}$$

The result follows from (6.7).

17. The change of variables (6.5), $v = x$ and $u = \mu x + \omega y$, converts the system into

$$\begin{aligned} \dot{x} &= F(x) - x(\mu x + \omega y) + \text{linear terms} \\ \dot{y} &= \mu[G(x) - F(x) + x(\mu x + \omega y)]/\omega. \end{aligned}$$

The result follows from (6.7).

18. The system undergoes Andronov-Hopf bifurcation when $F_v = -\mu G_u$ and $F_u G_v < -\mu G_u^2$. We perform all the steps from (6.4) to (6.7), disregarding linear terms (they do not influence $a$) and the terms of the order $o(\mu)$. Let $\omega = \sqrt{-\mu F_u G_v} + \mathcal{O}(\mu)$, then $u = (\mu G_u x - \omega y)/F_u = -\omega y/F_u + \mathcal{O}(\mu)$, and

$$f(x, y) = F(x, -\omega y/F_u + \mathcal{O}(\mu)) = F(x, 0) - F_u(x, 0)\omega y/F_u + \mathcal{O}(\mu)$$

and

$$g(x, y) = (\mu/\omega)[G_u F(x, 0) - F_u G(x, 0)] + \mathcal{O}(\mu).$$

The result follows from (6.7).

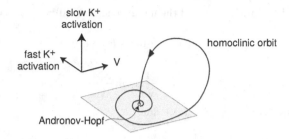

**Figure S.28:** Codimension-2 Shilnikov-Hopf bifurcation.

# Solutions for chapter 7

1. Take $c < 0$ so that the slow $w$-nullcline has a negative slope.

2. The quasi-threshold contains the union of canard solutions.

3. The change of variables $z = e^{i\omega t}u$ transforms the system into the form

$$\dot{u} = \varepsilon\{-u + e^{-i\omega t}I(t)\} ,$$

which can be averaged, yielding

$$\dot{u} = \varepsilon\{-u + I^*(\omega)\} .$$

Apparently, the stable equilibrium $u = I^*(\omega)$ corresponds to the sustained oscillation $z = e^{i\omega t}I^*(\omega)$.

4. The existence of damped oscillations with frequency $\omega$ implies that the system has a focus equilibrium with eigenvalues $-\varepsilon \pm i\omega$, where $\varepsilon > 0$. The local dynamics near the focus can be represented in the form (7.3). The rest of the proof is the same as the one for exercise 3.

5. Even though the slow and the fast nullclines in Fig.5.21 intersect in only one point, they continue to be close and parallel to each other in the voltage range 10 mV to 30 mV. Such a proximity creates a tunneling effect (Rush and Rinzel 1996) that prolongs the time spent near those nullclines.

6. (Shilnikov-Hopf bifurcation) The model is near a codimension-2 bifurcation having a homoclinic orbit to an equilibrium undergoing subcritical Andronov-Hopf bifurcation, as we illustrate in Fig.S.28. Many weird phenomena can happen near bifurcations of codimension-2 or higher.

# Solutions for chapter 8

1. Consider two coupled neurons firing together.

2. The equation

$$\dot{V} = c(b - b_{sn}) + a(V - V_{sn})^2$$

can be written in the form

$$\dot{V} = a(V - V_{rest})(V - V_{thresh})$$

with

$$V_{rest} = V_{sn} - \sqrt{c(b_{sn} - b)/a} \qquad \text{and} \qquad V_{thresh} = V_{sn} + \sqrt{c(b_{sn} - b)/a},$$

provided that $b < b_{sn}$.

3. The system $\dot{v} = b + v^2$ with $b > 0$ and the initial condition $v(0) = v_{\text{reset}}$ has the solution (check by differentiating)

$$v(t) = \sqrt{b}\tan(\sqrt{b}(t + t_0)),$$

where

$$t_0 = \frac{1}{\sqrt{b}}\operatorname{atan}\frac{v_{\text{reset}}}{\sqrt{b}}.$$

From the condition $v(T) = v_{\text{peak}} = 1$, we find

$$T = \frac{1}{\sqrt{b}}\operatorname{atan}\frac{1}{\sqrt{b}} - t_0 = \frac{1}{\sqrt{b}}\left(\operatorname{atan}\frac{1}{\sqrt{b}} - \operatorname{atan}\frac{v_{\text{reset}}}{\sqrt{b}}\right),$$

which alternatively can be written as

$$T = \frac{1}{\sqrt{b}}\operatorname{atan}\left(\sqrt{b}\frac{v_{\text{reset}} - 1}{v_{\text{reset}} + b}\right).$$

4. The system $\dot{v} = -|b| + v^2$ with the initial condition $v(0) = v_{\text{reset}} > \sqrt{|b|}$ has the solution (check by differentiating)

$$v(t) = \sqrt{|b|}\,\frac{1 + e^{2\sqrt{b}(t + t_0)}}{1 - e^{2\sqrt{b}(t + t_0)}},$$

where

$$t_0 = \frac{1}{2\sqrt{|b|}}\ln\frac{v_{\text{reset}} - \sqrt{|b|}}{v_{\text{reset}} + \sqrt{|b|}}.$$

From the condition $v(T) = 1$, we find

$$T = \frac{1}{2\sqrt{|b|}}\left(\ln\frac{1 - \sqrt{|b|}}{1 + \sqrt{|b|}} - \ln\frac{v_{\text{reset}} - \sqrt{|b|}}{v_{\text{reset}} + \sqrt{|b|}}\right).$$

5. The saddle-node bifurcation occurs when $b = 0$, regardless of the value of $v_{\text{reset}}$, which is a straight vertical line in Fig.8.3. If $v_{\text{reset}} < 0$, then the saddle-node bifurcation is on an invariant circle. When $b < 0$, the unstable node (saddle) equilibrium is at $v = \sqrt{|b|}$. Hence, the saddle homoclinic orbit bifurcation occurs when $v_{\text{reset}} = \sqrt{|b|}$.

6. The change of variables $v = g/2 + V$, $b = g^2/4 + B$ transforms $\dot{v} = b - gv + v^2$ to $\dot{V} = B + V^2$ with $V_{\text{reset}} = -\infty$ and $V_{\text{peak}} = +\infty$. It has the threshold $V = \sqrt{B}$, the rheobase $B = 0$, and the same F-I curve as in the original model with $g = 0$. In $v$-coordinates, the threshold is $v = g/2 + \sqrt{b - g^2/4}$, which is greater than $\sqrt{b}$, the new rheobase is $b = g^2/4$, which is greater than $b = 0$, and the new F-I curve is the same as the old one, just shifted to the right by $g^2/4$.

7. Let $b = \varepsilon r$ with $\varepsilon \ll 1$ be a small parameter. The change of variables

$$v = \sqrt{\varepsilon}\tan\frac{\vartheta}{2}$$

uniformly transforms (8.2) into the theta-neuron form

$$\dot{\vartheta} = \sqrt{\varepsilon}\{(1 - \cos\vartheta) + (1 + \cos\vartheta)r\}.$$

on the unit circle except for the small interval $|\vartheta - \pi| < 2\sqrt[4]{\varepsilon}$ corresponding to the action potential ($v > 1$); see Hoppensteadt and Izhikevich (1997) for more details.

8. Use the change of variables

$$v = \frac{\sqrt{\varepsilon}\vartheta}{1 - |\vartheta|} \ .$$

To obtain other theta neuron models, use the change of variables

$$v = \sqrt{\varepsilon}h(\vartheta) \ ,$$

where the monotone function $h$ maps $(-\pi, \pi)$ to $(-\infty, \infty)$ and scales like $1/(\vartheta \pm \pi)$ when $\vartheta \to \pm\pi$. The corresponding model has the form

$$\vartheta' = h^2(\vartheta)/h'(\vartheta) + r/h'(\vartheta) \ .$$

In particular, $h^2(\vartheta)/h'(\vartheta)$ exists, and is bounded and $1/h'(\vartheta) = 0$ when $\vartheta \to \pm\pi$. These imply a uniform velocity independent from the input $r$ when $\vartheta$ passes the value $\pm\pi$ corresponding to firing a spike.

9. The equilibrium $v = I/(b+1), u = bI/(b+1)$ has the Jacobian matrix

$$L = \begin{pmatrix} -1 & -1 \\ ab & -a \end{pmatrix}$$

with $\mathrm{tr}L = -(a+1)$ and $\det L = a(b+1)$. It is a stable node (integrator) when $b < (a+1)^2/(4a) - 1$ and a stable focus (resonator) otherwise.

10. The quadratic integrate-and-fire neuron with a dendritic compartment

$$\begin{aligned} \dot{V} &= B + V^2 + g_1(V_d - V) \\ \dot{V}_d &= g_{\mathrm{leak}}(E_{\mathrm{leak}} - V_d) + g_2(V - V_d) \end{aligned}$$

can be written in the form (8.3, 8.4), with $v = V - g_1/2$, $u = -g_1 V_d$, $I = B - g_1^2/4 - (g_1^2 g_2 + g_{\mathrm{leak}} E_{\mathrm{leak}})/(g_{\mathrm{leak}} + g_2)$, $a = g_{\mathrm{leak}} + g_2$, and $b = -g_1 g_2/a$.

11. A MATLAB program generating the figure is provided on the author's Web page (www.izhikevich.com).

12. An example is in Fig.S.29.

13. An example is in Fig.S.30.

# Solutions for chapter 9

1. (Planar burster) Izhikevich (2000a) suggested the system

$$\begin{aligned} \dot{x} &= x - x^3/3 - u + 4S(x)\cos 40u, \\ \dot{u} &= \mu x \ , \end{aligned}$$

with $S(x) = 1/(1 + e^{5(1-x)})$ and $\mu = 0.01$. It has a hedgehog limit cycle depicted in Fig.S.31.

2. (Noise-induced bursting) Noise can induce bursting in a two-dimensional system with coexistence of resting and spiking states. Indeed, noisy perturbations can randomly push the state of the system into the attraction domain of the resting state or into the attraction domain of the limit cycle attractor, as in Fig.S.32. The solution meanders between the states, exhibiting a random bursting pattern as in Fig.9.55 (right). Neocortical neurons of the RS and FS types, as well as stellate neurons of the entorhinal cortex, exhibit such bursting; see chapter 8.

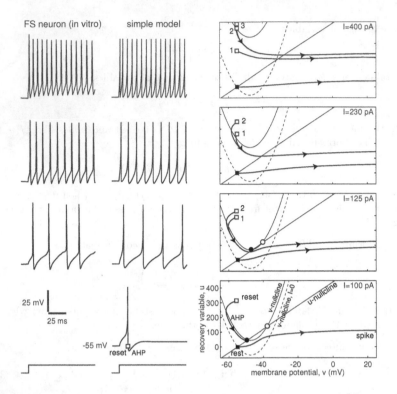

Figure S.29: Comparison of *in vitro* recordings of a fast spiking (FS) interneuron of layer 5 rat visual cortex with simulations of the simple model with linear slow nullcline $20\dot{v} = (v + 55)(v + 40) - u + I$, $\dot{u} = 0.15\{8(v + 55) - u\}$, if $v \geq 25$, then $v \leftarrow -55$, $u \leftarrow u + 200$.

3. (Noise-induced bursting) Bursting occurs because noisy perturbations push the trajectory into and out of the attraction domain of the limit cycle attractor, which coexists with the resting equilibrium; see the phase portrait in Fig.S.33.

4. (Rebound bursting in the FitzHugh-Nagumo oscillator) The oscillator is near the fold limit cycle bifurcation. The solution makes a few rotations along the ghost of the cycle before returning to rest; see Fig.S.34.

5. Yes, they can, at the end of a burst. Think of a "fold/Hopf" or "circle/Hopf" burster. The resting equilibrium is a stable focus immediately after the termination of a burst, and then it is transformed into a stable node to be ready for the circle or fold bifurcation. Even "circle/circle" bursters can exhibit such oscillations, if the resting equilibrium turns into a focus for a short period of time somewhere in the middle of a quiescent phase. In any case, the oscillations should disappear just before the transition to the spiking state.

6. (Hopf/Hopf bursting) Even though there is no coexistence of attractors, there is a hysteresis loop due to the slow passage effect through the supercritical Andronov-Hopf bifurcation; see Fig.S.35. The delayed transition to spiking creates the hysteresis loop and enables bursting.

7. (Hopf/Hopf canonical model) First, we restrict the fast subsystem to its center manifold and transform it into the normal form for supercritical Andronov-Hopf bifurcation, which after

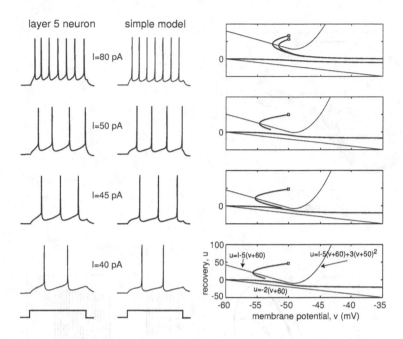

Figure S.30: Comparison of *in vitro* recordings of a regular spiking (RS) neuron with simulations of the simple model $100\dot{v} = I - 5(v+60) + 3(v+50)^2_+ - u$, $\dot{u} = 0.02\{-2(v+60) - u\}$, if $v \geq 35$, then $v \leftarrow -50$, $u \leftarrow u + 70$.

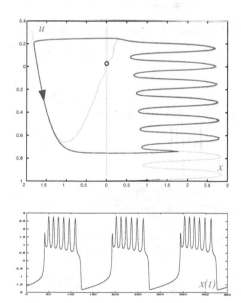

Figure S.31: Solution to exercise 1. Nullclines, a hedgehog limit cycle, and a bursting solution of a planar system. (Modified from Izhikevich 2000a.)

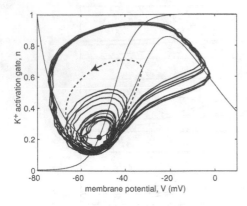

Figure S.32: Noise-induced bursting in two-dimensional system; See exercise 2.

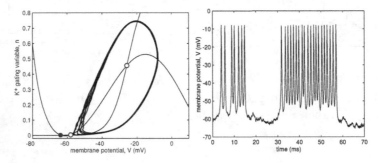

Figure S.33: Noise-induced bursting in a two-dimensional system with coexistence of an equilibrium and a limit cycle attractor; see exercise 3.

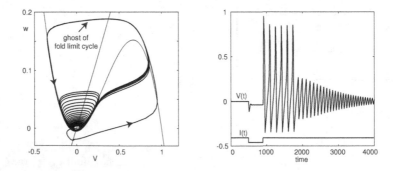

Figure S.34: Rebound bursting in the FitzHugh-Nagumo oscillator; see exercise 4.

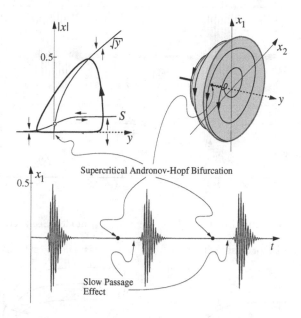

Figure S.35: Hopf/Hopf bursting without coexistence of attractors; see exercise 6. (Modified from Hoppensteadt and Izhikevich 1997.)

appropriate re-scaling, has the form

$$\dot{z} = (u + i\omega)z - z|z|^2 \ .$$

Here, $u$ is the deviation from the slow equilibrium $u_0$. The slow subsystem

$$\dot{u} = \mu g(ze^{i\omega t} + \text{complex-conjugate}, u)$$

can be averaged and transformed into the canonical form.

8. (Bursting in the $I_{\mathrm{Na,t}} + I_{\mathrm{Na,slow}}$-model) First, determine the parameters of the $I_{\mathrm{Na,t}}$-model corresponding to the subcritical Andronov-Hopf bifurcation, and hence the coexistence of the resting and spiking states. Then, add a slow high-threshold persistent Na$^+$ current that activates during spiking, depolarizes the membrane potential, and stops the spiking. During resting, the current deactivates, the membrane potential hyperpolarizes, and the neuron starts to fire again.

9. Replace the slow Na$^+$ current in the exercise above with a slow dendritic compartment with dendritic resting potential far below the somatic resting potential. As the dendritic compartment hyperpolarizes the somatic compartment, the soma starts to fire (due to the inhibition-induced firing described in section 7.2.8). As the somatic compartment fires, the dendritic compartment slowly depolarizes, removes the hyperpolarization and stops firing.

10. (Bursting in the $I_{\mathrm{Na,p}} + I_{\mathrm{K}} + I_{\mathrm{Na,slow}}$-model) The time constant $\tau_{\mathrm{slow}}(V)$ is relatively small in the voltage range corresponding to the spike after-hyperpolarization (AHP). Deactivation of the Na$^+$ current during each AHP is much stronger than its activation during the spike peak. As a result, the Na$^+$ current deactivates (turns off) during the burst, and then slowly reactivates to its baseline level during the resting period, as one can see in Fig.S.36.

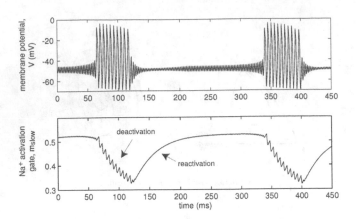

Figure S.36: Bursting in the $I_{Na,p}+I_K+I_{Na,slow}$-model. See exercise 10.

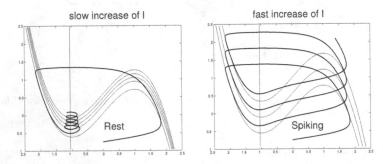

Figure S.37: The system has a unique attractor, equilibrium, yet it can exhibit repetitive spiking activity when the N-shaped nullcline is moved upward not very slowly.

11. The mechanism of spiking, illustrated in Fig.S.37, is closely related to the phenomenon of accommodation and anodal break excitation. The key feature is that this bursting is not fast-slow.

    The system has a unique attractor – a stable equilibrium – and the solution always converges to it. The slow variable $I$ controls the vertical position of the N-shaped nullcline. If $I$ increases, the nullcline slowly moves upward, and so does the solution, because it tracks the equilibrium. However, if the rate of change of $I$ is not small enough, the solution cannot catch up with the equilibrium and starts to oscillate with a large amplitude. Thus, the system exhibits spiking behavior even though it does not have a limit cycle attractor for any fixed $I$.

12. From the first equation, we find the equivalent voltage

$$|z|^2 = |1+u|_+ = \begin{cases} 1+u & \text{if } 1+u > 0\,, \\ 0 & \text{if } 1+u \le 0\,, \end{cases}$$

so that the reduced slow subsystem has the form

$$\begin{aligned} \dot{u} &= \mu[u - u^3 - w]\,, \\ \dot{w} &= \mu[|1+u|_+ - 1]\,, \end{aligned}$$

and it has essentially the same dynamics as the van der Pol oscillator.

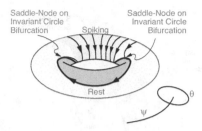

Figure S.38: Answer to exercise 13.

13. The fast equation

$$\dot{\vartheta} = 1 - \cos\vartheta + (1 + \cos\vartheta)r$$

is the Ermentrout-Kopell canonical model for Class 1 excitability, also known as the theta neuron (Ermentrout 1996). It is quiescent when $r < 0$ and fires spikes when $r > 0$. As $\psi$ oscillates with frequency $\omega$, the function $r = r(\psi)$ changes sign. The fast equation undergoes a saddle-node on invariant circle bifurcation; hence the system is a "circle/circle" burster of the slow-wave type; see Fig.S.38.

14. To understand the bursting dynamics of the canonical model, rewrite it in polar coordinates $z = re^{i\varphi}$:

$$
\begin{aligned}
\dot{r} &= ur + 2r^3 - r^5 \,, \\
\dot{u} &= \mu(a - r^2) \,, \\
\dot{\varphi} &= \omega \,.
\end{aligned}
$$

Apparently, it is enough to consider the first two equations, which determine the oscillation profile. Nontrivial ($r \neq 0$) equilibria of this system correspond to limit cycles of the canonical model, which may look like periodic (tonic) spiking with frequency $\omega$. Limit cycles of this system correspond to quasi-periodic solutions of the canonical model, which look like bursting; see Fig.9.37.

The first two equation above have a unique equilibrium,

$$\begin{pmatrix} r \\ u \end{pmatrix} = \begin{pmatrix} \sqrt{a} \\ a^2 - 2a \end{pmatrix}$$

for all $\mu$ and $a > 0$, which is stable when $a > 1$. When $a$ decreases and passes an $\mu$ neighborhood of $a = 1$, the equilibrium loses stability via Andronov-Hopf bifurcation. When $0 < a < 1$, the system has a limit cycle attractor. Therefore, the canonical model exhibits bursting behavior. The smaller the value of $a$, the longer the interburst period. When $a \to 0$, the interburst period becomes infinite.

15. Take $w = I - u$. Then (9.7) becomes

$$
\begin{aligned}
\dot{v} &= v^2 + w \,, \\
\dot{w} &= \mu(I - w) \approx \mu I \,.
\end{aligned}
$$

16. Let us sketch the derivation. Since the fast subsystem is near saddle-node homoclinic orbit bifurcation for some $u = u_0$, a small neighborhood of the saddle-node point $v_0$ is invariantly foliated by stable submanifolds, as in Fig.S.39. Because the contraction along the stable submanifolds is much stronger than the dynamics along the center manifold, the fast subsystem can be mapped into the normal form $\dot{v} = q(u) + p(v - v_0)^2$ by a continuous change of variables.

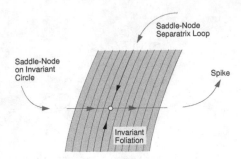

Figure S.39: A small neighborhood of the saddle-node point can be invariantly foliated by stable submanifolds.

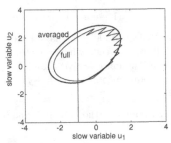

Figure S.40: exercise 18.

When $v$ escapes the small neighborhood of $v_0$, the neuron is said to fire a spike, and $v$ is reset to $v \leftarrow v_0 + c(u)$. Such a stereotypical spike also resets $u$ by a constant $d$. If $g(v_0, u_0) \approx 0$, then all functions are small, and linearization and appropriate re-scaling yield the canonical model. If $g(v_0, u_0) \neq 0$, then the canonical model has the same form as in the previous exercise.

17. The derivation proceeds as in the previous exercise, yielding

$$\begin{aligned} \dot{v} &= I + v^2 + (a, u) , \\ \dot{u} &= \mu A u . \end{aligned}$$

where $(a, u)$ is the scalar (dot) product of vectors $a, u \in \mathbb{R}^2$, and $A$ is the Jacobian matrix at the equilibrium of the slow subsystem. If the equilibrium is a node, it generically has two distinct eigenvalues and two real eigenvectors. In this case, the slow subsystem uncouples into two equations, each along the corresponding eigenvector. Appropriate re-scaling gives the first canonical model. If the equilibrium is a focus, the linear part can be made triangular in order to get the second canonical model.

18. The solution of the fast subsystem

$$\dot{v} = u + v^2 , \qquad v(0) = -1 ,$$

with fixed $u > 0$ is

$$v(t) = \sqrt{u} \tan \left( \sqrt{u}\, t - \operatorname{atan} \frac{1}{\sqrt{u}} \right) .$$

The interspike period, $T$, is defined by $v(T) = +\infty$, given by the formula

$$T(u) = \frac{1}{\sqrt{u}} \left( \frac{\pi}{2} + \operatorname{atan} \frac{1}{\sqrt{u}} \right) .$$

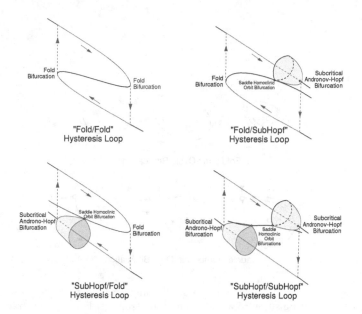

Figure S.41: Classification of point-point codimension-1 hysteresis loops.

The result follows from the integral

$$\frac{1}{T(u)} \int_0^{T(u)} d_i\, \delta(t - T(u))\, dt = \frac{d_1}{T(u)}$$

and the relationships

$$f(u) = \frac{1}{T(u)} \qquad \text{and} \qquad \operatorname{atan} \frac{1}{\sqrt{u}} = \operatorname{arcot} \sqrt{u}\,.$$

Periodic solutions of the averaged system (focus case) and the full system are depicted in Fig.S.40. The deviation is due to the finite size of the parameters $\mu_1$ and $\mu_2$ in Fig.9.35.

19. There are only two codimension-1 bifurcations of an equilibrium that result in transitions to another equilibrium: saddle-node *off* limit cycle and subcritical Andronov-Hopf bifurcation. Hence, there are four point-point hysteresis loops, depicted in Fig.S.41. More details are provided in Izhikevich (2000a).

20. These figures are modified from Izhikevich (2000a), where one can find two models exhibiting this phenomenon. The key feature is that the slow subsystem is not too slow, and the rate of attraction to the upper equilibrium is relatively weak. The spikes are actually damped oscillations that are generated by the fast subsystem while it converges to the equilibrium. Periodic bursting is generated via the point-point hysteresis loop.

21. There are only two codimension-1 bifurcations of a small limit cycle attractor (subthreshold oscillation) on a plane that result in sharp transitions to a large-amplitude limit cycle attractor (spiking): fold limit cycle bifurcation and saddle-homoclinic orbit bifurcation; see Fig.S.42. These two bifurcations paired with any of the four bifurcations of the large-amplitude limit cycle attractor result in eight planar codimension-1 cycle-cycle bursters; see Fig.S.43. More details are provided by Izhikevich (2000a).

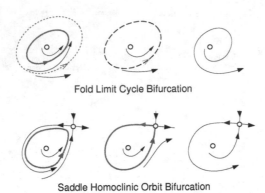

Fold Limit Cycle Bifurcation

Saddle Homoclinic Orbit Bifurcation

Figure S.42: Codimension-1 bifurcations of a stable limit cycle in planar systems that result in sharp loss of stability and transition to a large-amplitude (spiking) limit cycle attractor, not shown in the figure. Fold limit cycle: A stable limit cycle is approached by an unstable one, they coalesce, and then they disappear. Saddle homoclinic orbit: A limit cycle grows into a saddle. The unstable manifold of the saddle makes a loop and returns via the stable manifold (separatrix).

| *Bifurcations* | *Saddle-Node on Invariant* **Circle** | *Saddle* **Homoclinic** *Orbit* | *Supercritical Andronov-* **Hopf** | **Fold** *Limit* **Cycle** |
|---|---|---|---|---|
| **Fold** *Limit* **Cycle** | fold cycle/ circle | fold cycle/ homoclinic | fold cycle/ Hopf | fold cycle/ fold cycle |
| *Saddle* **Homoclinic** *Orbit* | homoclinic/ circle | homoclinic/ homoclinic | homoclinic/ Hopf | homoclinic/ fold cycle |

Figure S.43: Classification of codimension-1 cycle-cycle planar bursters.

# References

Acebron J. A., Bonilla L. L., Vincente C. J. P., Ritort F., Spigler R. (2005) The Kuramoto model: A simple paradigm for synchronization phenomena. Review of Modern Physics, 77:137–185 .

Alonso A. and Klink R. (1993) Differential electroresponsiveness of stellate and pyramidal-like cells of medial entorhinal cortex layer II. Journal of Neurophysiology, 70:128–143.

Alonso A. and Llinas R. R. (1989) Subthreshold $Na^+$-dependent theta-like rhythmicity in stellate cells of entorhinal cortex layer II. Nature, 342:175–177.

Amini B., Clark J. W. Jr., and Canavier C. C. (1999) Calcium dynamics underlying pacemaker-like and burst firing oscillations in midbrain dopaminergic neurons: A computational study. Journal of Neurophysiology, 82:2249-2261.

Amir R., Michaelis M., and Devor M. (2002) Burst discharge in primary sensory neurons: Triggered by subthreshold oscillations, maintained by depolarizing afterpotentials. Journal of Neuroscience, 22:1187–1198.

Armstrong C. M. and Hille B. (1998) Voltage-gated ion channels and electrical excitability. Neuron 20:371–380.

Arnold V. I. (1965) Small denominators. I. Mappings of the circumference onto itself. Transactions of the AMS series 2, 46:213–284.

Arnold V. I., Afrajmovich V. S., Il'yashenko Yu. S., and Shil'nikov L.P. (1994) Dynamical Systems V. Bifurcation Theory and Catastrophe Theory. Berlin and New York: Springer-Verlag.

Aronson D. G., Ermentrout G. B., and Kopell N. (1990) Amplitude response of coupled oscillators. Physica D, 41:403–449.

Arshavsky Y. I., Berkinblit M. B., Kovalev S. A., Smolyaninov V. V., and Chaylakhyan L. M. (1971) An analysis of the functional properties of dendrites in relation to their structure, in: I. M. Gelfand, V.S. Gurfinkel, S.V. Fomin, M.L. Zetlin (Eds.), Models of the Structural and Functional Organization of Certain Biological Systems, pp. 25-71, Cambridge, Mass: MIT Press.

Bacci A., Rudolph U., Huguenard J. R., and Prince D.A. (2003a) Major differences in inhibitory synaptic transmission onto two neocortical interneuron subclasses. Journal of Neuroscience, 23:9664–9674.

Bacci A., Huguenard J. R., Prince D. A. (2003b) Long-lasting self-inhibition of neocortical interneurons mediated by endocannabinoids. Nature, 431:312–316.

Baer S. M., Erneux T., and Rinzel J. (1989) The slow passage through a Hopf bifurcation: Delay, memory effects, and resonances. SIAM Journal on Applied Mathematics, 49:55–71.

Baer S. M., Rinzel J., and Carrillo H. (1995) Analysis of an autonomous phase model for neuronal parabolic bursting. Journal of Mathematical Biology, 33:309–333.

Baesens C., Guckenheimer J., Kim S., and MacKay R. S. (1991) Three coupled oscillators: Mode-locking, global bifurcations and toroidal chaos. Physica D, 49:387–475.

Baker M. D. and Bostock H. (1997) Low-threshold, persistent sodium current in rat large dorsal root ganglion neurons in culture. Journal of Neurophysiology, 77:1503–1513.

Baker M. D. and Bostock H. (1998) Inactivation of macroscopic late $Na^+$ current and characteristics of unitary late $Na^+$ currents in sensory neurons. Journal of Neurophysiology, 80:2538–2549.

Bautin N. N. (1949) The behavior of dynamical systems near to the boundaries of stability. Gostekhizdat., Moscow-Leningrad, 2nd ed., Moscow: Nauka, (1984) [in Russian].

Beierlein M., Gibson J. R., and Connors B. W. (2003) Two dynamically distinct inhibitory networks in layer 4 of the neocortex. Journal of Neurophysiology, 90:2987–3000.

Bekkers J. M. (2000) Properties of voltage-gated potassium currents in nucleated patches from large layer 5 pyramidal neurons of the rat. Journal of Physiology, 525:593-609.

Benoit E. (1984) Canards de $\mathbb{R}^3$. These d'etat, Universite de Nice.

Benoit E., Callot J.-L., Diener F., and Diener M. (1981) Chasse au canards. Collectanea Mathematica, 31–32(1–3):37–119.

Bertram R., Butte M. J., Kiemel T., and Sherman A. (1995) Topological and phenomenological classification of bursting oscillations. Bulletin of Mathematical Biology 57:413–439.

Blechman I. I. (1971) Synchronization of Dynamical Systems. [in Russian: "Sinchronizatzia Dinamicheskich Sistem", Moscow:Nauka].

Bower J. M. and Beeman D. (1995) The Book of GENESIS. New York: Springer-Verlag.

Bressloff P. C. and Coombes S. (2000) Dynamics of strongly coupled spiking neurons. Neural Computation, 12:91–129.

Brizzi L., Meunier C., Zytnicki D., Donnet M., Hansel D., Lamotte d'Incamps B., and van Vreeswijk C. (2004) How shunting inhibition affects the discharge of lumbar motoneurons: a dynamic clamp study in anaesthetized cats. Journal of Physiology, 558:671–683.

Brown E., Moehlis J., and Holmes P. (2004) On the phase reduction and response dynamics of neural oscillator populations. Neural Computation, 16:673–715.

Brown T. G. (1911) The intrinsic factors in the act of progression in the mammal. Proceedings of Royal Society London B, 84:308-319.

Brunel N., Hakim V., and Richardson M. J. (2003) Firing-rate resonance in a generalized integrate-and-fire neuron with subthreshold resonance. Physical Review E, 67:051916.

Bryant H. L. and Segundo J. P. (1976) Spike initiation by transmembrane current: a white-noise analysis. Journal of Physiology, 260:279–314.

Butera R. J., Rinzel J., and Smith J. C. (1999) Models of respiratory rhythm generation in the pre-Botzinger complex. I. Bursting pacemaker neurons. Journal of Neurophysiology, 82:382–397.

Canavier C. C., Clark J. W., and Byrne J. H. (1991) Simulation of the bursting activity of neuron R15 in Aplysia: Role of ionic currents, calcium balance, and modulatory transmitters. Journal of Neurophysiology, 66:2107-2124.

Carnevale N. T. and Hines M. L. (2006) The NEURON Book. Cambridge: Cambridge University Press.

Cartwright M. L. and Littlewood J. E. (1945) On nonlinear differential equations of the second order: I. The equation $\ddot{y} - k(1 - y^2)\dot{y} + y = b\lambda k \cos(\lambda t + \alpha)$, $k$ large. Journal of London Mathematical Society, 20:180–189.

del Castillo J. and Morales T. (1967) The electrical and mechanical activity of the esophageal cell of ascaris lumbricoides. The Journal of General Physiology, 50:603–629.

Chay T. R. and Cook D. L. (1988) Endogenous bursting patterns in excitable cells. Mathematical Biosciences, 90:139 –153.

Chay T. R. and Keizer J. (1983) Minimal model for membrane oscillations in the pancreatic $\beta$-cell. Biophysical Journal, 42:181-190.

Chow C. C. and Kopell N. (2000) Dynamics of spiking neurons with electrical coupling. Neural Computation, 12:1643-1678.

Chu Z., Galarreta M., and Hestrin S. (2003) Synaptic Interactions of Late-Spiking Neocortical Neurons in Layer 1, 23:96–102

Clay J. R. (1998) Excitability of the squid giant axon revisited. Journal of Neurophysiology, 80:903–913.

Cohen A. H., Holmes P. J., and Rand R. H. (1982) The nature of the coupling between segmental oscillators of the lamprey spinal generator for locomotion: A mathematical model. Journal of Mathematical Biology, 13:345–369.

Cole K. S., Guttman R., and Bezanilla F. (1970) Nerve excitation without threshold. Proceedings of the National Academy of Sciences, 65:884–891.

Collins J. J. and Stewart I. (1994) A group-theoretic approach to rings of coupled biological oscillators. Biological Cybernetics, 71:95-103.

Collins J. J. and Stewart I. (1993) Coupled nonlinear oscillators and the symmetries of animal gaits. Journal of Nonlinear Science,. 3:349–392.

Connor J. A., Walter D., and McKown R. (1977) Modifications of the Hodgkin-Huxley axon suggested by experimental results from crustacean axons. Biophysical Journal, 18:81–102.

Connors B. W. and Gutnick M. J. (1990) Intrinsic firing patterns of diverse neocortical neurons. Trends in Neuroscience, 13:99–104.

Coombes S. and Bressloff P. C. (2005) Bursting: The genesis of rhythm in the nervous system. World Scientific.

Daido H. (1996) Onset of cooperative entrainment in limit-cycle oscillators with uniform all-to-all interactions: Bifurcation of the order function. Physica D, 91:24–66.

Dayan P. and Abbott L.F. (2001) Theoretical Neuroscience. The MIT Press.

Del Negro C. A., Hsiao C.-F., Chandler S. H., and Garfinkel A. (1998) Evidence for a novel bursting mechanism in rodent trigeminal neurons. Biophysical Journal, 75:174–182.

Denjoy A. (1932) Sur les courbes definies par les equations differentielles a la surface du tore.

J. Math. Pures et Appl. 11:333-375.

Destexhe A. , Contreras D., Sejnowski T. J., and Steriade M. (1994) A model of spindle rhythmicity in the isolated thalamic reticular nucleus. Journal of Neurophysiology, 72:803–818.

Destexhe A. and Gaspard P. (1993) Bursting oscillations from a homoclinic tangency in a time delay system. Physics Letters A, 173:386–391.

Destexhe A., Rudolph M., Fellous J.M., and Sejnowski T.J. (2001) Fluctuating synaptic conductances recreate in vivo-like activity in neocortical neurons. Neuroscience, 107:13–24.

de Vries G. (1998) Multiple bifurcations in a polynomial model of bursting oscillations. Journal of Nonlinear Science, 8:281–316.

Dickson C. T., Magistretti J., Shalinsky M. H., Fransen E., Hasselmo M. E., and Alonso A. (2000) Properties and role of $I_h$ in the pacing of subthreshold oscillations in entorhinal cortex layer II neurons. Journal of Neurophysiology, 83:2562–2579.

Doiron B., Laing C., Longtin A, and Maler L. (2002) Ghostbursting: A novel neuronal burst mechanism. Journal of Computational Neuroscience, 12:5–25.

Doiron B., Chacron M. J., Maler L., Longtin A., and Bastian J. (2003) Inhibitory feedback required for network oscillatory responses to communication but not prey stimuli. Nature, 421:539-543.

Dong C.-J. and Werblin F. S. (1995) Inwardly rectifying potassium conductance can accelerate the hyperpolarization response in retinal horizontal cells. Journal of Neurophysiology, 74:2258–2265

Eckhaus W. (1983) Relaxation oscillations including a standard chase of French ducks. Lecture Notes in Mathematics, 985:432–449.

Erisir A., Lau D., Rudy B., Leonard C. S. (1999) Function of specific $K^+$ channels in sustained high-frequency firing of fast-spiking neocortical interneurons. Journal of Neurophysiology, 82:2476–2489.

Ermentrout G. B. (1981) $n : m$ phase-locking of weakly coupled oscillators. Journal of Mathematical Biology, 12:327–342.

Ermentrout G. B. (1986) Losing amplitude and saving phase. In Othmer H. G., (ed.), Nonlinear Oscillations in Biology and Chemistry. Springer-Verlag.

Ermentrout G. B. (1992) Stable periodic solutions to discrete and continuum arrays of weakly coupled nonlinear oscillators. SIAM Journal on Applied Mathematics, 52:1665–1687.

Ermentrout G. B. (1994) An introduction to neural oscillators. In Neural Modeling and Neural Networks, F. Ventriglia, (ed.), Pergamon Press, Oxford, pp.79–110.

Ermentrout G. B. (1996) Type I membranes, phase resetting curves, and synchrony. Neural Computation, 8:979–1001.

Ermentrout G. B. (1998) Linearization of F-I curves by adaptation. Neural Computation, 10:1721–1729.

Ermentrout G. B. (2002) Simulating, Analyzing, and Animating Dynamical Systems: A Guide to XPPAUT for Researchers and Students (Software, Environments, Tools). SIAM.

Ermentrout G. B. (2003) Dynamical consequences of fast-rising, slow-decaying synapses in neuronal networks. Neural Computation, 15:2483-2522

Ermentrout G. B. and Kopell N. (1984) Frequency plateaus in a chain of weakly coupled oscillators, I. SIAM Journal on Mathematical Analysis, 15:215–237.

Ermentrout G. B. and Kopell N. (1986a) Parabolic bursting in an excitable system coupled with a slow oscillation. SIAM Journal on Applied Mathematics 46:233–253.

Ermentrout G. B. and Kopell N. (1986b) Subcellular oscillations and bursting. Mathematical Biosciences, 78:265–291.

Ermentrout G. B. and Kopell N. (1990) Oscillator death in systems of coupled neural oscillators. SIAM Journal on Applied Mathematics, 50:125–146.

Ermentrout G. B. and Kopell N. (1991) Multiple pulse interactions and averaging in systems of coupled neural oscillators. Journal of Mathematical Biology, 29:195–217.

Ermentrout G. B. and Kopell N. (1994) Learning of phase lags in coupled neural oscillators. Neural Computation, 6:225–241.

FitzHugh R. (1955) Mathematical models of threshold phenomena in the nerve membrane. Bulletin of Mathematical Biophysics, 7:252–278.

FitzHugh R. (1960) Threshold and plateaus in the Hodgkin-Huxley nerve equations. The Journal of General Physiology. 43:867–896.

FitzHugh R. A. (1961) Impulses and physiological states in theoretical models of nerve membrane. Biophysical Journal, 1:445–466.

FitzHugh R. (1969) Mathematical models of excitation and propagation in nerve. In Schwan (ed.) Biological Engineering, New York: McGraw-Hill.

FitzHugh R. (1976) Anodal excitation in the Hodgkin-Huxley nerve model. Biophysical Journal, 16:209–226.

Fourcaud-Trocme N., Hansel D., van Vreeswijk C., and Brunel N. (2003) How spike generation mechanisms determine the neuronal response to fluctuating inputs. Journal of Neuroscience, 23:11628–11640.

Frankel P. and Kiemel T. (1993) Relative phase behavior of two slowly coupled oscillators. SIAM Journal on Applied Mathematics, 53:1436–1446.

Gabbiani F, Metzner W, Wessel R, and Koch C. (1996) From stimulus encoding to feature extraction in weakly electric fish. Nature. 384:564–567.

Geiger J. R. P. and Jonas P. (2000) Dynamic control of presynaptic $Ca^{2+}$ inflow by fastInactivating $K^+$ channels in hippocampal mossy fiber boutons. Neuron, 28:927–939.

Gerstner W. and Kistler W. M. (2002) Spiking Neuron Models: Single Neurons, Populations, Plasticity. Cambridge: Cambridge University Press.

Gibson J. R., Belerlein M., and Connors B. W. (1999) Two networks of electrically coupled inhibitory neurons in neocortex. Nature, 402:75–79.

Glass L. and MacKey M. C. (1988) From Clocks to Chaos. Princeton, N.J.: Princeton University Press.

Goel P. and Ermentrout B. (2002) Synchrony, stability, and firing patterns in pulse-coupled oscillators. Physica D, 163:191–216.

Golomb D., Yue C., and Yaari Y. (2006) Contribution of persistent Na$^+$ current and M-type K$^+$ current to somatic bursting in CA1 pyramidal cells: combined experimental and modeling study. J. Neurophys., 96:1912–1926.

Golubitsky M., Josic K. and Kaper T. J. (2001) An unfolding theory approach to bursting in fast-slow systems. In: *Global Analysis of Dynamical Systems: Festschrift Dedicated to Floris Takens on the Occasion of his 60th Birthday.* (H. W. Broer B. Krauskopf, and G. Vegter, eds.) Institute of Physics, 277–308.

Golubitsky M. and Stewart I. (2002) Patterns of oscillation in coupled cell systems. In: Geometry, Dynamics, and Mechanics: 60th Birthday Volume for J. E. Marsden. P. Newton, P. Holmes, and A. Weinstein, (eds.), Springer-Verlag, 243–286.

Gray C. M. and McCormick D. A. (1996) Chattering cells: Superficial pyramidal neurons contributing to the generation of synchronous oscillations in the visual cortex. Science. 274:109-113.

Grundfest H. (1971) Biophysics and Physiology of Excitable Membranes. W. J. Adelman (ed.), New York: Van Nostrand Reinhold.

Guckenheimer J. (1975) Isochrons and phaseless sets. Journal of Mathematical Biology, 1:259–273.

Guckenheimer J, Harris-Warrick R, Peck J, and Willms A. (1997) Bifurcation, bursting, and spike frequency adaptation. Journal of Computational Neuroscience, 4:257–277.

Guckenheimer J. and Holmes D. (1983) Nonlinear Oscillations, Dynamical Systems, and Bifurcations of Vector Fields. New York: Springer-Verlag.

Guevara M. R. and Glass L. (1982) Phase locking, periodic doubling bifurcations and chaos in a mathematical model of a periodically driven oscillator: a theory for the entrainment of biological oscillators and the generation of cardiac dysrhythmias. Journal of Mathematical Biology, 14:1–23.

Guttman R., Lewis S., and Rinzel J. (1980) Control of repetitive firing in squid axon membrane as a model for a neuroneoscillator. Journal of Physiology, 305:377–395.

Hansel D., Mato G., and Meunier C. (1995) Synchrony in excitatory neural networks. Neural Computations, 7:307–335.

Hansel D., Mato G., Meunier C., and Neltner L. (1998) On numerical simulations of integrate-and-fire neural networks. Neural Computation, 10:467–483.

Hansel D. and Mato G. (2003) Asynchronous states and the emergence of synchrony in large networks of interacting excitatory and inhibitory neurons. Neural Computation, 15:1–56.

Harris-Warrick R. M. and Flamm R. E. (1987) Multiple mechanisms of bursting in a conditional bursting neuron. Journal of Neuroscience, 7:2113–2128.

Hastings J. W. and Sweeney B. M. (1958) A persistent diurnal rhythms of luminescence in *Gonyaulax polyedra.* Biological Bulletin, 115:440–458.

Hausser M. and Mel B. (2003) Dendrites: bug or feature? Current Opinion in Neurobiology, 13:372–383.

Hausser M., Spruston N., and Stuart G. J. (2000) Diversity and dynamics of dendritic signaling. Science, 290:739–744.

Heyward P., Ennis M., Keller A., and Shipley M. T. (2001) Membrane bistability in olfactory bulb mitral cells. Journal of Neuroscience, 21:5311–5320.

Hille B. (2001) Ion Channels of Excitable Membranes. (3nd ed.) Sunderland, Mass: Sinauer.

Hindmarsh J. L. and Rose R. M. (1982) A model of the nerve impulse using two first-order differential equations. Nature 296:162–164.

Hines M. A. (1989) Program for simulation of nerve equations with branching geometries. International Journal of Biomedical Computing, 24:55–68.

Hodgkin A. L. (1948) The local electric changes associated with repetitive action in a non-medulated axon. Journal of Physiology, 107:165–181.

Hodgkin A. L. and Huxley A. F. (1952) A quantitative description of membrane current and application to conduction and excitation in nerve. Journal of Physiology, 117:500–544.

Holden L. and Erneux T. (1993a) Slow passage through a Hopf bifurcation: form oscillatory to steady state solutions. SIAM Journal on Applied Mathematics, 53:1045–1058.

Holden L. and Erneux T. (1993b) Understanding bursting oscillations as periodic slow passages through bifurcation and limit points. Journal of Mathematical Biology, 31:351–365.

Hopf E. (1942) Abzweigung einer periodischen Losung von einer stationaren Losung eines Differetialsystems. Ber. Math.-Phys. Kl. Sachs, Aca. Wiss. Leipzig, 94:1–22.

Hoppensteadt F. C. (1997) An Introduction to the Mathematics of Neurons. Modeling in the Frequency Domain. 2nd ed. Cambridge: Cambridge University Press.

Hoppensteadt F. C. (2000) Analysis and Simulations of Chaotic Systems. 2nd ed. New York: Springer-Verlag.

Hoppensteadt F. C. and Izhikevich E. M. (1996a) Synaptic organizations and dynamical properties of weakly connected neural oscillators: I. Analysis of canonical model. Biological Cybernetics, 75:117–127.

Hoppensteadt F. C. and Izhikevich E. M. (1996b) Synaptic organizations and dynamical properties of weakly connected neural oscillators. II. Learning of phase information. Biological Cybernetics, 75:129–135.

Hoppensteadt F. C. and Izhikevich E. M. (1997) Weakly Connected Neural Networks. New York: Springer-Verlag.

Hoppensteadt F. C. and Keener J. P. (1982) Phase locking of biological clocks. Journal of Mathematical Biology, 15:339–349.

Hoppensteadt F. C. and Peskin C. S.(2002) Modeling and Simulation in Medicine and the Life Sciences. 2nd ed. New York: Springer-Verlag.

Hughes S. W., Cope D. W., Toth T. L., Williams S. R., and Crunelli V. (1999) All thalamocortical neurones possess a T-type $Ca^{2+}$ 'window' current that enables the expression of bistability-mediated activities. Journal of Physiology, 517:805–815.

Huguenard J. R. and McCormick D. A. (1992) Simulation of the currents involved in rhythmic oscillations in thalamic relay neurons. Journal of Neurophysiology, 68:1373–1383.

Hutcheon B., Miura R.M., and Puil E., (1996). Subthreshold membrane resonance in neocortical neurons. Journal of Neurophysiology, 76:683–697.

Izhikevich E. M. (1998) Phase models with explicit time delays. Physical Review E, 58:905–908.

Izhikevich E. M. (1999) Class 1 neural excitability, conventional synapses, weakly connected networks, and mathematical foundations of pulse-coupled models. IEEE Transactions On Neural Networks,10:499–507.

Izhikevich E. M. (1999) Weakly connected quasiperiodic oscillators, FM interactions, and multiplexing in the brain. SIAM Journal on Applied Mathematics, 59:2193–2223.

Izhikevich E. M. (2000a) Neural excitability, spiking, and bursting. International Journal of Bifurcation and Chaos, 10:1171–1266.

Izhikevich E. M. (2000b) Phase equations for relaxation oscillators. SIAM Journal on Applied Mathematics, 60:1789–1805.

Izhikevich E. M. (2001a) Resonate-and-fire neurons. Neural Networks, 14:883–894

Izhikevich E. M. (2001b) Synchronization of elliptic bursters. SIAM Review, 43:315–344.

Izhikevich E. M. (2002) Resonance and selective communication via bursts in neurons having subthreshold oscillations. BioSystems, 67:95–102.

Izhikevich E. M. (2003) Simple Model of Spiking Neurons. IEEE Transactions on Neural Networks, 14:1569–1572.

Izhikevich E. M. (2004) Which model to use for cortical spiking neurons? IEEE Transactions on Neural Networks, 15:1063–1070.

Izhikevich E. M. (2006) Bursting. Scholarpedia, 1(3):1300.

Izhikevich E. M., Desai N. S., Walcott E. C., and Hoppensteadt F. C. (2003) Bursts as a unit of neural information: selective communication via resonance . Trends in Neuroscience, 26:161–167.

Izhikevich E. M. and FitzHugh R. (2006) FitzHugh-Nagumo model. Scholarpedia, 1(9):1349.

Izhikevich E. M. and Hoppensteadt F. C. (2003) Slowly coupled oscillators: Phase dynamics and synchronization. SIAM Journal on Applied Mathematics, 63:1935–1953.

Izhikevich E. M. and Hoppensteadt F. C. (2004) Classification of bursting mappings. International Journal of Bifurcation and Chaos, 14:3847–3854.

Izhikevich E. M. and Kuramoto Y. (2006) Weakly coupled oscillators. Encyclopedia of Mathematical Physics, Elsevier, 5:448.

Jahnsen H. and Llinas R. (1984) Electrophysiological properties of guinea-pig thalamic neurons: An in vitro study. Journal of Physiology London, 349:205–226.

Jensen M. S., Azouz R., and Yaari Y. (1994) Variant firing patterns in rat hippocampal pyramidal cells modulated by extracellular potassium. Journal of Neurophysiology, 71:831–839.

Jian Z., Xing J.L., Yang G.S., and Hu S.J. (2004) A novel bursting mechanism of type A neurons in injured dorsal root ganglia. NeuroSignals, 13:150–156.

Johnson C. H. (1999) Forty years of PRC – what have we learned?. Chronobiology International, 16:711–743.

Johnston D. and Wu S. M. (1995) Foundations of Cellular Neurophysiology. Cambridge, Mass: MIT Press.

Katriel G. (2005) Stability of synchronized oscillations in networks of phase-oscillators. Discrete and Continuous Dynamical Systems-Series B, 5:353–364.

Kawaguchi Y. (1995) Physiological subgroups of nonpyramidal cells with specific morphological characteristics in layer II/III of rat frontal cortex. Journal of Neuroscience, 15:2638–2655.

Kawaguchi Y. and Kubota Y. (1997) GABAergic cell subtypes and their synaptic connections in rat frontal cortex. Cerebral Cortex, 7:476–486.

Kay A. R., Sugimori M., and Llinas R. (1998) Kinetic and stochastic properties of a persistent sodium current in mature guinea pig cerebellar Purkinje Cells. Journal of Neurophysiology, 80:1167–1179.

Keener J. and Sneyd J. (1998) Mathematical Physiology. New York: Springer-Verlag.

Kepler T. B., Abbott L. F., and Marder E. (1992) Reduction of conductance based neuron models. Biological Cybernetics, 66:381–387.

Kinard T. A., de Vries G., Sherman A., and Satin L. S. (1999) Modulation of the bursting properties of single mouse pancreatic beta-cells by artificial conductances. Biophysical Journal, 76:1423-35

Klink R. and Alonso A. (1993) Ionic Mechanisms for the subthreshold oscillations and differential electroresponsiveness of medial entorhinal cortex layer II neurons. Journal of Neurophysiology, 70:144–157.

Koch C. (1999) Biophysics of Computation: Information Processing in Single Neurons. New York: Oxford University Press.

Kopell N. (1986) Coupled oscillators and locomotion by fish. In Othmer H. G. (Ed.) Nonlinear Oscillations in Biology and Chemistry. Lecture Notes in Biomathematics, New York: Springer-Verlag.

Kopell N. (1995) Chains of coupled oscillators. In Arbib M. A. (Ed.) Brain Theory and Neural Networks, Cambridge, Mass: MIT press.

Kopell N. and Ermentrout G. B. (1990) Phase transitions and other phenomena in chains of coupled oscillators. SIAM Journal on Applied Mathematics 50:1014–1052.

Kopell N., Ermentrout G. B., Williams T. L. (1991) On chains of oscillators forced at one end. SIAM Journal on Applied Mathematics, 51:1397–1417.

Kopell N. and Somers D. (1995) Anti-phase solutions in relaxation oscillators coupled through excitatory interactions. Journal of Mathematical Biology, 33:261–280.

Korngreen A. and Sakmann B. (2000) Voltage-gated $K^+$ channels in layer 5 neocortical pyramidal neurones from young rats: Subtypes and gradients. Journal of Physiology, 525.3:621–639.

Krinskii V.I. and Kokoz Yu.M. (1973) Analysis of equations of excitable membranes - I. Reduction of the Hodgkin-Huxley equations to a second order system. Biofizika, 18:506–511.

Kuramoto Y. (1975) in H. Araki (Ed.) International Symposium on Mathematical Problems in Theoretical Physics, Lecture Notes in Physics, 39:420–422, New York: Springer-Verlag.

Kuramoto Y. (1984) Chemical Oscillations, Waves, and Turbulence. New York: Springer-Verlag.

Kuznetsov Yu. (1995) Elements of Applied Bifurcation Theory. New York: Springer-Verlag.

Lapicque L. (1907) Recherches quantitatives sur l'excitation electrique des nerfs traitee comme une polarization. J Physiol Pathol Gen 9:620-635.

Latham P. E., Richmond B. J., Nelson P. G., and Nirenberg S. (2000) Intrinsic dynamics in neuronal networks. I. Theory. Journal of Neurophysiology, 83:808–27.

Lesica N. A and Stanley G. B. (2004) Encoding of natural scene movies by tonic and burst spikes in the lateral geniculate nucleus. Journal of Neuroscience, 24:10731–10740.

Levitan E. S., Kramer R. H., and Levitan I. B. (1987) Augmentation of bursting pacemaker activity by egg-laying hormone in Aplysia neuron R15 is mediated by a cyclic AMP-dependent increase in Ca2+ and K+ currents. Proceedings of National Academy of Sciences. 84 :6307–6311.

Levitan E. S. and Livitan I. B. (1988) A cyclic GMP analog decreases the currents underlying bursting activity in the Aplysia neuron R15. Journal of Neuroscience, 8:1162–1171.

Li J., Bickford M. E., and Guido W. (2003) Distinct firing properties of higher order thalamic relay neurons. Journal of Neurophysiology, 90: 291–299.

Lienard A. (1928) Etude des oscillations entretenues, Rev. Gen. Elec. 23:901–954.

Lisman J. (1997) Bursts as a unit of neural information: making unreliable synapses reliable. Trends in Neuroscience, 20:38–43.

Lopatin A. N., Makhina E. N., and Nichols C. G. (1994) Potassium channel block by cytoplasmic polyamines as the mechanism of intrinsic rectification. Nature, 373:366–369.

Luk W. K. and Aihara K. (2000) Synchronization and sensitivity enhancement of the Hodgkin-Huxley neurons due to inhibitory inputs. Biological Cybernetics, 82:455–467.

Magee J. C. (1998) Dendritic hyperpolarization-activated currents modify the integrative properties of hippocampal CA1 pyramidal neurons. Journal of Neuroscience, 18:7613–7624.

Magee J. C. and Carruth M. (1999) Dendritic voltage-gated ion channels regulate the action potential firing mode of hippocampal CA1 pyramidal neurons. Journal of Neurophysiology, 82:1895–1901.

Magistretti J. and Alonso A. (1999) Biophysical properties and slow voltage- dependent Inactivation of a sustained sodium current in entorhinal cortex layer-II principal neurons. Journal of General Physiology, 114:491–509.

Mainen Z. F. and Sejnowski T. J. (1995) Reliability of spike timing in neocortical neurons. Science, 268:1503–1506.

Mainen Z. F. and Sejnowski T. J. (1996) Influence of dendritic structure on firing pattern in model neocortical neurons. Nature, 382:363–366.

Malkin I. G. (1949) Methods of Poincare and Liapunov in theory of non-linear oscillations. [in Russian: "Metodi Puankare i Liapunova v teorii nelineinix kolebanii" Moscow: Gostexizdat].

Malkin I. G. (1956) Some Problems in Nonlinear Oscillation Theory. [in Russian: "Nekotorye zadachi teorii nelineinix kolebanii" Moscow: Gostexizdat].

Marder E. and Bucher D. (2001) Central pattern generators and the control of rhythmic movements. Current Biology, 11:986–996.

Markram H, Toledo-Rodriguez M, Wang Y, Gupta A, Silberberg G, and Wu C. (2004) Interneurons of the neocortical inhibitory system. Nature Review Neuroscience, 5:793–807

Medvedev G. (2005) Reduction of a model of an excitable cell to a one-dimensional map. Physica D, 202:37–59.

McCormick D. A. (2004) Membrane properties and neurotransmitter actions, in Shepherd G.M. The Synaptic Organization of the Brain. 5th ed. New York: Oxford University Press.

McCormick D. A. and Huguenard J. R. (1992) A Model of the electrophysiological properties of thalamocortical relay neurons. Journal of Neurophysiology, 68:1384–1400.

McCormick D. A. and Pape H.-C. (1990) Properties of a hyperpolarization-activated cation current and its role in rhythmic oscillation in thalamic relay neurones. Journal of Physiology, 431:291–318.

Melnikov V. K. (1963) On the stability of the center for time periodic perturbations. Transactions of Moscow Mathematical Society, 12:1–57.

Mines, G. R. (1914) On circulating excitations on heart muscles and their possible relation to tachycardia and fibrillation. Transactions of Royal Society Canada, 4:43–53.

Mirollo R. E. and Strogatz S. H. (1990) Synchronization of pulse-coupled biological oscillators. SIAM Journal on Applied Mathematics, 50:1645–1662.

Mishchenko E. F., Kolesov Yu. S., Kolesov A. Yu., and Rozov N. K. (1994) Asymptotic Methods in Singularly Perturbed Systems. New York and London: Consultants Bureau.

Morris C. and Lecar H. (1981) Voltage oscillations in the barnacle giant muscle fiber. Biophysical Journal, 35:193–213.

Murray J. D. (1993). Mathematical Biology. New York: Springer-Verlag.

Nagumo J., Arimoto S., and Yoshizawa S. (1962) An active pulse transmission line simulating nerve axon. Proc. IRE. 50:2061–2070.

Nejshtadt A. (1985) Asymptotic investigation of the loss of stability by an equilibrium as a pair of eigenvalues slowly crosses the imaginary axis. Usp. Mat. Nauk 40:190–191.

Neu J. C. (1979) Coupled chemical oscillators. SIAM Journal of Applied Mathematics, 37:307–315.

Nisenbaum E. S., Xu Z. C., and Wilson C. J. (1994) Contribution of a slowly inactivating potassium current to the transition to firing of neostriatal spiny projection neurons. Journal of Neurophysiology, 71:1174–1189.

Noble D. (1966) Applications of Hodgkin-Huxley equations to excitable tissues. Physiological Review, 46:1–50.

Nowak L. G., Azouz R., Sanchez-Vives M. V., Gray C. M., and McCormick D. A. (2003) Electrophysiological classes of cat primary visual cortical neurons in vivo as revealed by quantitative analyses. Journal of Neurophysiology, 89: 1541–1566.

Oswald A. M., Chacron M. J., Doiron B., Bastian J., and Maler L. (2004) Parallel processing of sensory input by bursts and isolated spikes. Journal of Neuroscience, 24:4351–62.

Pape H.-C., and McCormick D. A. (1995) Electrophysiological and pharmacological properties of interneurons in the cat dorsal lateral geniculate nucleus. Neuroscience, 68: 1105–1125.

Parri H. R. and Crunelli V. (1998) Sodium current in rat and cat thalamocortical neurons: Role of a non-inactivating component in tonic and burst firing, Journal of Neuroscience,

18:854–867.

Pedroarena C. and Llinas R. (1997) Dendritic calcium conductances generate high frequency oscillation in thalamocortical neurons. Proceedings of the National Academy of Sciences, 94:724–728.

Perko L. (1996) Differential Equations and Dynamical Systems, New York: Springer-Verlag.

Pernarowski M. (1994) Fast subsystem bifurcations in a slowly varied Lienard system exhibiting bursting. SIAM Journal on Applied Mathematics, 54:814–832.

Pernarowski M., Miura R. M., and Kevorkian J. (1992) Perturbation techniques for models of bursting electrical activity in pancreatic $\beta$-cells. SIAM Journal on Applied Mathematics, 52:1627–1650.

Pfeuty B., Mato G., Golomb D., Hansel D. (2003) Electrical synapses and synchrony: The role of intrinsic currents. Journal of Neuroscience, 23:6280–6294.

Pikovsky A., Rosenblum M., Kurths J. (2001) Synchronization: A Universal Concept in Nonlinear Science. Cambridge: Cambridge University Press.

Pinsky P. and Rinzel J. (1994) Intrinsic and network rhythmogenesis in a reduced Traub model of CA3 neurons. Journal of Computational Neuroscience, 1:39–60.

Pirchio M., Turner J. P., Williams S. R., Asprodini E., and Crunelli V. (1997) Postnatal development of membrane properties and delta oscillations in thalamocortical neurons of the cat dorsal lateral geniculate nucleus. Journal of Neuroscience, 17 :5428–5444.

Plant R. E. (1981) Bifurcation and resonance in a model for bursting nerve cells. Journal of Mathematical Biology, 11:15–32.

Pontryagin L. S. and Rodygin L. V. (1960) Periodic solution of a system of ordinary differential equations with a small parameter in the terms containing derivatives Sov. Math. Dokl. 1: 611–614.

Rall W. (1959) Branching dendritic trees and motoneuron membrane resistivity. Experimental Neurology, 1:491–527.

Reinagel P, Godwin D, Sherman S. M., and Koch C. (1999) Encoding of visual information by LGN bursts. Journal of Neurophysiology, 81:2558–2569.

Reuben J. P., Werman R., and Grundfest H. (1961) The ionic mechanisms of hyperpolarizing responses in lobster muscle fibers. Journal of General Physiology, 45:243–265.

Reyes A. D. and Fetz E. E. (1993) Two modes of interspike interval shortening by brief transient depolarizations in cat neocortical neurons. Journal of Neurophysiology, 69: 1661–1672.

Richardson, M. J. E., Brunel, N. and Hakim, V. (2003) From subthreshold to firing-rate resonance. Journal of Neurophysiology, 89:2538–2554.

Rinzel J. and Ermentrout G. B. (1989) Analysis of neural excitability and oscillations. In Koch C., Segev I. (eds) Methods in Neuronal Modeling, Cambridge, Mass: MIT Press.

Rinzel J. (1978) On repetitive activity in nerve. Federation Proceedings, 37:2793–2802.

Rinzel J. (1985) Bursting oscillations in an excitable membrane model. In: Sleeman B. D., Jarvis R. J., (Eds.) *Ordinary and Partial Differential Equations Proceedings of the 8th Dundee Conference*, Lecture Notes in Mathematics, 1151. Berlin: Springer, 304–316.

Rinzel J. (1987) A formal classification of bursting mechanisms in excitable systems. In: E. Teramoto, M. Yamaguti, eds. Mathematical Topics in Population Biology, Morphogenesis, and Neurosciences, vol. 71 of Lecture Notes in Biomathematics, Berlin: Springer-Verlag.

Rinzel J. and Lee Y.S. (1986) On different mechanisms for membrane potential bursting. In Othmer H.G. (Ed) Nonlinear Oscillations in Biology and Chemistry. Lecture Notes in Biomathematics, no. 66, Berlin and New York: Springer-Verlag.

Rinzel J. and Lee Y. S. (1987) Dissection of a model for neuronal parabolic bursting. Journal of Mathematical Biology, 25:653–675.

Robbins J., Trouslard J., Marsh S. J., and Brown D. A. (1992) Kinetic and pharmacological properties of the M-current in rodent neuroblastoma × glioma hybrid cells, Journal of Physiology, 451:159–185.

Rosenblum M. G. and Pikovsky A. S. (2001) Detecting direction of coupling in interacting oscillators. Physical Review E, 64, p. 045202.

Roy J. P., Clercq M., Steriade M., and Deschenes M. (1984) Electrophysiology of neurons of lateral thalamic nuclei in cat: mechanisms of long-lasting hyperpolarizations. Journal of Neurophysiology, 51:1220–1235.

Rubin J. and Terman D. (2000) Analysis of clustered firing patterns in synaptically coupled networks of oscillators. Journal of Mathematical Biology, 41:513–545.

Rubin J. and Terman D. (2002) Geometric singular perturbation analysis of neuronal dynamics. Handbook of Dynamical systems, vol. 2: Toward Applications (B. Fiedler and G. Iooss, eds.) Amsterdam: Elsevier.

Rush M. E. and Rinzel J. (1995) The potassium A-Current, low firing rates and rebound excitation in Hodgkin-Huxley models. Bulletin of Mathematical Biology, 57:899–929.

Rush M. E. and Rinzel J. (1994) Analysis of bursting in a thalamic neuron model. Biological Cybernetics, 71:281–291.

Samborskij S. N. (1985) Limit trajectories of singularly perturbed differential equations. Dokl. Akad. Nauk Ukr. SSR., A, 9:22–25.

Sanabria E. R. G., Su H., and Yaari Y. (2001) Initiation of network bursts by $Ca^{2+}$-dependent intrinsic bursting in the rat pilocarpine model of temporal lobe epilepsy. Journal of Physiology, 532:205–216.

Sharp A. A., O'Neil M. B., Abbott L. F., Marder E. (1993) Dynamic clamp: computer-generated conductances in real neurons. Journal of Neurophysiology, 69:992–995.

Shepherd G. M. (2004) The Synaptic Organization of the Brain. 5th ed. New York: Oxford University Press.

Sherman S. M. (2001) Tonic and burst firing: Dual modes of thalamocortical relay. Trends in Neuroscience, 24:122–126.

Shilnikov A. L., Calabrese R., and Cymbalyuk G. (2005) Mechanism of bi-stability: Tonic spiking and bursting in a neuron model. Physics Review E, 71, 056214.

Shilnikov A. L. and Cymbalyuk G. (2005) Transition between tonic spiking and bursting in a neuron model via the blue-sky catastrophe. Physical Review Letters, 94, 048101.

Shilnikov A. L. and Cymbalyuk G (2004) Homoclinic bifurcations of periodic orbits en a route from tonic spiking to bursting in neuron models. Regular and Chaotic Dynamics, vol. 9, [2004-11-19]

Shilnikov L. P., Shilnikov A. L., Turaev D., Chua L. O. (2001) Methods of qualitative theory in nonlinear dynamics. Part II, Singapore: World Scientific.

Shilnikov L. P., Shilnikov A. L., Turaev D., Chua L.O. (1998) Methods of qualitative theory in nonlinear dynamics. Part I, Singapore: World Scientific.

Shilnikov, A. L. and Shilnikov, L. P, (1995) Dangerous and safe stability boundaries of equilibria and periodic orbits" in NDES'95, University College Dublin, Ireland, 55-63.

Shishkova M. A. (1973) Investigation of a system of differential equations with a small parameter in highest derivatives. Dokl. Adad. Nauk SSSR 209. No.3, 576–579. English transl. Sov. Math., Dokl. 14,483–487

Skinner F. K., Kopell N., Marder E. (1994) Mechanisms for oscillation and frequency control in reciprocal inhibitory model neural networks. Journal of Computational Neuroscience, 1:69–87.

Smolen P., Terman D., and Rinzel J. (1993) Properties of a bursting model with two slow inhibitory variables. SIAM Journal on Applied Mathematics, 53:861–892.

Somers D. and Kopell N. (1993) Rapid synchronization through fast threshold modulation. Biological Cybernetics, 68:393–407.

Somers D. and Kopell N. (1995) Waves and synchrony in networks of oscillators or relaxation and non-relaxation type. Physica D, 89:169–183.

Stanford I. M., Traub R. D., and Jefferys J. G. R. (1998) Limbic gamma rhythms. II. Synaptic and intrinsic mechanisms underlying spike doublets in oscillating subicular neurons. Journal of Neurophysiology, 80:162–171.

Stein R.B. (1967) Some models of neuronal variability. Biophysical Journal, 7: 37–68.

Steriade M. (2003) Neuronal Substrates of Sleep and Epilepsy. Cambridge: Cambridge University Press.

Steriade M. (2004) Neocortical cell classes are flexible entities. Nature Reviews Neuroscience, 5:121–134.

Strogatz S. H. (1994) Nonlinear Dynamics and Chaos. Readings, Mass: Addison-Wesley.

Strogatz S. H. (2000) From Kuramoto to Crawford: Exploring the onset of synchronization in populations of coupled oscillators. Physica D, 143:1–20.

Stuart G., Spruston N., Hausser M. (1999) Dendrites. New York: Oxford University Press.

Su H, Alroy G, Kirson ED, and Yaari Y. (2001) Extracellular calcium modulates persistent sodium current-dependent burst-firing in hippocampal pyramidal neurons. Journal of Neuroscience, 21:4173–4182.

Szmolyan P. and Wechselberger M. (2001) Canards in $\mathbb{R}^3$. Journal of Differential Equations, 177:419–453.

Szmolyan P. and Wechselberger M. (2004) Relaxation oscillations in $\mathbb{R}^3$. Journal of Differential Equations, 200:69–104.

Tateno T., Harsch A., and Robinson H. P. C. (2004) Threshold firing frequency-current relationships of neurons in rat somatosensor cortex: type 1 and type 2 dynamics. Journal of Neurophysiology 92:2283–2294.

Tennigkeit F., Ries C.R., Schwarz D.W.F., and Puil E. (1997) Isoflurane attenuates resonant responses of auditory thalamic neurons. Journal Neurophysiology, 78:591–596.

Terman D. (1991) Chaotic spikes arising from a model of bursting in excitable membranes. SIAM Journal on Applied Mathematics, 51:1418–1450.

Timofeev I., Grenier F., Bazhenov M., Sejnowski T. J. and Steriade M. (2000) Origin of slow cortical oscillations in deafferented cortical slabs. Cerebral Cortex, 10:1185–1199.

Toledo-Rodriguez M., Blumenfeld B., Wu C., Luo J, Attali B., Goodman P., and Markram H. (2004) Correlation maps allow neuronal electrical properties to be predicted from single-cell gene expression profiles in rat neocortex. Cerebral Cortex, 14:1310–1327.

Traub R. D., Wong R. K., Miles R., and Michelson H. (1991) A model of a CA3 hippocampal pyramidal neuron incorporating voltage-clamp data on intrinsic conductances. Journal of Neurophysiology, 66:635–650.

Tuckwell H. C. (1988) Introduction to Theoretical Neurobiology. Cambridge: Cambridge University Press.

Uhlenbeck G.E. and Ornstein L.S. (1930) On the theory of the Brownian motion. Physical Review, 36:823–841.

Van Hemmen J. L. and Wreszinski W. F. (1993) Lyapunov function for the Kuramoto model of nonlinearly coupled oscillators. Journal of Statistical Physics, 72:145–166.

van Vreeswijk C. (2000) Analysis of the asynchronous state in networks of strongly coupled oscillators. Physical Review Letters, 84:5110–5113.

van Vreeswijk C., Abbott L. F., Ermentrout G. B. (1994) When inhibition not excitation synchronizes neural firing. Journal of Computational Neuroscience, 1:313–321.

van Vreeswijk C. and Hansel D. (2001) Patterns of synchrony in neural networks with spike adaptation. Neural Computation, 13:959–992.

Wang X.-J. (1999) Fast burst firing and short-term synaptic plasticity: a model of neocortical chattering neurons. Neuroscience, 89:347–362.

Wang X.-J. and Rinzel J. (1992) Alternating and synchronous rhythms in reciprocally inhibitory model neurons. Neural Computation, 4:84–97.

Wang X.-J. and Rinzel, J. (1995) Oscillatory and bursting properties of neurons, In Brain Theory and Neural Networks. Ed. Arbib, M. A. Cambridge, Mass: MIT press.

Wechselberger M. (2005) Existence and bifurcation of Canards in $\mathbb{R}^3$ in the case of a folded node. SIAM Journal on Applied Dynamical Systems, 4:101–139.

Wessel R., Kristan W.B., and Kleinfeld D. (1999) Supralinear summation of synaptic inputs by an invertebrate neuron: Dendritic gain is mediated by an "inward rectifier" $K^+$ current. Journal of Neuroscience, 19:5875–5888.

White J. A., Rubinstein J. T., and Kay A. R. (2000) Channel noise in neurons. Trends in Neuroscience, 23:131–137.

Williams J. T., North R. A., and Tokimasa T. (1988) Inward rectification of resting and opiate-activated potassium currents in rat locus coeruleus neurons. Journal of Neuroscience, 8:4299–4306.

Williams S. R. and Stuart G. J. (2003) Role of dendritic synapse location in the control of action potential. Trends in Neuroscience, 26:147–154.

Willms A. R., Baro D. J., Harris-Warrick R. M., and Guckenheimer J. (1999) An improved parameter estimation method for Hodgkin-Huxley models, Journal of Computational Neuroscience, 6:145–168.

Wilson C. J. (1993) The generation of natural firing patterns in neostriatal neurons. In Progress in Brain Research. Arbuthnott G. and Emson P. C. (eds), 277–297, Amsterdam: Elsevier.

Wilson C. J. and Groves P. M. (1981) Spontaneous firing patterns of identified spiny neurons in the rat neostriatum. Brain Research, 220:67–80.

Wilson H. R. (1999) Spikes, Decisions, and Actions: The dynamical Foundations of Neuroscience. New York: Oxford University Press.

Wilson H. R. and Cowan J. D. (1972) Excitatory and inhibitory interaction in localized populations of model neurons. Biophys J 12:1–24.

Wilson H. R. and Cowan J. D. (1973) A Mathematical theory of the functional dynamics of cortical and thalamic nervous tissue. Kybernetik, 13:55–80.

Winfree A. (1967) Biological rhythms and the behavior of populations of coupled oscillators. Journal of Theoretical Biology, 16:15–42.

Winfree A. (1974) Patterns of phase compromise in biological cycles. Journal of Mathematical Biology, 1:73–95.

Winfree A. (2001) The Geometry of Biological Time. 2nd ed. New York: Springer-Verlag.

Wolfram S. (2002) A New Kind of Science. Wolfram Media.

Wu N., Hsiao C.-F., Chandler S. (2001) Membrane resonance and subthreshold membrane oscillations in mesencephalic V neurons: participants in burst generation. Journal of Neuroscience, 21:3729–3739.

Young G. (1937) Psychometrika, 2:103.

Yuan A., Dourado M., Butler A., Walton N., Wei A., Salkoff L. (2000) SLO-2, a $K^+$ channel with an unusual $Cl^-$ dependence. Nature Neuroscience, 3:771–779.

Yuan A., Santi C. M., Wei A., Wang Z. W., Pollak K., Nonet M., Kaczmarek L., Crowder C. M., and Salkoff L. (2003) The sodium-activated potassium channel is encoded by a member of the SLO gene family. Neuron. 37:765–773.

Yue C., Remy S., Su H., Beck H., and Yaari Y. (2005) Proximal persistent $Na^+$ channels drive spike afterdepolarizations and associated bursting in adult CA1 pyramidal cells. Journal of Neuroscience, 25:9704–9720.

Yue C. and Yaari Y. (2004) KCNQ/M channels control spike afterdepolarization and burst generation in hippocampal neurons. Journal of Neuroscience, 24:4614–4624.

Zhan X. J., Cox C. L., Rinzel J., and Sherman S. M. (1999) Current clamp and modeling studies of low-threshold calcium spikes in cells of the cat's lateral geniculate nucleus. Journal of Neurophysiology, 81:2360–2373.

# Index

$o(\varepsilon)$, 458
$p$:$q$-phase-locking, 456

accommodation, 222
action potential, *see* spike
activation, 33, 34
adaptation variable, 8
adapting interspike frequency, 236
adjoint equation, 462
afterdepolarization (ADP), 260
afterhyperpolarization, 41, 260, 296
AHP, *see* afterhyperpolarization
amplifying gate, 129
Andronov-Hopf bifurcation, *see* bifurcation
anodal break excitation, *see* postinhibitory
         spike, *see* postinhibitory
Arnold tongue, 456
attraction domain, 16, 62, 108
attractor, 9, 60
    coexistence, 13, 66
    ghost, 75, 478
    global, 63
    limit cycle, 10, 97
autonomous dynamical system, 58
averaging, 339

basal ganglia, 311
basin of attraction, *see* attraction domain
Bendixson's criterion, 126
bifurcation, 11, 70, 216
    Andronov-Hopf, 13, 116, 168, 181, 199,
        286
    Bautin, 200, 362
    big saddle homoclinic, 189
    blue-sky, 192
    Bogdanov-Takens, 194, 251, 284
    circle, 348
    codimension, 75, 163, 169, 192
    cusp, 192

diagram, 77
equilibrium, 159
flip, 190, 454
fold, 454
fold limit cycle, 181
fold limit cycle on homoclinic torus,
        192
fold-Hopf, 194
homoclinic, *see* saddle homoclinic
limit cycle, 178
Neimark-Sacker, 192
pitchfork, 194
saddle homoclinic orbit, 279, 482, 496
saddle-focus homoclinic, 190
saddle-node, 11, 74, 78, 113, 162, 271
saddle-node homoclinic orbit, 201, 483
saddle-node on invariant circle, 13, 164,
        180, 272, 279, 284, 306, 477
subcritical, 209
subHopf, 348
supercritical, 209
to bursting, 344
transcritical, 209
bistability, 14, 66, 72, 82, 108, 226, 248,
        286, 299, 316, 328, 368
black hole, 451
blue-sky catastrophe, 192
Boltzmann function, 38, 45
Bonhoeffer–van der Pol, *see* model
brainstem, 313
bursting, 288, 296, 325
    $m+k$ type, 336
    autonomous, 328
    circle/circle, 354
    classification, 347
    conditional, 328
    dissection, 336
    excitability, 328, 343

fast-slow, 335
fold/circle, 366
fold/fold cycle, 364
fold/homoclinic, 350
fold/Hopf, 365
forced, 327
hedgehog, 377
Hopf/Hopf, 380
hysteresis loop, 343, 352, 359, 363
intrinsic, 328
minimal model, 332
oscillation, 486
planar, 348
point-cycle, 348
point-point, 382
slow-wave, 344, 356
subHopf/fold cycle, 299, 359
synchronization, 373, 487

cable equation, 42
canard, 199, 241, 497
central pattern generator (CPG), 334, 472
CH (chattering), *see* neuron
chain of oscillators, 471
channels, 25
cobweb diagram, 452
coherent state, 474
coincidence detection, 233
complex spike, 343
compression function, 486
conductance, 27, 32
conductance-based, *see* model
cortex, 281
coupled bursters, 486
coupled oscillators, 465
coupled relaxation oscillators, 470, 484
coupling
    delayed, 480
    gap-junction, 479
    pulsed, 444, 477
    synaptic, 481
    weak, 480
current, 27
    $K^+$, 46
    $Na^+$, 45
    amplifying, 55, 129, 147

cation, 47
hyperpolarization-activated, 47
Ohmic, 28, 53
persistent, 33, 45
ramp, 221
resonant, 55, 130, 147, 270, 330
rheobase, 155, 242
transient, 33, 35, 45
zap, 232
current threshold, *see* rheobase
current-voltage relation, *see* I-V
cycle slipping, 457, 470

DAP, *see* afterdepolarization
deactivation, 33
deinactivation, 33
delay, 480
delay loss of stability, *see* stability
dendrite, 43, 292
dendritic compartment, 43, 292
dendritic-somatic ping pong, 290
depolarization, 29, 41
desynchronization, 374
determinant, 103
Dirac delta function, 444
direction field, *see* vector field
dissection of bursting, 336
down-state, 316
drifting, 470
dynamic clamp, 288
dynamical system, 8, 57

eigenvalue, 61, 102
eigenvector, 102
elliptic bursting, *see* bursting, subHopf/fold
        cycle
energy function, 474
entorhinal cortex, 314
entrainment, 467
equilibrium, 60, 99
    classification, 103
    focus, 104
    hyperbolic, 69, 103
    node, 103
    saddle, 104
    stable, 60, 100, 161
    unstable, 61

equivalent circuit, 28
equivalent voltage, 151, 341
Euler method, 58
excitability, 9, 11, 81, 215
    Class 1/2, 221, 228
    Class 3, 222
    class of, 218, 449
    Hodgkin's classification, 14, 218
excitation block, 118
excitation variable, 8
exponential integrate-and-fire, *see* model

F-I curve, 15, 188, 218, 227, 255, 321
fast threshold modulation (FTM), 484
fast-slow dynamics, 329, 335
firing threshold, 3
FitzHugh-Nagumo model, *see* model
fixed point, 453
Floquet multiplier, 454
focus, *see* equilibrium
FRB (fast rhythmic bursting), *see* neuron,
    CH
French duck, *see* canard
frequency
    acceleration, 255
    adaptation, 255
    mismatch, 470
    plateaus, 472
    preference, 232, 237, 265
frequency-current curve, *see* F-I
frequency-locking, 467
FS (fast spiking), *see* neuron

gap-junction, 44, 467, 479
Gaussian function, 38
GENESIS, 6, 24, 44
geometrical analysis, 59
ghost
    seeattractor, 478
gradient system, 474

half-center oscillator, 334
hard loss, *see* stability
Hartman-Grobman, *see* theorem
hedgehog burster, 377
heteroclinic trajectory, *see* trajectory
Hindmarsh-Rose, *see* model

hippocampus, 308
Hodgkin-Frankenhaeuser layer, 331
Hodgkin-Huxley, *see* model
homoclinic trajectory, *see* trajectory
Hopf bifurcation, *see* bifurcation, Andronov-
    Hopf
hyperbolic equilibrium, *see* equilibrium, 103
hyperpolarization, 29
hyperpolarization-activated channels, 36, 131,
    136
hysteresis, 13, 67, 259, 342, 382

I-V relation, 30, 54, 77, 151, 155, 161, 256,
    316
    instantaneous, 31, 152
    multiple scales, 257
    steady-state, 31, 34, 59, 99, 152, 162
IB (intrinsically bursting), *see* neuron
impedance, 233
in vivo, 287
inactivation, 33, 35
incoherent state, 474
infinitesimal PRC, 459
inhibition-induced spiking, 244
input conductance, 29
input resistance, 29, 155
instantaneous voltage threshold, 282
integrate-and-fire, *see* model
integrator, 13, 55, 81, 119, 229, 240, 269,
    272, 284, 316, 368
interneuron, *see* neuron
intra-burst, *see* interspike
ions, 25
isochron, 445

Jacobian matrix, 102, 473

Kirchhoff's law, 28
Kuramoto phase model, *see* model
Kuramoto synchronization index, 474

Landau $o(\varepsilon)$, 458
latency, *see* spike
Liapunov coefficient, 200
limit cycle, 10, 96
    Bendixson's criterion, 126
linear analysis, 101

low-threshold, *see* spike
LS (late spiking), *see* neuron
LTS (low-threshold spiking), *see* neuron

manifold
    stable, 109, 445
    threshold, 240
    unstable, 109
MATLAB, 6, 24, 51, 58, 274, 322, 367, 446,
        448, 462, 494, 498, 501
mean-field approximation, 474
membrane potentia, *see* potential
membrane voltage, *see* potential
mesencephalic V, *see* neuron
minimal model, *see* model
mitral, *see* neuron
model
    $I_A$, 142
    $I_{Ca}+I_K$, 6
    $I_{Cl}+I_K$, 158
    $I_K+I_{Kir}$, 140
    $I_{Na,p}+E_{Na}([Na^+]_{in/out})$, 158
    $I_{Na,p}+I_K$, 6, 9, 89, 128, 132, 163, 172,
        182, 201, 225, 257, 327
    $I_{Na,p}+I_K+I_{K(M)}$, 253, 327
    $I_{Na,p}+I_h$, 136
    $I_{Na,t}$, 129, 133
    $I_{Na}+I_K$, 452
    $I_h+I_{Kir}$, 138
    Bonhoeffer–van der Pol, 123, 381
    canonical, 278, 353, 357, 363
    conductance-based, 43
    Emrentrout-Kopell, 357
    exponential integrate-and-fire, 81
    FitzHugh-Nagumo, 21, 106, 223
    Hindmarsh-Rose, 123
    Hodgkin-Huxley, 37, 128, 147, 334
    integrate-and-fire, 268, 275, 493
    irreducible, *see* minimal
    Kuramoto, 467, 474
    minimal, 127
        $Ca^{2+}$-gated, 147
    minimal for bursting, 332
    Morris-Lecar, 6, 89, 132
    phase, 279
    planar, 89

quadratic integrate-and-fire, 80, 203,
        270, 279, 353, 477, 483, 494
    reduction, 147
    resonate-and-fire, 269
    simple, 153, 272
    theta, 320, 322
    van der Pol, 123
modulation
    slow, 252
monostable dynamics, 14
Morris-Lecar, *see* model
multistability, *see* bistability

neocortex, 281
neostriatum, 311
Nernst, *see* potential
neurocomputational property, 367
NEURON, 6, 24, 44
neuron, 1
    basal ganglia, 311
    BSNP, 297
    CH, 281, 294, 351
    FS, 281, 298
    hippocampal, 308, 328
    IB, 281, 288, 351
    inhibitory, 301
    LS, 282, 300
    LTS, 281, 296
    mesencephalic V, 313
    mitral, 248, 316
    neostriatal, 311
    Purkinje, 319
    RS, 281, 282
    RSNP, 296
    RTN, 306
    stellate, 314
    TC, 305
    theta, 320
node, *see* equilibrium
noise, 177
normal form, 75, 170, 271
nullcline, 92

olfactory bulb, 316
orbit, *see* trajectory
order parameter, 474
oscillation, 177

homoclinic, 482
interburst, 329
intraburst, 329
multifrequency, 468
phase, 444
quasi-periodic, 468
slow, 232
SNIC, 477
subthreshold, 13, 177, 230, 286, 298,
316
slow, 258
oscillator, 385
Andronov-Hopf, 451, 492
half-center, 334
relaxation, 98, 107, 198, 470
oscillator death, 492

pacemaker, 9
parabolic bursting, *see* bursting, circle/circle
partial synchronization, 474
period, 97, 445
periodic orbit, 10
persistent current, *see* current
phase, *see* oscillation
phase deviation, 466
phase drifting, 468
phase lag, 468
phase lead, 468
phase line, 58
phase model, *see* model
coupled oscillators, 465
Kuramoto reduction, 460, 476
linear response, 459
Malkin reduction, 461, 476
Winfree reduction, 459, 476
phase oscillator, 475
phase portrait, 9, 67, 108
geometrical analysis, 59
local equivalence, 69
topological equivalence, 68
phase space, 58
phase transition curve, *see* PTC
phase trapping, 468
phase walk-through, 470
phase-locking, 456
phase-resetting curve, *see* PRC

phaseless set, 451
ping-pong, 262, 290
Poincare phase map, 452
postinhibitory
depression, 260
facilitation, 243, 260
spike, 5, 242, 252, 259, 314
postsynaptic potential, 2
potential
equivalent, 151, 341
Nernst, 26, 32
resting, 29
reverse, 32
PRC, 446, 459, 462
PSP, *see* postsynaptic potential
PTC, 450
Purkinje neuron, 248

quadratic integrate-and-fire, *see* model
quasi-threshold, 241

radial isochron clock, 446
Rall's branching law, 43
ramp input, 224
rebound, *see* postinhibitory
recovery variable, 8
refractory period, 41, 269
regular point, 73
relaxation oscillator, *see* oscillator, 484
repeller, 62, 97
repolarization, 41
resonance, 5, 232
resonant gate, 130
resonator, 13, 55, 119, 229, 241, 313, 316,
368, 372
rest point, *see* equilibrium
resting potential, *see* potential
reverse potential, *see* potential
rheobase, 4, 155, 242
rotation number, 467
RS (regular spiking), *see* neuron
RTN (reticular thalamic nucleus), *see* neuron
saddle, 18, *see* equilibrium
saddle quantity, 185
saddle-node bifurcation, *see* bifurcation

saddle-node equilibrium, 104
saddle-node of periodics, *see* bifurcation, fold limit cycle
saddle-node on invariant circle bifurcation, *see* bifurcation
sag, *see* voltage
self-ignition, 492
separatrix, 18, 109, 240
shock input, 224
simple model, *see* model
slow modulation, 252
slow passage effect, 175, 361
slow subthreshold oscillation, 258
slow transition, 75
slow-wave bursting, *see* bursting
SNIC, *see* bifurcation, saddle-node on invariant circle
SNLC, *see* bifurcation, saddle-node on invariant circle
soft loss, *see* stability
somatic-dendritic ping-pong, 262
spike, 2, 41, 63
    all-or-none, 4, 95, 268
    complex, 343
    dendritic, 43, 261, 292
    doublet, 236
    frequency modulation, 255
    inhibition-induced, 244
    latency, 4, 18, 75, 242, 246, 284, 312
    low-threshold, 5, 306
    postinhibitory, 298
    potassium, 140
    propagation, 42
    rebound, *see* postinhibitory
    synchronization, 374, 486
    upside-down, 145
    upstroke, 41
spike time response curve, *see* PRC
square-wave bursting, *see* bursting, fold/homoclinic
squid axon, 14
stability, 60
    asymptotic, 60, 97, 100, 453
    delay loss, 175, 361
    exponential, 100, 103
    loss, hard/soft, 204

    neutral, 100
stable manifold, *see* manifold
state line, *see* phase line
state space, *see* phase space
stellate cell, *see* neuron
step input, 224
striatum, 311
stroboscopic map, 452
stutter, 227, 301, 316
subcritical Andronov-Hopf, *see* bifurcation
subthreshold, 63
subthreshold oscillation, *see* oscillation
supercritical Andronov-Hopf, *see* bifurcation
superthreshold, 63
suprathreshold, *see* superthreshold
synapse, 2
synaptic coupling, 481
synchronization, 385, 443, 454, 467
    anti-phase, 454
    in-phase, 454
    of bursts, 373, 487
    of spikes, 486
    out-of-phase, 454

TC (thalamocortical), *see* neuron
thalamic
    relay neuron, 305
thalamic burst mode, 306
thalamic interneuron, 308
thalamic relay mode, 305
thalamus, 304
theorem
    averaging, 340
    Ermentrout, 473
    Hartman-Grobman, 69, 103
    Malkin, 462
    Pontryagin–Rodygin, 341
theta-neuron, *see* model
threshold, 3, 63, 95, 111, 238, 268
    current threshold, *see* rheobase
    firing, 3
    manifold, 240
    quasi-, 241
time crystal, 451
topological equivalence, 68

topological normal form, *see* normal form
torus knot, 467
trace, 103
trajectory, 94
    canard, 199
    heteroclinic, 111
    homoclinic, 111
    periodic, 96
transient current, *see* current
transmembrane potential, *see* potential
traveling wave, 471
type of excitability, *see* excitability

unstable equilibrium, 62
unstable manifold, *see* manifold
up-state, 316

van der Pol, *see* model
vector field
    planar, 89
velocity field, *see* vector field
voltage sag, 259, 284, 314
voltage-clamp, 30
voltage-gated channels, 33

wave, 471
weak coupling, 458

XPP, 6, 24

Printed in the United States
by Baker & Taylor Publisher Services